NEW
PARENTS

NEW PARENTS

A GUIDE TO PREGNANCY, BABY AND CHILD CARE FOR TODAY'S MOTHERS AND FATHERS

Consultant Editor

DR DAVID HARVEY
Consultant Paediatrician
Queen Charlotte's Maternity Hospital, London

CONTENTS

The Authors

Miss Mary Anderson
Consultant Obstetrician
at the Lewisham Hospital, London

Dr Kate Costeloe
Consultant Paediatrician
and Senior Lecturer in Child Health, Department of
Neonatal Medicine, Homerton Hospital, London

Caroline Flint
Senior Midwife
and Member of the Royal College of Midwives

Dr Catherine James
formerly Consultant Obstetrician and Gynaecologist,
St Thomas' Hospital, London

Dr Sue Jenkins
Senior Clinical Medical Officer
in Paddington District Health Authority

Dr Josephine Likierman
General Practitioner

Mrs Margaret Polden
Senior Obstetric Physiotherapist,
Hammersmith Hospital, London

Dr Leon Polnay
Consultant Paediatrician,
Nottingham Community Health Service and
University Hospital, Nottingham

Dr Diane Smyth
Consultant Paediatrician in the Child Development Unit,
Paddington Green Children's Hospital, London

Dr John Stroobant
Consultant Paediatrician
at Whipps Cross Hospital, London

Acknowledgments
Editor: Nicky Adamson
Art Editor: Pat Sumner
Designer: Annie Tomlin
Production: Shane Lask and Audrey Johnston

Illustrations by Elaine Anderson and Kathy Wyatt
Special photography by Ron Sutherland

The publishers would like to thank the following for their
kind permission to use photographs in the book: Ace
Photo Agency/Michael Bluestone 17; Ace Photo Agency/
Anthony Price 227; Ace Photo Agency/Gabe Palmer half
title page; Bubbles Photo Library/Loisjoy Thurstun 33;
Bubbles Photo Library/Julie Fisher 51, 104, 289; Sally
and Richard Greenhill 59, 189, 237; Susan Griggs Agency
Limited 249; Jerrican/Clement title page; Camilla Jessel
106, 128, 133, 199, 231; Steve Lyne 117, 124-125; Tony
Stone Photo Library 9, 103, 110, 225; Jennie
Woodcock 137; Tim Woodcock 163.

This edition specially produced for
The Leisure Circle Limited
by the Hamlyn Publishing Group Limited
a division of the Octopus Publishing Group
Michelin House, 81 Fulham Road
London SW3 6RB

Introduction

I first saw the birth of a baby thirty years ago, when I was a medical student. Even today, I still find the event just as exciting and amazing. The fetus, which has been totally dependent inside the mother's womb, suddenly makes a cry and becomes a separate human being. The word 'miracle' may be overworked, but it is really needed for that moment.

The problem is that the birth of a baby is not only exciting and wonderful; it also causes many anxieties for the parents. I believe that parents should be given as much information as possible about pregnancy and child development, so that they can fully understand what may happen – that is the reason for this book. At one time, it was common for doctors and midwives to surround their work with a sort of mist. Some people say that this was partly because of a wish to protect their professions; I think they also thought their patients would be worried by too much information. We now realize that this was very misguided; parents and professionals can work together much more successfully if the parents understand what the problems are and how they might be managed.

It is very easy to imagine that medical decisions are clear cut. In fact, they are a long way from that; anyone who joins a medical ward round or meeting finds out how much more we need to know and even how much doubt there may be. The right course of action is not always obvious but is chosen after balancing a number of advantages and disadvantages. Of course, a normal process like childbirth may proceed without any hitch, but sometimes there are important choices to be made to improve the outcome for the baby or mother.

Books on pregnancy and child care at one time only stressed the normal. This was a little naïve because it ignored genuine problems which do arise; it was also a symptom of the wish to cloud medicine from the public. For example, it was common to leave out any mention of serious illness in the first few days after birth. In fact, about ten per cent of newborn babies need what is called 'special care'. This means that they have to be admitted to a special unit for observation and treatment. Some of them need intensive care using modern life-saving equipment, such as ventilators to keep them breathing. In this book we have not shied away from describing the illnesses that affect some babies and what you might expect if your baby is among the one in ten to be admitted to the special care unit. I hope that you will have the chance to visit the unit in your own hospital fairly early in pregnancy, so that you are familiar with the surroundings if your baby is unlucky enough to go there.

Our plan has been to make this a book for both parents. I am very pleased and impressed by the number of fathers who come to out-patient clinics today, and in Britain about 90 per cent of women have their partners with them at the birth of the baby. It was not always like that. We often think how idyllic it used to be for a baby to be born at home; even allowing for the risks that have to be taken into account, I suspect that the emotional side of the delivery was not always well looked after. I am amused to see old films from the 1930s and 1940s in which the doctor comes out of a bedroom to tell the father that he has a girl or a boy; it is clear that he had been kept away from the birth.

One of the major advances in the last decade has been the discovery of the importance of the relationship between parents and their newborn baby – one could probably say *rediscovery*, since many of the concepts are really a reiteration of the virtue of being kind and caring. I always avoid the word 'bonding' since it seems to imply a sort of glue between the mother and her baby. However, I feel that we must not get too carried away in our enthusiasm for the rediscovery. For example, skin-to-skin contact between the mother and her baby is clearly a very good thing if it is possible immediately after birth; it seems to promote a special feeling between the two of them and is also good for breast feeding. If it is not possible, however, it would be sad for a mother to feel that irreparable damage has been done. After all, babies can be adopted very satisfactorily, so it is clearly not essential for normal human life. Unfortunately, it sometimes cannot happen because the baby is not well. For instance, urgent treatment may be needed to make sure that breathing has started, or the baby may have been born very prematurely allowing you only time to give a quick cuddle before the baby is taken to the special care baby unit. We have tried to explain all such issues much more than in the past.

Each one of us knows that a hospital can be an unnerving and even frightening place. Feelings are very important in medicine and midwifery, so caring for the emotions is as necessary as caring for the body. We have not set out to be frightening, but have planned the book to be realistic. I hope we have succeeded in finding a middle way between the extremes of giving no explanation except a rose-tinted view of natural childbirth and a fearsome account implying that all childbirth is abnormal.

Every year brings new advances and problems. We were anxious that the book should be really up to date, because modern obstetrics and paediatrics produce many questions which need to be answered. Ultrasound and fetal monitoring were unknown a couple of decades ago, and such modern technology is bound to raise questions about safety and whether they interfere with the normal course of a pregnancy. It will be important for new methods to be carefully evaluated, not only to be certain that they work and are safe, but also that they do not have hidden side-effects such as producing unnecessary distress for parents. In order to tell parents what is likely to happen in obstetrics, I am sad to include a short section on AIDS. The developing epidemic is bound to affect all our lives: it is very unfortunate that it has been sensational-ized by the newspapers, but we cannot deny that it is a great threat with very serious consequences for mothers and babies. The infection has so far affected only a few women in the United Kingdom, but in parts of New York City 1 in 60 women have been infected by the virus before pregnancy.

The book is not only about pregnancy. The first few months and years of a child's life are tremendous fun, but also a period of worry. The main thing that parents need is common sense. The approach *you* feel you should adopt in looking after your baby will almost certainly be the best; other members of the family can be helpful with advice and support, but don't let them take over. The first baby is always more of a worry because you don't known what to expect, so we have tried to set a framework of what is normal. The information in the book comes from the experience of many people, both professionals and parents, and we hope it is presented in such a way that you have plenty of objective advice to lean on. I cannot stress too much that each baby is an individual and that you, as parents, are the right people to judge what is best for your baby.

After a year or two, it seems extraordinary that the toddler ever was a helpless baby. The rapid development that occurs was one of the main things that attracted me to paediatrics. It is exciting to see children starting to talk and walk; but babies are not stupid even at birth – they can communicate with us if we give them the chance.

As we get old, all of us will depend more and more on the young to look after us: they are the investment for our future. But that should not be the only reason for giving them the best possible care. We all have a responsibility to care for children, who depend on adults for their protection. There are so many things we can do. For instance, if you seriously believe that you know a child who is being abused, you should do something about it. Doctors are always sad to see children who have been physically injured by their parents and recently we have come to realize that sexual abuse is much more prevalent than we thought. Both of these can cause serious damage to a child's health and, indeed, entire future development. We decided not to put a long section about them in the book, but the most important thing to emphasize is that they should never happen. If you feel that you are about to injure or abuse your child, go and seek profes-sional advice at once.

A baby is protected against many infections during most of the first year, but the second and third years are a time of frequent illnesses. Very often these can be treated simply, but you will want to know when to consult a doctor. Recent years have seen a reduction in the immunization rates in many communities, very often because of publicity about the possible side-effects of the vaccines. There is no procedure which does not have a risk, but the risks of not immunizing are often not stressed. We have tried to give a balanced account of what modern medicine can offer children. There are many occasions when no drugs are necessary and it is then sensible to avoid them, but in some diseases it is possible to cure, and this book emphasizes how we can offer the best medical care. This not only involves medicines and surgery, but other obvious things, too, like making it possible for parents to stay in hospital with their children.

Like so many authors, we have struggled with the question of whether to use 'he' or 'she' for the baby. All of us have an aversion to 'it' or 'he/she'. We have decided to let the author of each chapter choose which pronoun they prefer, and believe that this has produced a comfortable mix.

The three decades since I started training in medicine have been an exciting time. During this period, the survival of small premature babies has become a reality and tremendous advances have been made in the treatment of many children's illnesses, such as cancer. Of course, so much remains to be done – such as urgent action to reduce deaths and disability from accidents. But one of the major advances has been the rediscovery that professionals and parents can produce the best results if they work together as a team.

DR DAVID HARVEY

CHAPTER ONE

BEGINNINGS

The physiology of reproduction and how to prepare yourself for pregnancy

Having a baby is always a major event, whether it is the first, or third, or even the sixth child in a family. From early pregnancy on, this new person places physical and emotional demands on his or her parents which, as any grandparent knows, continue well into adulthood. Yet parenthood is uniquely rewarding, bringing with it the uncomplicated and unquestioning love of the young child.

For many parents, however, taking on the responsibility of parenthood means careful planning and difficult decision-making. Many babies are still unexpected, though none the less loved, but for other couples, deciding to have a baby means facing up to serious discussions about timing, career prospects, financial considerations, housing, the effect on their relationship, and simple apprehension about the loss of personal freedom. After all, the first baby increases the family unit by 50 per cent.

Becoming a parent changes your life permanently, so preparing yourselves for it both emotionally and practically does pay dividends. No-one can really describe how any individual person is going to feel when he or she becomes a parent – it is a new experience every time. However, before you start, there are pointers which can help you make decisions about your well-being, your chances of conceiving and your ability to bring a healthy child into the world.

THE REPRODUCTIVE PROCESS

The potential for reproduction is something which is determined in its broadest terms from the time of a person's own conception – for it is at this moment that the genetic sex is decided and a chain of events is set in motion which will eventually lead to development into men and women of the human species. The many changes and adaptations which are involved in the production of such fundamentally different beings are so subtle and complex as to seem miraculous indeed, but the ways in which these two such apparently disparate bodies are so perfectly designed to generate new life is perhaps the most fascinating of all. To set the scene for

successful pregnancy everyone has to undergo a long period of development and maturation until the body's anatomy and physiology, whether it be male or female, is in full working order for this complicated function.

BASIC ANATOMY

In men the external organs of reproduction are the penis and testes (testicles). The testes are contained in a bag of skin called the scrotum, lying outside the body cavity in the genital region. Although two testes are the norm, reproduction is still possible when only one is present. The testes produce the spermatozoa (sperm) which are required to fertilize the female ovum (egg) – the first step in the formation of a new life – and they also produce the male hormone testosterone. Testosterone is responsible for male development at puberty and the maintenance of sexual function thereafter.

The testes have a rich nerve and blood supply and are very sensitive to painful stimuli, as is well known. It may seem rather illogical that these delicate structures which are so vital for reproduction should have evolved to occupy such a vulnerable position, when the ovary, the equivalent structure in the female, is well protected within the bony pelvis. As with many things in nature, there is, however a sensible explanation – the sperm could not survive if exposed to the heat within the body cavity, and require a lower environmental temperature for optimum development. Abnormalities in the scrotum can raise the temperature, reducing sperm production and causing male infertility.

Lying alongside the testis, is the epididymis, which is the main storehouse of the sperms and in which they become more motile (active) and mature. Arising from the epididymis is the vas deferens (sperm tube) by which sperms are transported to the seminal vesicles, structures which lie just behind the bladder and prostate gland. (It is this sperm tube which is divided for male sterilization in

Being a parent can be uniquely rewarding, but careful preparation is always invaluable.

the operation of vasectomy, when further pregnancies are not desired.) The seminal vesicles are also involved in the short term storage of sperm but their main function is to provide the sticky fluid which forms much of the volume of the ejaculated semen.

The penis is a flaccid cylindrical structure which is capable, under appropriate stimulation, of becoming hard and erect, because of its ability to be engorged with blood. At the moment of orgasm seminal fluid is ejaculated from the penis via the urethra, the hollow tube which runs along its length from the bladder and to which the seminal vesicles are connected, thus allowing the deposition of sperm into the female vagina. Both processes are fundamentally controlled by complex nerve pathways under the influence of some of the highest centres in the brain, and as such are very much affected by psychological and emotional factors.

Sperm are being constantly formed in the male from puberty onwards until their production declines in old age. Each mature sperm is about $\frac{1}{25}$ of a millimetre long and consists of a head, neck, body and tail. The tail gives motion to the sperm and allows it to make swimming movements from the vagina up into the uterus and Fallopian tube. In any one ejaculate there will be on average about 200 million sperm contained in 2-4 ml of fluid.

In women the organs of reproduction are all contained within the bony pelvis and consist of the vagina, the uterus and cervix, the Fallopian tubes and ovaries. Surrounding the entrance to the vagina there are external folds of skin known as the labia (lips) and just inside the vagina are the openings of tiny glands which produce the mucus secretions required for lubrication during intercourse. The vagina itself is an elastic muscular canal about 8-10cm (3-4in) long into the top portion of which protrudes the cervix (neck of the womb).

The cervix is an integral part of the uterus (womb) and together they are usually directed forwards at almost a right angle to the length of the vagina, to take up what is called a position of anteversion. The cervix plays a special part in the process of conception by producing mucus which, at the time of ovulation (egg production), is particularly favourable to the passage of sperm.

The uterus is capable of enormous expansion – in its pre-pregnant state it is similar in size to an egg, but by the end of pregnancy it occupies the whole of the abdomen and its weight has increased more than tenfold. Attached to the upper part of the uterus are the Fallopian tubes – these are delicate hollow structures whose frond-like ends (fimbriae) are closely applied to the ovaries. Fertilization of the ovum (egg) by the sperm takes place in the Fallopian tube and its gentle squeezing movements transport the newly formed embryo into the uterine cavity where it will implant and grow.

The ovaries are the female equivalent of the testes – they lie in close relation to the outer ends of the Fallopian tubes and produce the mature ova (eggs) which are essential to reproduction. In a newborn baby girl the ovaries contain thousands of ova, but these remain undeveloped until the time of puberty.

THE MENSTRUAL CYCLE

As a result of complex hormonal mechanisms at puberty, the ovaries begin to function in a monthly cycle, ripening and releasing one ovum each time. This menstrual cycle, as it is called, is regulated by interdependent hormones produced not only by the ovaries but also by the pituitary gland and the hypothalamus in the brain. At the start of a cycle one or other ovary will start to develop a follicle which contains the ovum designated to mature that month. This stimulates the production of the hormone oestrogen from the ovary, which in turn influences the follicle to rupture (ovulation) and releases the ovum, which passes into the Fallopian tube. In a normal 28 day cycle this would take place on the fourteenth day from the beginning of menstruation.

The ruptured follicle now becomes known as the corpus luteum; as well as oestrogen, it produces another hormone called progesterone. This hormone helps to prepare the lining of the womb (endometrium) for an ensuing pregnancy. If fertilization of the egg does not take place, then the corpus luteum disintegrates after approximately fourteen days and the endometrium is shed with the four to five days of bleeding we recognize as menstruation (monthly or menstrual period).

This regular process of monthly preparation for pregnancy goes on for many years, but is not always totally efficient. Sometimes ovulation does not take place regularly, and this is particularly likely in the early years just after periods start, in middle age (the late thirties and early forties) as the menopause approaches, immediately after a pregnancy, and after stopping the oral contraceptive pill. Without ovulation pregnancy cannot occur and this is one of the many reasons for infertility.

CONCEPTION

During the act of sexual intercourse, sperm contained in the seminal fluid are deposited in the upper part of the vagina, by the mechanisms already described. There could be as many as 400 million in any one ejaculate and they immediately start on their journey, using their tail structures to swim up

THE WOMAN'S REPRODUCTIVE ORGANS

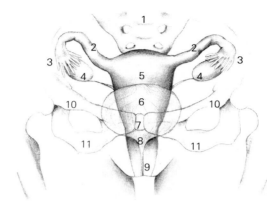

1 Sacrum

2 Fallopian tubes

3 Fimbriae

4 Ovaries

5 Uterus

6 Bladder (in front of uterus)

7 Symphysis pubis

8 Cervix

9 Vagina

10 Pelvic girdle

11 Ischial tuberosities

THE MAN'S REPRODUCTIVE ORGANS

1 Seminal vesicles

2 Pelvic girdle

3 Bladder

4 Prostate gland (below bladder)

5 Vas deferens

6 Cowper's gland

7 Urethra

8 Penis (containing erectile tissue)

9 Testes

through the cervix towards the Fallopian tubes, which they reach in about 30 minutes. Many sperms are lost on the way and only a few thousand actually reach their destination. Only one sperm will succeed in fertilizing the ovum which has been released from the ovary and once this has happened the activity of all the other sperm is inhibited.

The survival times of ova and spermatozoa are very short; for a pregnancy to result, intercourse has to be carefully timed to the monthly cycle. The ovum survives for only about 24 hours after it has been released so, ideally, sperm should be already present in the Fallopian tube to fertilize it. A sperm can survive a little longer than the ovum, up to 48 hours, so if pregnancy is planned, your best chance of success is to have intercourse around the time of ovulation – the day before being the very best of all.

You can calculate when you ovulate from observation of your monthly cycle. Ovulation takes place about fourteen days before your next period would start; if you have fairly regular cycles you can work out your most fertile time of the month from the calendar. You can also examine the nature of the mucus produced by your cervix. The change that takes place in this around the time of ovulation has already been mentioned and it is quite easy to notice in your normal vaginal secretions – the mucus becomes clear and rather 'tacky'. If your periods tend to be irregular it is more difficult to predict when an egg will be released and you may have to use the temperature method to check when ovulation has occurred. Because of effects of the hormone progesterone, body temperature rises by about 1°C (2°F) after ovulation and this change can be seen if you take your temperature each day. Using this method can be quite difficult and it is not necessary unless you are having fertility problems.

PRE-PREGNANCY PREPARATION

The early months of pregnancy are a time of great importance in a baby's development – it is during this time that the organs are formed and when very rapid growth is taking place. However, for many couples, the possibility of pregnancy may be unsuspected until this formative time is well under way. We know there are harmful influences which can effect a baby at this time and that these risks can be reduced if they have been considered before the baby is conceived. For this reason many prospective parents like to prepare ahead for pregnancy – a little like getting fit for a race or planning your holiday. Of course many pregnancies are not premeditated and are no less successful because of that, but a little forward thinking will make you feel even more confident.

When discussing pre-pregnancy counselling it is logical to think in terms of advice that is generally useful to all, and then to consider couples who may have specific problems or needs. Often the first decision that has to be made is when to stop using contraception. If you are using a barrier method or intrauterine device, then once its use has been discontinued you can try to conceive straight away. If you are using the contraceptive pill, however, it is best to stop this two or three months before you plan a pregnancy and use an alternative method such as the cap or sheath. This gap allows restoration of your natural menstrual cycle and the resumption of ovulation already referred to. It also makes it easier to calculate the baby's due date when you become pregnant again (see below).

If you are planning your pregnancy in order to have your baby at a particular time of year, perhaps to fit with work schedules or older children's school holidays, it is perhaps appropriate here to explain how doctors and midwives talk about the duration of a pregnancy. They nearly always refer to the length of a pregnancy in weeks, it being more accurate than to talk of months (see p. 14). (To illustrate this point – a pregnancy lasts on average 40 weeks, a length usually equated with nine months in popular parlance. However, many people would calculate one month to equal four weeks, because this is the cycle associated with 'monthly periods', which would then make the average pregnancy ten months long – so you can see how confusion may arise!)

For medical purposes, duration of pregnancy is always calculated from the first day of the last menstrual period and not from the time of conception, so what is referred to as 'four weeks' pregnant' is about the time when the majority of women would be missing their first period, rather than being four weeks from the time they have conceived. Unfortunately, the last menstrual period is only an accurate guide to the duration of pregnancy provided the cycle is regular each month, with ovulation occurring on day fourteen. If periods are erratic then the length of pregnancy may have to be calculated by ultrasound. In this book, any discussion about lengths of pregnancy follows the medical convention of weeks from the last period, with the assumption of conception two weeks later.

You may also want to take into account financial and career considerations in deciding the age at which your pregnancy is planned. With modern obstetric care, even the older mother can expect a relatively trouble-free time if she is generally fit and healthy, but the most favourable decade for having your family from the point of view of medical risk is between 20 and 30 years.

PRE-PREGNANCY AVERAGE WEIGHT FOR WOMEN					
Height without shoes (m)	Women Weight without clothes (kg) Acceptable average	Acceptable weight range	Height without shoes (ft, in)	Women Weight without clothes (lb) Acceptable average	Acceptable weight range
1.45	46.0	42–53	4 10	102	92–119
1.48	46.5	42–54	4 11	104	94–122
1.50	47.0	43–55	5 0	107	96–125
1.52	48.5	44–57	5 1	110	99–128
1.54	49.5	44–58	5 2	113	102–131
1.56	50.4	45–58	5 3	116	105–134
1.58	51.3	46–59	5 4	120	108–138
1.60	52.6	48–61	5 5	123	111–142
1.62	54.0	49–62	5 6	128	114–146
1.64	55.4	50–64	5 7	132	118–150
1.66	56.8	51–65	5 8	136	122–154
1.68	58.1	52–66	5 9	140	126–158
1.70	60.0	53–67	5 10	144	130–163
1.72	61.3	55–69	5 11	148	134–168
1.74	62.6	56–70	6 0	152	138–173
1.76	64.0	58–72			
1.78	65.3	59–74	Bray, 1979; based on Metropolitan Life Insurance tables		

HEALTH, WEIGHT AND DIET

Having once decided when you want to have your baby, before you start trying there are a number of things you should check. It is important to discover your immunity to rubella (German measles). Rubella is a viral illness which is very mild in adults but can cause severe damage to a fetus particularly during the first three months of pregnancy, resulting in severe disabilities such as heart problems, deafness and blindness. Your immunity can be checked by a simple blood test and if it is found that you are not immune then you can be immunized by your doctor. Pregnancy should be avoided for three months after this but then you can be confident that you are no longer at risk, as immunity usually lasts for life, except in very rare circumstances where the injection does not 'take'. You may have been told you have already had the infection in the past but it is very difficult to be certain about this, as a rubella

illness can be very like other viral infections. It is now usual to invite girls approaching puberty (age eleven to thirteen) to be immunized at school, so you may well have the immunity already. However, not everyone takes up the offer, or you may have already left school before this became national policy in Britain.

Unless you are certain you have already been immunized the blood test is advisable and can be arranged through your doctor or family planning clinic.

As a potential mother you should also pay some consideration to your weight and diet. Of the many factors which may influence the course and outcome of pregnancy, nutritional status around the time of conception is one of the most important. You should check your weight against the chart which defines the ideal range for your height and body build given above. If you find that you are very much over or under the weight range recommended then it would be sensible to correct this before pregnancy, as either state increases the likelihood of pregnancy complications. In particular pregnancy is no time for dieting.

As well as starting your pregnancy at the optimum weight it is important to eat a healthy and balanced diet to provide all the vitamins and nutrients essential for the baby's growth. There has been much debate about the advisability of taking vitamin and mineral supplements in the pre-pregnancy period and as yet their value for general use remains unproven, although they are almost certainly not harmful. More to the point are the general principles of healthy diet – eating enough to maintain an appropriate weight for height, choosing unrefined foods like wholemeal bread and cereals, taking some fresh food daily and selecting a wide range of foods from the four main groups: meat and fish, bread and cereals, milk and dairy products, and fruit and vegetables.

AVOIDING SMOKING

There are of course some habits, dietary and otherwise, which are best avoided when planning a pregnancy, the most important of which are smoking and alcohol consumption. We all know of people who have smoked heavily and consumed large quantities of alcohol all through pregnancies and had perfectly healthy, well grown babies but the medical evidence is overwhelming that indulging in these habits puts the baby at more risk. It is best if possible to give up smoking altogether, but the information about alcohol is not quite so clear. Obviously if you can avoid drinking then you are taking no risk but the occasional glass of beer or wine is probably not harmful. This advice applies to *both partners* trying for a successful pregnancy since excessive alcohol and tobacco consumption can affect male fertility by depressing sperm production and motility, as well as damaging the fertilized ovum.

Do try and avoid taking any pills, medicines or other drugs around the time of conception; if you are receiving regular medication it is sensible to discuss your plans for pregnancy with your doctor in case a change is needed. Seeing your doctor is also a good opportunity to have your blood pressure checked and to have a pelvic examination and cervical smear test if these have not been done recently at your family planning clinic. At this time you can also find out about your local facilities for antenatal supervision and delivery, discover whether your GP offers shared care, and obtain information on useful books and pamphlets for further reading (see p. 15). For some specific

medical conditions such as diabetes, kidney disease, heart disease and high blood pressure pre-pregnancy advice and preparation is very important.

SPECIALIZED ADVICE

For some couples, rather more specialized advice may be required. One of the commoner situations in which this may arise is in counselling the older woman about the risks of having a baby with a chromosomal congenital abnormality – the one most often encountered being Down's syndrome (once known as mongolism). The chances of having an affected baby increase with maternal age as shown in the graph on page 27. Although you will be counselled again in pregnancy it is easier to have thought through your response to the question of antenatal diagnosis, should you be in the at risk age group, particularly now that chorion villus sampling can be used for diagnosis as early as eight to ten weeks from the last period (see p. 28). Other situations where pre-pregnancy information may be needed is for those couples who are at risk of carrying a haemoglobinopathy (see p. 26) who can be checked by means of a simple blood test, those who have had problems in previous pregnancies, and those where there is a family history of inherited disease for whom it is possible to arrange genetic counselling. If you think that you may need advice of this kind then your doctor should be consulted.

GENETIC COUNSELLING

Many parents who have a relative with a handicapped child, or who have one themselves (see p. 22), worry about the same problem occurring with future children. If this is your situation, then the advice and reassurance of a genetic counsellor could help to sort out your anxieties.

Genes are carried on chromosomes and are the fundamental basis of all inherited characteristics. At conception each person inherits thousands of genes from their parents. Sometimes one or two of these are harmful and can cause disease or handicap. The possibility of this happening is greater if the parents are related before marriage, such as cousins, for it is more likely they will carry the same genes because they inherited them from a common ancestor.

Genetic counselling can help parents in different ways. Not all parents want all that the service can offer. That does not matter. The doctor or clinical geneticist who gives the advice must first make an accurate diagnosis of affected family members and this may involve them being examined, some investigations and acquisition of relevant reports.

The correct diagnosis then allows the geneticist to calculate the risks of recurrence in subsequent children, or of recurrence in other family members. He or she can give advice about the cause and course of the disease, the risk to future children and ways to prevent it happening again. Help and support can also be provided in making difficult decisions once the facts are established.

PROBLEMS WITH FERTILITY

It is by no means usual for a couple to achieve a pregnancy the first time they try, even when intercourse has been perfectly timed, and it may take several months before success is accomplished. Most doctors would not regard a couple as subfertile until they have been trying for a pregnancy for at least a year. Sadly, however, infertility can occur and is known to affect about one in ten couples in the Western world. Failure to conceive can be due to one or more reasons affecting the man, the woman or both.

MALE INFERTILITY

The only true test of a man's fertility is his ability to father a child. Short of this, some indication of male fertility or infertility is given by the sperm count, which reports on the number of sperm present, their shape and motility. Fertile men usually produce between 50 million and 150 million sperm per millilitre of ejaculated fluid. Men with sperm counts under ten million per millilitre are usually infertile. But the quality of the sperm matters as much as the number produced. Men are occasionally fertile despite low sperm counts and, conversely, men with high counts may not always be fertile.

Some men produce no sperm at all – this may follow infections such as some venereal diseases and mumps, sterilization by vasectomy, radiation therapy for cancers in the genital region or such men may have a rare disorder of their chromosomes (genetic make-up). Sperm counts may also be greatly reduced in men who smoke tobacco or marijuana, and also those who drink alcohol heavily.

The treatment of male infertility is largely angled at removing the cause – stopping excessive smoking and drinking, reversing a vasectomy, tying off abnormal scrotal veins and so on. Sometimes powerful hormone injections may improve sperm production, with steroid drugs to decrease the effects of an antibody interference.

Sometimes normal sperm may be rendered inactive when they arrive at the cervix, because the mucus through which they must pass there is thick, acid and therefore hostile. This may be counter-acted by treating any infection present which might cause this, and by giving the woman oestrogen tablets to make the mucus flow clear and plentiful at the time of ovulation.

FEMALE INFERTILITY

One of the most common causes of female infertility is ovulation failure. Ovulation can be achieved by giving the woman tablets which help the pituitary gland stimulate egg ripening or by powerful injections of hormones which stimulate the ovaries directly. In this case there is an increased likelihood of multiple births. By and large, however, the treatment for ovulation problems using closely monitored modern medical techniques is successful. Multiple births are usually limited to twins.

Another frequent cause of female infertility is blockage of the Fallopian tubes, which prevents fertilization of the ovum. Tube damage may follow severe pelvic infections or the formation of adhesions (bands or scar tissue) after surgical operations. Fallopian tubes may also be artificially blocked for sterilization.

The unblocking of Fallopian tubes is relatively straightforward, thanks to up-to-date microsurgical techniques. The blocked portions are removed and the ends joined up again. However, if the lining of the remaining pieces of Fallopian tube has been damaged by previous infection, then the fertilized ovum will not be sustained and nourished in the tube as usual and a pregnancy will not develop, despite the tubes being open again.

A neat way of by-passing the tubes is by in vitro fertilization (IVF) – the test tube baby approach. In this technique eggs are removed from the woman's stimulated ovaries and mixed with her partner's sperm in a dish, under specially controlled conditions. The fertilized eggs are then placed inside her uterus some hours later. Their development is then monitored – usually only one embryo survives to grow into a healthy baby, and the pregnancy proceeds in the normal way. It should be stressed, however, that IVF requires considerable motivation on the part of both prospective parents and that the number of women suited to this treatment is very small.

INVESTIGATING INFERTILITY

If you are worried about your fertility, talk it over with your general practitioner who can give you general advice, explain what special tests may be necessary and refer you to a specialist. There are also self-help groups who can support you with counselling and advice.

ANTENATAL CARE

The pattern of pregnancy care and its importance for the health and well-being of you and your baby

Pregnancy is not an illness. The majority of mothers-to-be are healthy women who go through the normal process of bearing a child without any problems beyond the minor discomforts associated with the development of the fetus in the uterus. Occasional problems can occur, however, which may threaten the health of the baby or the mother, or both. And some women with existing conditions, such as diabetes or some form of physical disability, need extra help during pregnancy. For these reasons, regular antenatal check-ups are important – to reassure you that all is well and to act quickly when it is not.

THE LENGTH OF PREGNANCY

You usually have your first full antenatal check-up between the tenth and twelfth weeks of pregnancy, during what is sometimes known as the first trimester. 'Trimester' is a term used by doctors to mean a three month period: for convenience pregnancy is divided into three trimesters (weeks 1 to 12, 13 to 28 and 29 to 40). These divisions are not particularly significant.

People have traditionally thought of pregnancy as being nine months long, but doctors and midwives prefer to use a more accurate method to establish the estimated date of delivery (EDD). The average pregnancy lasts 38 weeks from conception, which for most women will take place in the middle of their menstrual cycle (see p. 10). However, since this assumes that all women have a regular 28 day cycle, which is by no means the case, your EDD is usually calculated from the first day of your last menstrual period. A simple way to find this out is to add 40 weeks from the date of the start of your last period, or alternatively to add seven days to the first day of your last period and then add nine months to that. For example, if your last period started on 14 June, add seven days (21 June), then add nine months (21 March) which becomes your EDD. Bear in mind that these dates are only estimates: a normal pregnancy can be anything from 38 to 42 weeks long.

If for some reason you don't know or can't remember the date of your last period, or if your cycle is very irregular, during your first antenatal check-up the doctor or midwife will try to establish the size and therefore the age of the fetus by measuring the size of your uterus during an internal examination (see p. 23), or you will be given an ultrasound scan (see p. 25).

CONFIRMING THE PREGNANCY

The first sign of pregnancy for most women is a missed menstrual period (known as amenorrhoea) which is a sign that the developing embryo has embedded in the endometrium (see p. 39). However, if your periods are irregular you may notice other signs first (see p. 43). In fact, if you have partially suppressed periods for a month or two, you may not even know that you are pregnant for a while.

Your breasts may enlarge and become quite tender. You also notice that the nipples and areola (the area round the nipples) become darker, and the areola will develop small protuberances, called Montgomery's tubercles, glands which help to keep the nipples supple. Some women experience nausea (morning sickness) right from the start, though this usually develops over the first six weeks or so, subsiding at about twelve to fourteen weeks (see p. 44). You may also notice a need to urinate more often, and you might also become aware of increasing tiredness.

You can confirm the pregnancy before you see your GP by having a urine test. Family planning clinics and health centres may offer pregnancy testing, and chemists can also arrange a urine test for a small charge. Alternatively you could try a home pregnancy testing kit.

VISITING YOUR GP

When you think you may be pregnant, visit your family doctor as soon as possible. Unless you have a particular condition which requires urgent decision-making, or you or your doctor think your pregnancy may already be fairly far advanced, your doctor is unlikely to do more at this stage than to

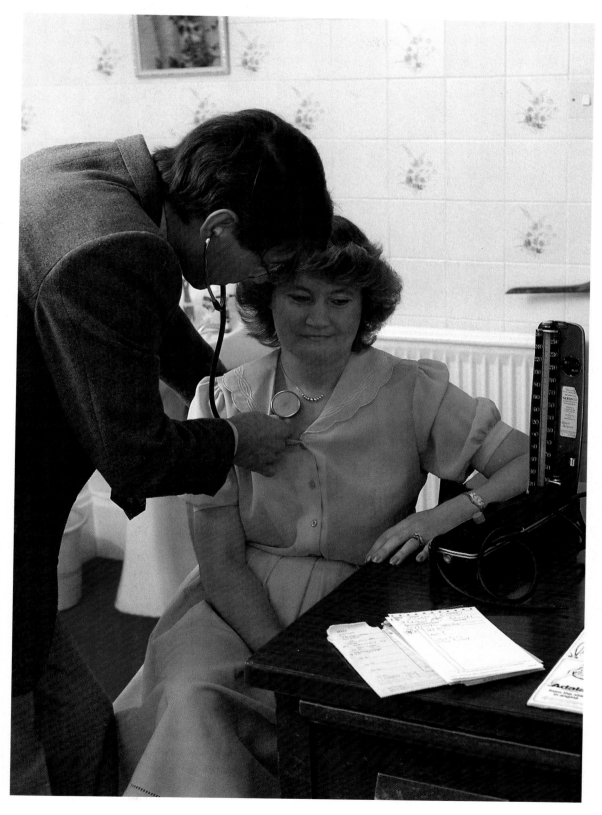

congratulate you, check that you are generally well and make arrangements for antenatal care, depending on where you want to have your baby.

It is worth thinking about birth options before you have this discussion with your doctor. If you are not sure, talk about it with your GP and defer the decision for a few days, after which you can make the necessary arrangements through your doctor at another consultation. The information given in the next few pages about pregnancy care and the pros and cons of hospital or home births may help you make up your mind.

PREGNANCY CARE

Pregnancy care varies in different parts of the country; in some areas you will have a wide range of choices, in others very few. Three different care givers can provide antenatal care – your GP, a midwife, or a specialist doctor at the hospital, called an obstetrician.

A GP does antenatal check-ups in the surgery. Obstetricians usually give their care in the hospital antenatal clinic – but a few go out to a clinic in the community so that women do not always have to travel to the hospital. Midwives are able to be much more flexible than obstetricians or GPs, as they can work in and out of the hospital or the community, giving antenatal care either in the local health centre, in the GP's surgery, in the hospital or in your own home. Midwives are the experts in normal childbirth, and if all goes well with your pregnancy and birth it will be a midwife who delivers your baby, as she does for 76 per cent of pregnant women, and who provides most of your pregnancy care.

There are many combinations of antenatal care. If they opt for a hospital delivery, some women go to the hospital antenatal clinic for all their appointments where they are examined by an obstetrician or a midwife. Hospital antenatal clinics are busy places and although you will nominally be under the care of a consultant obstetrician, in practice you may not always see the same doctor or midwife at every visit.

Even though they may be giving birth in hospital, some women go to their GP or community midwife for all their antenatal care, apart from one or two hospital visits at the start of pregnancy and towards the end. Some of these 'shared care' arrangements also fit another hospital visit in at about 30 weeks.

More rarely, you may be able to have all or most of your antenatal care in your own home with a midwife, with perhaps two or three visits only to your GP. This is most likely to happen if you have a home delivery through your GP or take on the services of an independent midwife.

WHERE TO HAVE THE BABY

You can either have your baby at home or in hospital. Most women in the UK have their babies in hospital and there is some controversy about the relative merits of a home or hospital delivery. Increasing evidence shows that if you are healthy and want to have your baby at home, there is no reason why you shouldn't. The difficulty nowadays is to find a doctor and community or independent midwife in your area who are willing to offer this service, as health authorities tend to concentrate resources for pregnancy and childbirth on hospital care, and many doctors are not convinced of the safety of home deliveries. At the same time, many hospital maternity units are trying to relax their atmosphere to make it as comfortable for mothers as possible.

HOME DELIVERIES

If you decide to have your baby at home, you will need to find a midwife who can look after you. Find her either at your GP's surgery or write to the Nursing Officer at your local hospital maternity unit and ask her to send a midwife to see you.

When you talk to your GP about your preferences, find out if he or she is prepared to be involved in a home delivery as well. Some doctors are unable or unwilling to offer this service, particularly to first-time mothers. If so, the Nursing Officer should have a list of doctors who are willing to do this. Some midwives have claimed that a doctor isn't necessary at all, but this would be unwise.

In some areas there is a midwife in private practice who delivers babies at home and provides all your antenatal and postnatal care for a fee. You can find out if there are any practising near you through the Independent Midwives Association. You could also ask the local branch of the Association for the Improvement of the Maternity Services (AIMS), the National Childbirth Trust (NCT), or the Society to Support Home Confinements. (All these addresses are given on pages 297-299). Joining a local branch of any of these organizations will enable you to meet other women who had their babies at home so you can find out first hand how to go about it in your area.

HOSPITAL DELIVERIES

Having a hospital delivery does not necessarily mean having a long stay in the postnatal ward nowadays. There is a tendency for mothers to leave hospital earlier nowadays, both because of pressure on beds and because it is not medically necessary for them to stay longer. Some women go into hospital when labour starts and stay there for about a week after the baby is born; others, especially if they have a child or children already, only stay for 48 hours or less and then go home to be looked after by their family and friends and the community midwife (see p. 132).

THE DOMINO SYSTEM

Many women feel that a hospital delivery is very impersonal; in a busy unit you are unlikely to know the midwife who delivers you before you go into labour. With the 'Domiciliary In and Out' (Domino) system, the community midwife who has been looking after you during pregnancy comes to your home as soon as you are in labour. She then decides when it is appropriate for you to go to hospital, calls the ambulance and travels there with you. There she delivers the baby and returns home with you a few hours after the baby is born.

THE GP UNIT

In some parts of the country there are small hospitals or hospital departments known as GP Units. Ask your doctor if he or she is involved in one of these. The unit may be a separate small hospital, or based in a larger hospital, either housed separately in the grounds or contained within the main building. GP units are usually more intimate and community-based than large maternity units in general hospitals. Sometimes the doctor may deliver babies himself, or his community midwife will supervise the delivery and the doctor will just come in to check your progress if necessary.

PROS AND CONS

The main risks of a home delivery are usually defined as excessive bleeding of the mother or problems with the baby's breathing at birth, which are difficult to deal with safely outside hospital. However, midwives usually carry drugs to help the uterus contract in case of bleeding and also carry the equipment to administer intravenous fluids to increase blood volume. Midwives also carry resuscitation equipment for the baby if there is any difficulty with breathing.

If any emergency crops up during a home delivery the mother can be transferred to hospital just as if she was having a 'domino' delivery, or a specially equipped ambulance can be called, bringing a doctor and midwife (called a 'flying squad') to help the midwife at home. 'Flying squads' are mainly attached to large hospitals and may be some distance

from your home. About one in ten of women having a first baby at home end up having a 'domino' delivery instead, but fewer women having their second or third babies at home end up in hospital.

Women having babies at home feel that they are taking responsibility for their birth and for their babies right from the start. For many women, a home delivery is relaxing and intimate: only your immediate family and a midwife or doctor that you know will be present and you do not have to interrupt the progress of your labour with a journey to the hospital.

THE RISKS OF HOME BIRTHS

Most doctors advise against home deliveries for a first baby. There are also valid arguments against having a baby at home if you have any medical problems such as kidney disease, very high blood pressure, a heart condition or diabetes. Women who have had a Caesarean section in the past have a 1 in 100 chance that the scar on their uterus could give way during a subsequent labour, so many doctors and midwives feel that the risk is too great and are very reluctant to agree to a home delivery for a woman who has had a previous Caesarean section. In addition, if your height is 157cm (5ft 2in) or less, you have an increased chance of needing a Caesarean section, so you will probably be safer if you arrange for a hospital delivery. You would be safer with a hospital delivery if you are having twins, and if your baby is breech you will be advised to go into hospital, even if you had arranged a home birth originally.

It is always a good idea to ask your mother how she gave birth to you and your brothers and sisters. If she gave birth normally, your pelvis is probably like hers and you will be able to give birth normally too. If she needed a Caesarean delivery it may mean that her pelvis was narrow at some points and you may have inherited that. If she had a forceps delivery it may have been for the same reason.

In many areas it is very difficult to organize a home delivery, and a hospital delivery is inevitable. Many women prefer this anyway; they like the security of knowing that if anything goes wrong at the last minute there will be up-to-date equipment and specialist staff available immediately to deal with the emergency. Some women, especially first time mothers, prefer to have a few days in the postnatal ward to get used to their babies and to have the option to call on a midwife day or night to advise them. It is also an opportunity to meet other mothers, some of whom may be more experienced. And although it may be a wrench to leave older children at home, some second or third time mothers like the fact that even 36 hours in hospital gives them the opportunity to be alone with the new baby without the extra pressures of family life.

THE RISKS OF HOSPITAL BIRTHS

The risks to women of having a baby in hospital are not often discussed because most women have their babies there, but they do exist. They are usually seen as being two-fold – the risk of infection due to the large number of people using the hospital, and the risk from interference in a normal physiological experience which may have an adverse effect on labour. For instance, in hospital you are more likely to be electronically monitored (see p.81). Although monitoring may be necessary it sometimes is not, and, unless there is a 'remote control' facility, it does mean that the mother cannot move around as she would normally do in labour. As a result the pain she feels may be more intense because she is unable to do anything physical to relieve it. This in turn may lead to the use of more painkillers which may affect not only the way the baby is delivered but also the baby's condition.

In addition to these possible inconveniences during labour, a few hospitals still remove babies from their mothers to a nursery, especially at night. This may not worry some mothers who would be glad to hand over responsibility to the staff in the hospital, especially if they are very tired after a difficult labour. But it is not particularly pleasant for a mother who feels well and wants to keep her baby with her all the time to be denied that choice.

A hospital is a large institution catering for a wide section of the population, and like all large institutions it cannot always fit in with every individual's needs even though everyone working there does their best, whereas if you are at home you are probably the centre of attention. If you are fortunate to have the choice of several different types of service for your antenatal care and birth, weigh up all the pros and cons according to your own feelings and expectations. These expectations may not always be possible to fulfill – every labour is different and things can change at the very last minute, but at least you will feel that you have made the initial decisions.

THE FIRST ANTENATAL CHECK-UP

If you decide to have your baby at the hospital, your doctor will give you a letter of referral which you can either take or send to the antenatal appointments office. Telephone the hospital first if you are unsure of the procedure. The appointments office will then send you an appointment for the 'booking clinic',

along with information about the hospital and any special instructions, such as whether to bring a urine sample.

Your doctor will have indicated in the introductory letter whether there is any particular reason for urgency, such as a history of previous miscarriage. If so, you will be given an appointment as soon as possible; otherwise you can expect it to be around the twelfth week of pregnancy.

THE BOOKING CLINIC

Your first antenatal visit to the hospital will be to the booking clinic. This clinic usually takes a long time, as the hospital needs to gather a great deal of information about you, especially if you are expecting your first child. Depending on the appointments system and the number of women to be seen, you could be at the hospital for about three hours on this visit. Go prepared with a drink and something to while away the time: if you don't have a long wait after all, that will be a bonus.

The order in which things happen in a booking clinic may vary from hospital to hospital, but they all cover the same basic procedures. What follows is a typical routine. All the information will be entered into your notes which are the hospital's permanent record of your pregnancy. You may be given your notes to look at – more usually the hospital keeps the notes and gives you a co-operation card in which the same information is entered in abbreviated form. It is a good idea to keep this card with you at all times. If you are having shared care your family doctor or community midwife will want to see what the hospital has put into it and will enter his or her own observations as well at subsequent antenatal check-ups in the surgery. If you are having all your care at the hospital, your co-op card (as it is usually known) is helpful if you ever require emergency treatment.

When you arrive at the clinic, you will probably be weighed and your height measured. You will be weighed at every subsequent antenatal visit. Weight gain is one indication of the progress of labour – excessive weight gain can cause problems, but it is also important that you put on enough weight, according to your height and build (see p. 46).

THE URINE TEST

You will be asked to bring a clean sample of urine to every antenatal visit, and will probably be given a special container. At the booking clinic you will be asked to provide a 'mid-stream specimen of urine' (MSU) for testing. This is a specimen uncontaminated by mucus or discharge, and you will be given a

Blood pressure is a useful indicator of the health of your pregnancy and will be measured by the midwife or doctor at every antenatal check-up.

special sterile cleansing pack with instructions for use. Sterile water and cotton wool swabs are provided to clean your genital area; you then pass a small amount of urine into the lavatory, stopping the flow in 'mid-stream', catching the next part of the stream in the jar provided. You take this to the midwife or assistant for testing. Some women find they can stop and start the flow of urine with ease because of the strength of their pelvic floor muscles (see p. 32), while others find it more difficult. It is worth persevering since the midwife may ask you for another sample if the first is contaminated. Your urine sample will be checked immediately for the presence of protein and sugar, and also be cultured for infection.

These tests give important signals about your health and the progress of your pregnancy, which is why you are asked to bring a sample every time. Protein in urine may indicate kidney infection, or, later in pregnancy, may be a symptom of pre-eclampsia (see p. 70), especially if associated with high blood pressure. Sugar in urine is a possible sign of diabetes, but many non-diabetic women have sugar in their urine during pregnancy due to hormonal changes. This will be double-checked with your blood test (see later). Your urine will also

be checked for the presence of ketones (also known as acetones) which appear when the body is short of glucose. This could be due to dietary deficiency, excessive nausea or dehydration, and you will receive treatment for it.

BLOOD PRESSURE

At this first and every subsequent antenatal visit your blood pressure and pulse will be measured, using a special instrument called a sphygmomano-meter.

Blood pressure is an important gauge of the health of your pregnancy. It is measured in terms of the pressure at the peak of a heartbeat (systolic pressure) and when the heart is most relaxed (diastolic pressure). Normal blood pressure can range from 90/60 to 130/85, and the systolic pressure can vary widely according to how active you are being at the time. The diastolic level should, however, remain about the same. Blood pressure should drop as your pregnancy advances due to the action of the hormone progesterone. If the diastolic level rises more than a certain amount, it may be a symptom of pre-eclampsia and you will probably be advised to have bed rest (see p. 70).

BLOOD TESTS

At some point during your first visit you will be asked to give a blood sample. This may be taken by a doctor or midwife, or, more likely, you will have to go to a special department to have the sample taken by a specialist technician called a phlebotomist. This first sample is very important as it gives a lot of important information about your health and the health of your baby. It will be used to establish your blood group (A, B, O or AB). The haemoglobin level (Hb) of your blood will also be checked to see if you are anaemic, and you may be given iron and folic acid tablets to prevent anaemia (see p. 52).

Your blood will also be tested for the rhesus factor. If like most of the population your blood contains this, you are 'rhesus positive', and have no further problems. If however you are 'rhesus negative' (no rhesus factor), there may be future difficulties if your baby has rhesus positive blood. Rhesus positive and rhesus negative blood are incompatible, and if during pregnancy or birth some of the baby's blood crosses from the placenta into the mother's bloodstream the mother may develop antibodies which would destroy the rhesus factor in the blood of a subsequent baby. The baby could be born severely anaemic, requiring an exchange blood transfusion (see p. 122).

Fortunately this situation is now very rare since the condition can be treated. If you are found to be rhesus negative, you may be given a dose of rhesus antibody (immunoglobulin Anti-D) after the birth. In some circumstances you may be given this during pregnancy, for instance after an amniocentesis or an antepartum haemorrhage (see p. 62). Some units even give it routinely at 36 weeks to rhesus negative women.

Your blood will also be tested to see if you are immune to rubella (German measles), which can have a catastrophic effect on the baby if contracted during pregnancy (see p. 13). If you are not immune you will be offered immunization after the birth. (Never be inoculated during pregnancy. Rubella immunization involves a 'live' vaccine, so it could have the same effect on your unborn baby as the disease itself.)

Your blood will also be screened for sexually transmitted diseases, especially syphilis. Although very few women now have this disease, those who do may not know it and it can be transmitted to the fetus after about 20 weeks. If the disease is found before 20 weeks, it can be successfully treated. Blood is not automatically screened for AIDS at the moment, but if you think you may be at risk from this disease you can ask the doctor to arrange this for you (see also p. 29).

THE INTERVIEW

Apart from the physical examination by the doctor, which is usually the last item in the booking clinic schedule, by far the longest time will be spent on your 'booking history'. This is taken by a midwife in the form of an informal interview conducted in private. It consists of a long series of personal and medical details about yourself, your family and your partner which gives the medical staff information which may be helpful in the management of your pregnancy and birth, and possibly in the subsequent care of your baby. This information is confidential so don't be shy about giving complete details of your medical history, particularly any gynaecological details such as a termination of pregnancy (abortion), pelvic infection or sexually transmitted disease.

The most important questions the midwife will ask you concern the progress of your present pregnancy and that of any earlier pregnancies, even if they ended in miscarriage or termination. She will want to know the date of your last period, its duration and what it is usually like. She will record whether you are suffering from headaches, nausea or other discomforts. She will ask at what week of pregnancy any previous children were born, or when miscarriages took place, and about any abnormal deliveries.

The midwife will want to know social details of your life as well. She will ask about your past health and that of your partner, and of your parents and grandparents. She will want to know if any handicapped babies have been born to either family (if you don't know it's worth enquiring of relatives before you go to hospital), and she will want to know how your mother gave birth to you and your brothers and sisters. She will also want to know whether you were breast or bottle fed and whether you have decided which method of feeding your prefer for your own baby.

She will also ask you about your medical history and that of your partner; whether you suffer from any chronic condition, what infectious diseases you and your partner have had, and whether either of you has had heart disease, tuberculosis, mental illness or allergies, or whether there are any members of your families who suffer or suffered from these conditions. Don't worry if you don't know all the answers to these questions, but if you find out subsequently tell the midwife at your next antenatal check-up.

The midwife will give you the relevant forms for obtaining free medication and dental treatment until one year after the baby's birth, and will also tell you how to apply for maternity benefit.

symphysis pubis

uterus

ovary

urethra

bladder

vagina

anus

cervix

rectum

bowel

coccyx

To check the size and position of the uterus, the doctor inserts two fingers into the vagina while pressing on the abdomen with the other hand.

The midwife may well ask you if there is anything special you were thinking about for labour – any special way you want to be looked after, or would prefer to be delivered if possible. If she doesn't talk about this, raise the topic yourself. You may well be shell-shocked by this 'interrogation' but this is a good time to ask questions if you have any, and your partner may like to as well if he is with you. If you haven't decided about how you want to conduct your labour yet, you can have this part filled in at a later visit, but it is best to discuss it as early in your pregnancy as possible so that it can be recorded in your notes, rather than leaving it to the last minute. Trying to make special requests in a busy labour ward can make communication difficult.

THE PHYSICAL EXAMINATION

At the first antenatal visit, the physical examination is always carried out by an obstetrician (or your GP if he or she is looking after your antenatal care).

There may well be another long wait before you see the doctor. If you especially want to see a woman doctor, you should always ask and the midwife will try and arrange it. However, it isn't always possible since there are far fewer female obstetricians than male. If the pregnancy proceeds normally, you will be examined by a midwife at future visits at least until the last few weeks of pregnancy. You are usually seen by the doctor at certain important times, such as 28 and 36 weeks, and thereafter until full-term.

The doctor will examine your breasts and nipples and give advice on their care if you intend to breastfeed. He or she will listen to your heart and lungs and ask you if you smoke. If you do you will be advised to give it up (see p. 46).

THE INTERNAL EXAMINATION

The most important part of this first examination is the palpation of your abdomen and the internal examination. You will be asked to lie on the couch and the doctor will press (palpate) your abdomen to feel whether the uterus has grown big enough to be felt above the symphisis pubis (see p. 41). This does not happen until about the twelfth week of pregnancy, so it is a useful guide to the exact stage of your pregnancy. The doctor will then give you an internal examination to assess the size of the uterus by pressing on your abdomen with one hand and feeling the position of the cervix with the other. This is particularly useful if you were not sure of the date of your last menstrual period, and you may find that you are further on with the pregnancy than you thought. If this is the case the doctor is likely to arrange for you to have an ultrasound scan as soon as possible to confirm his or her own findings.

You may also have a cervical smear taken if you have not had one done recently. The doctor will insert a speculum into your vagina and gently scrape a few cells from your cervix to be examined for abnormal cells by a specialist cytologist in the laboratory. You will probably get the result at your next appointment, but any treatment required will probably be left until after the birth.

If you already have a history of miscarriage the doctor may decide to avoid making an internal examination until later in your pregnancy, perhaps at about fifteen or sixteen weeks, after the vulnerable period for early miscarriage has passed. In this case he will almost certainly refer you for an early ultrasound scan as well.

FATHERS AT THE ANTENATAL CLINIC

Your partner will always be made welcome at the antenatal clinic – it is useful for him to know how your pregnancy is progressing first hand. Fathers are invariably invited into the consulting room, and may have useful information to contribute to the booking history about their families' medical history and their own feelings concerning the forthcoming birth. Your partner will also be able to give an outsider's view of how you have been during your pregnancy – whether you have been more irritable or more emotional than usual. He will also be able to hear for himself advice about diet, giving up smoking and reducing alcohol – it could help you both to stop or cut down on these.

Your partner may also be better able to remember the questions you wanted to ask, and take in more of the information and advice given to you towards the end of your pregnancy when your concentration begins to waver. It is useful to have someone with you with whom to discuss the conversations afterwards. And a final important benefit for fathers in the antenatal clinic is the insight it will give them into the whole process of childbirth. Most hospitals welcome fathers into the labour ward nowadays, and most women want to have their partners with them during labour and birth. However there are still some men who are reluctant or diffident about

being there. Attending antenatal check-ups with their partners can help to demystify childbirth for them and prepare them just as it does mothers, especially if these visits are combined with preparation classes (see p. 30).

OTHER ADVICE

Before you leave the booking clinic you may well be invited to talk to one or two other health workers who are there to help you. Many hospitals invite couples to an introductory talk on parentcraft in which midwives and physiotherapists give advice on how to stay healthy and fit during pregnancy. They will also tell you how to join regular classes on parentcraft and preparation for childbirth (see p. 30).

There is usually a hospital dietician attached to the antenatal clinic who will advise you about healthy eating during pregnancy (see p. 46). If you are a vegan (a vegetarian who eats no animal produce at all) she will make sure that a midwife supplies you with extra Vitamin B12 supplements, since this vitamin is essential for the healthy growth of your baby and is only present in animal products. In some hospitals Asian women are advised to take extra Vitamin D. Vitamin D is usually produced through the action of the sun shining on skin; because many Asian women wear clothes which cover them almost completely they may not make enough Vitamin D for their needs. This is not a problem for Afro-Caribbean women.

If the midwife has reason to believe from your interview with her that you need special financial or welfare assistance, she may suggest you talk to the hospital social worker. This is particularly helpful if you are a single parent or if either you or your partner is unemployed or have housing problems. It is a good idea to set the wheels in motion early in pregnancy in order to make your life easier once the baby is born. The social worker can help you assess your rights to the various benefits (see pp. 294-295) both before and after the birth.

SPECIAL ANTENATAL TESTS

Most women require no more than the routine antenatal checks described above throughout their pregnancies. If however the midwife or doctor has any reason to be concerned about the health of yourself or the fetus, or if you are among a small minority of women who might be at risk of passing on certain inherited diseases or abnormalities to your baby (see p. 15), then you may be offered one of a number of special screening tests which help to diagnose such problems as early as possible.

ULTRASOUND

The use of ultrasound scanners in obstetric care is one of the most beneficial technical advances of the past twenty years. Almost all maternity units have this facility, and some of the machines in use are extremely sophisticated. Ultrasound was developed during the First World War as a means of detecting submarines under water; it works by bouncing very high frequency sound waves off solid objects which show up as a picture on a visual display unit. It is mainly used to check fetal age and health, since accurate measurements can be taken of the diameter of the head, the length of the spine or thigh bone, all of which can be used to compute fetal age. Position and presentation of the fetus can be ascertained, multiple pregnancies can be diagnosed with certainty at a very early stage, and a skilled operator can often distinguish the sex of the fetus (although they won't usually tell you!).

In addition more sophisticated machines can check the position and health of the placenta and the cervix, enabling early diagnosis of such conditions as placenta praevia or cervical incompetence (see pp. 60 and 63). Ultrasound can also be used to detect fetal abnormalities such as spina bifida, and uterine abnormalities such as fibroids. It can also be used to diagnose whether a miscarriage is likely to be inevitable as early as six or seven weeks of pregnancy, and is also used for amniocentesis and chorion villus sampling (see p. 28).

The ultrasound machine is completely harmless to the mother – indeed it avoids the need for an internal examination in many cases so can be seen as positively beneficial. It is also extremely interesting for both parents to see the baby on the screen, literally bringing the pregnancy to life. This can be particularly meaningful for fathers who sometimes feel excluded from the excitement of the pregnancy because they have no direct physical involvement. Some hospitals will provide you with a photograph of the image as a keepsake.

There is no evidence that the use of ultrasound use in pregnancy harms the fetus, although this has not yet been proven with certainty by long term research. Many hospital consultants confine routine scanning to a single appointment at about sixteen or seventeen weeks, others prefer to have a second scan done routinely later in pregnancy at perhaps 30 or 32 weeks. Occasionally you may be scanned more frequently if your doctor wants to check something specific, particularly if you experience any bleeding or if the doctor or midwife wants to check that the baby is growing properly (see p. 72).

In early pregnancy you will probably be asked to come to an ultrasound appointment with a full bladder. This can cause some discomfort if you are kept waiting, but it does help to give the radiographer a better view of your uterus on the screen. To be scanned, you lie on a couch in a darkened room. Your abdomen is smeared with warm oil or a special gel which allows the transducer (the scanning probe) to pass across your abdomen with ease and to give a clear image with less interference to

Most pregnant women are now given a routine ultrasound scan at sixteen to seventeen weeks to check the size, gestational age and health of the fetus and placenta. Ultrasound is also used to help diagnostic techniques, such as amniocentesis and chorion villus sampling, and to look for problems such as placenta praevia or perhaps the presence of more than one baby.

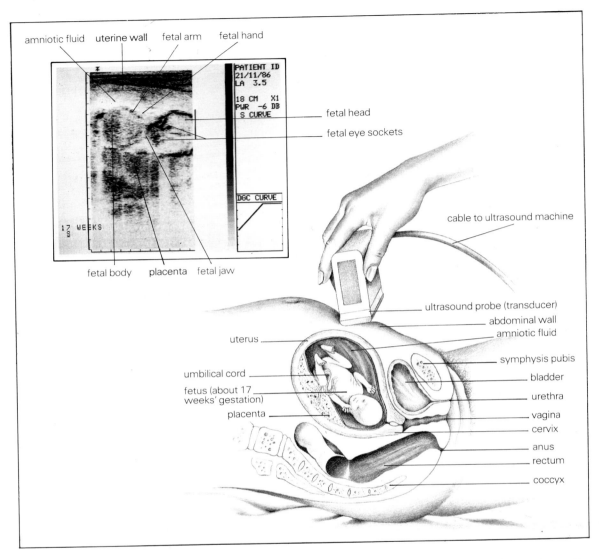

amniotic fluid uterine wall fetal arm fetal hand

PATIENT ID
21/11/86
LA 3.5

18 CM X1
PWR -6 DB
S CURVE

fetal head

fetal eye sockets

DGC CURVE

17 WEEKS

fetal body placenta fetal jaw

cable to ultrasound machine

ultrasound probe (transducer)
abdominal wall
amniotic fluid

uterus

symphysis pubis

umbilical cord

bladder

fetus (about 17 weeks' gestation)

urethra

placenta

vagina
cervix
anus
rectum
coccyx

Top: *The film positive taken from an ultrasound scan of a fetus of seventeen weeks' gestation.*
Above: *A cross-section of the mother's uterus, with a seventeen-week fetus. Ultrasound can now show congenital abnormalities of internal organs at this stage.*

the sound waves. The radiographer (sometimes called an ultrasonographer), moves the transducer across to produce the image on the screen which can then be interpreted.

SPECIAL BLOOD TESTS

In addition to the routine blood tests requested from all mothers at antenatal booking, some women will be tested for a specific group of blood disorders

which are passed on by inheritance – these disorders are known as 'haemoglobinopathies', and include sickle cell anaemia and thalassaemia. They are caused by an abnormality of haemoglobin, the substance that gives blood its red colour and carries oxygen round the body in the red blood cells. The type of haemoglobin you make depends on the genetic material you inherit from your parents. Sometimes an unusual haemoglobin may be inherited from only one parent (a 'carrier state' or 'trait'), or, more rarely, from both, when it can cause a serious and disabling illness. People with the 'trait' are not ill but could pass on the full blown condition to their children if their partners were similarly affected.

For couples at such risk antenatal diagnosis is possible and counselling can be made available.

Sickle cell disease is particularly common among people from West Africa or the Caribbean, while people of Mediterranean origin are more likely to have types of thalassaemia. Other races such as Arabs and those from the Indian sub-continent have a lesser but significant incidence. If you come from any of these parts of the world, or you are descended from someone who did, it is important that you have the simple blood screening test performed. If you are not offered it at the antenatal clinic please ask your midwife or doctor. It can even be done before pregnancy if you so wish.

Another blood test may be offered to certain women at about fifteen weeks of pregnancy which measures alpha feto protein (AFP) levels. Alpha feto protein is a substance in the blood of babies in the uterus which can spill over into the mother's bloodstream. If the level of AFP is very high, it can indicate that the baby has spina bifida (a defect in which the skin of the back does not close properly, leaving the spinal column exposed), so if found an ultrasound or amniocentesis may be suggested as confirmation. The AFP test is not 100 per cent accurate – high levels may not mean abnormality at all (they are one sign of a multiple birth, for instance) and as many as one in five women may be found to have high AFP levels but their babies are perfectly all right. Conversely a negative AFP test is not unfortunately a guarantee that no abnormality is present.

AMNIOCENTESIS

Amniocentesis is the name given to the procedure by which a sample of amniotic fluid is drawn from the uterus by means of a hollow needle inserted through the abdominal wall. Before the needle is inserted, an ultrasound scan is made to find the position of the fetus and the placenta so that the needle can be inserted in a safe place. A local anaesthetic is given in the abdominal wall so that you will feel no pain. It is advisable to rest for a day or so after an amniocentesis as the technique may irritate the uterus. If you feel any pain, experience any bleeding or leakage of fluid from the vagina after an amniocentesis, contact the hospital at once.

Amniocentesis is only used where it is considered important to check the chemical content of the fluid, or fetal cells floating in it for chromosomal abnormalities, especially those indicating Down's syndrome (which used to be called mongolism). If any abnormality is found the mother may then be offered a termination of pregnancy. This is a difficult and distressing decision for any couple to have to face and you will be given sympathetic counselling to help you. If you would not want a termination of

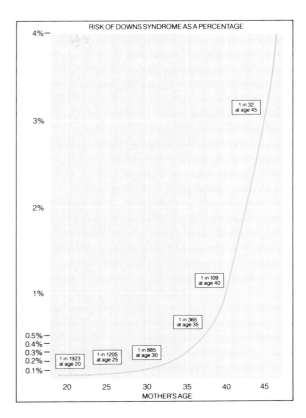

This graph shows how the risk of having a Down's syndrome baby rises steeply in women over the age of 35. Most maternity units will now offer amniocentesis to detect this condition to all pregnant women over the age of 37. However it should be remembered that 50 per cent of Down's babies are born to women under that age, simply because proportionately more women have babies then than between the ages of 35 and 45.

pregnancy under any circumstances, you do not have to accept an amniocentesis if it is offered. On the other hand, if you do have an amniocentesis and the result shows an abnormality you may find that even so you cannot face a termination. In this case every effort will be made to help you prepare yourself for the future (see p. 280).

Statistically, the older the mother the greater is the risk of chromosomal abnormalities occurring, so most of the larger hospitals offer amniocentesis to all women over 37. These women have a higher risk of producing a Down's syndrome baby, and by the age of 39 or over, the risk – about one per cent – is as great as the chance of miscarrying as a result of the amniocentesis itself. It is difficult to weigh up the risk of miscarriage against the risk of bearing an abnormal baby – the graph above may help you.

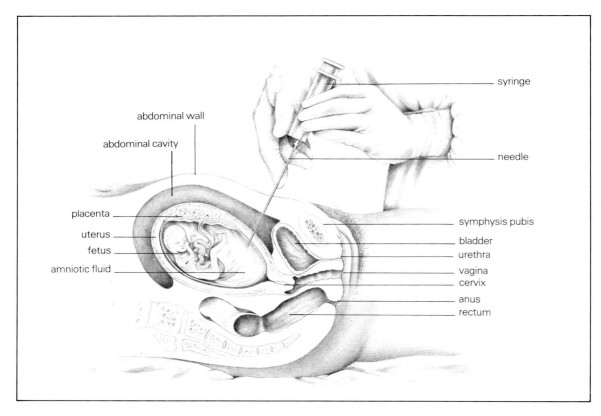

For amniocentesis, the skin of the abdomen is anaesthetized and a fine needle is inserted with ultrasound guidance into the top of the uterus. Amniotic fluid is then drawn out with a syringe.

Remember also that no test has yet been developed which can discover all types of congenital abnormality; amniocentesis only helps rule out some of the most distressing. And statistics can always be looked at another way – even when a mother is as old as 49, the chance of her having a normal healthy baby is as high as 91 per cent.

The earliest the test can be done is about fifteen weeks. Waiting for the result can be an anxious time as it can take as long as four weeks for the results of the amniocentesis to come through from the laboratory, by which time you may well be able to feel your baby moving. As a result many women who have amniocentesis do not let themselves become involved in the pregnancy until they have the result – they detach themselves as much as possible from their growing baby and keep their feelings suppressed. This of course does not mean they are any less upset if they have to have their pregnancies terminated; it is always a terrible decision to make.

If you are unlucky enough to have an unfavourable result after an amniocentesis and you opt for a termination of pregnancy, you may find that your doctor recommends inducing a premature labour, rather than an operation. However, in the former case you will of course be given all the pain relief you want.

CHORIONIC VILLUS SAMPLING

Most ways of detecting inherited diseases or congenital abnormalities cannot be performed until well into the second trimester. However, chorionic villus sampling is a new technique, only available in a few centres, which enables the doctors to find out as early as nine to eleven weeks whether a baby is likely to be affected.

Chorion villus sampling is used to examine fetal chromosomes and detect genetic disorders such as Down's syndrome, Tay Sachs disease, thalassaemia and cystic fibrosis. The early stage at which it can be performed means that if anything abnormal is found the parents can have the option of an early termination of pregnancy, if they so wish. However, the technique has not yet been perfected and there is a fairly high risk of miscarriage attached to it, although this is now well under ten per cent, and for this reason, it is only offered to women whose babies are most at risk from these congenital

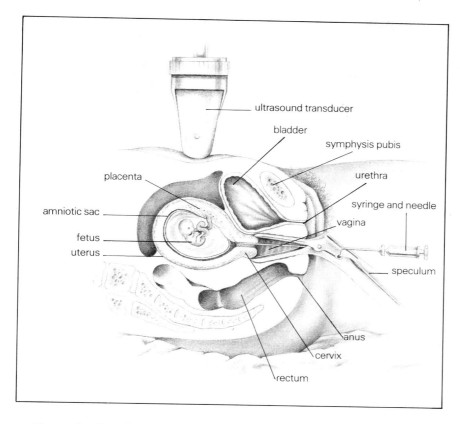

Chorion villus sampling is usually achieved by inserting a fine needle through the vagina and cervix with ultrasound guidance which removes a tiny sample of the villi near the internal os (neck of the uterus).

Labels on diagram: ultrasound transducer, bladder, symphysis pubis, urethra, placenta, syringe and needle, amniotic sac, vagina, fetus, uterus, speculum, anus, cervix, rectum

problems. On the other hand, since many miscarriages happen spontaneously at this stage of pregnancy, often because the fetus is abnormal, it is difficult for doctors always to be sure that a miscarriage associated with chorionic villus sampling would not have happened anyway.

Chorion villus sampling is performed with the help of ultrasound. Using a fine tube inserted either through the abdominal wall or through the cervix, the doctor guides it towards the chorionic villi, tiny root-like projections which eventually bed into the uterine wall to become the placenta (see p. 39). A few of these tiny projections are drawn out by a syringe and sent to the laboratory for testing. Although they are not part of the fetus, they have the same genetic make-up. It usually takes between seven and ten days to obtain the result – occasionally as much as two weeks – but even so, the waiting time is much less than that required for the result of an amniocentesis.

AIDS IN PREGNANCY

You will no doubt have heard a lot about this condition recently and may be anxious about its relevance to you and your baby. AIDS is a disease caused by a virus named the human immune deficiency virus (HIV) for which at present there is no cure. Acquisition of this virus means that the body's defence mechanism against disease becomes impaired and in many sufferers this leads to death from overwhelming infections. Not all people infected with the AIDS virus, however, have symptoms – some just carry it in their blood, but they could infect others under appropriate circumstances.

The disease is spread in three ways: by transmission in the blood, by sexual contact with an infected person, and from an infected mother to her baby. Although first reported in homosexual communities it is now clear that the disease can equally be spread by heterosexual partnerships.

AIDS is especially serious if associated with pregnancy because not only is there a strong possibility that the mother's disease may worsen, but there is a 60-70 per cent chance that the baby will acquire the infection in the womb and a 50 per cent chance that the child will die as a result. Because these risks are so great, women who are known to be infected are strongly advised to avoid pregnancy and should they become pregnant termination of pregnancy is recommended.

In the light of this it is now the policy of many obstetric units to offer antenatal screening for AIDS to certain mothers who are recognized to be in 'high risk' groups. The test is simple, involving only the taking of a blood sample, and the table summarizes those at risk. This 'at risk' group of the population is very small, so for most pregnant women AIDS will not be an issue they have to face. However, if you are at all anxious that you may be a carrier of infection for whatever reason then talk it over with your midwife and doctor who can easily arrange the screening test for you, if necessary.

You may be particularly worried about blood transfusions as it is recognized that this has been a way of transmitting the virus in the past, although very rarely in Britain. Nowadays, you can be reassured that all blood collected for transfusion in Britain is now screened, so if you have the misfortune to require a blood transfusion in your pregnancy you will not acquire AIDS.

FURTHER ANTENATAL VISITS

Most women in the UK have about fourteen antenatal appointments. Up to 28 weeks of pregnancy your antenatal checks will be at four-weekly intervals, unless there is some special reason to make them more frequent. From 28 to 36 weeks the appointments will be fortnightly, and from 36 weeks to birth the midwife or doctor will want to see you every week.

At each visit you will be asked to give a sample of urine, you will be weighed and your blood pressure taken. The size of the fetus will be measured by palpation, and the fetal heart rate monitored either through a Pinard's stethoscope (which is like a small ear trumpet) or with a portable ultrasound which amplifies the sound of the baby's heartbeat. If your partner comes with you to later antenatal appointments, he may be able to listen to the baby's

heartbeat through the stethoscope as well. You will notice that the fetal heartbeat is about twice as fast as yours – between 120 and 160 beats a minute.

The midwife will want to know when you first feel fetal movements (usually around the twentieth week for a first baby, but earlier for mothers who have had several children). Towards the end of pregnancy the presentation and position of the fetus will be checked, and any complications will be dealt with immediately they crop up.

If you have any worries between your antenatal appointments don't be afraid to call the clinic sister or your community midwife for advice, or go and see your own doctor at an ordinary appointment. If you have any queries about the minor discomforts of pregnancy (see pp. 44 and 50) it is a good idea to write them down so that you remember to mention them to the midwife at your next appointment.

PREPARATION CLASSES

As you approach the end of your pregnancy it is worth thinking about labour and how you want to deal with it so that you can discuss it with the midwife at the antenatal clinic, if you haven't already done so. Do you want your partner with you or some other person, like your mother, sister or a close friend? Decisions about positions for labour and delivery cannot always be made in advance, and many a firm resolve falters once labour starts. However you can discuss the options with your midwife and your partner beforehand, so that you can let the hospital know that you are thinking about squatting or using a birthing chair, or having an epidural anaesthetic.

All these topics are covered in the preparation classes that are provided by most hospitals, or sometimes in health clinics or doctors' surgeries. Some classes are also run by organizations like the National Childbirth Trust and take place in the homes of trained instructors. Hospital or clinic classes are usually run by midwives with the help of obstetric physiotherapists who are skilled in dealing with the physical aspects of pregnancy, birth and the puerperium.

Wherever the classes are held, and whatever they are called, they have the same aims and function. They give you an opportunity to get to know other people in your area who are expecting babies at the same sort of time as you are. This is more important than might appear at first – there is nothing more isolating especially for first-time parents than suddenly finding yourselves at home with a baby when you don't know other people close by with whom you can share experiences. Preparation classes teach you about what happens in labour, about pain

Antenatal classes welcome both mothers and fathers to prepare for labour and birth and offer an opportunity for questions and advice.

relief, about feeding, changing, bathing and other aspects of parentcraft. Classes are usually held informally, so they give an opportunity to ask questions and air your views. Fathers are welcome to all sessions, but as classes are usually held in the day time, there is often a special evening 'fathers session' at some point during the course to which you should try to take your partner.

In nearly all classes you will learn some type of relaxation. This is very important not just for your labour but for your life in the future. Babies can cause a great deal of stress and tension as well as joy, and learning to relax will help you cope with the stress more easily.

ANTENATAL EXERCISES

Preparation classes which involve obstetric physio-therapists may include some basic antenatal exercises to keep mothers more comfortable during pregnancy and to prepare them for labour. Even if you don't normally take any special form of exercise, it pays to be aware of the changes in your body which affect your muscles, ligaments, joints and posture. As your pregnancy progresses, and your growing uterus and baby rise out of your pelvis, your

abdominal muscles stretch and may separate (see p. 135). You may find yourself leaning back to compensate, which can affect your back. Even if you have never suffered from back pain before, the action of progesterone makes your joints more vulnerable during pregnancy (see p. 53). Your pelvic floor hammock, too, is taking the extra strain of up to 6kg (12-14lb) of extra weight by the end of your pregnancy, and with the increased pressure on your bladder this could lead to stress incontinence (see p. 55) unless you pay attention to exercising these muscles. All these points, and more, are usually covered by the physiotherapists, but if you haven't the opportunity to join a class the following basic exercises will help.

FEET AND LEGS

To improve the circulation in your legs and help prevent swelling and varicose veins, pump your feet up and down vigorously 30 times several times a day. This can be done sitting on a chair with your legs stretched out on a foot-stool. If you don't have a foot-stool, do one leg at a time, but do not cross your legs. If your ankles swell, do the exercises lying down with your legs raised on a stool so that they are higher than your head. In addition, you can circle your ankles ten times in each direction – this has a nice mobilizing feeling as well as being good for your circulation.

PELVIC TILTING

Pelvic tilting is a simple movement which, once you have learned it, can be done as you go about your daily routine, whether sitting, standing, kneeling or lying down. It helps to strengthen the abdominal muscles, helps correct your posture and gives relief to the backache that often accompanies postural problems during pregnancy. More specific advice on coping with sacro-iliac back pain (a particular problem of pregnancy) is given on page 55.

To practise pelvic tilting, start off by sitting on the edge of a chair with your knees apart and your hands resting on them. Rock backwards on your 'sitting' bones (the ischial tuberosities, as they are called, which are part of the pelvic girdle), drawing your abdominal muscles firmly in and rounding your back. Then gently rock the other way, releasing your abdominal muscles and curving your back the other way. This can be done slowly, holding the abdomen well pulled in while you count up to twelve, or as a small, faster movement to loosen a stiff back after you have been sitting still for a while.

Pelvic tilting on all fours is probably the best position for strengthening the abdominal muscles and relieving a tired back. Do the movement slowly and carefully, holding the abdominal muscles in for a count of twelve and then gently releasing them while allowing your back to hollow out as much as is comfortable.

The pelvic tilt done while standing corrects the posture as well as being good for the abdominal muscles and back. Stand with feet slightly apart and lift your ribs away from where your waist used to be. (Make sure your shoulders are relaxed and that you are not holding your breath.) Tilt the pelvis backwards and forwards, drawing your abdominal muscles in and your buttocks under, before relaxing to allow your back to arch slightly behind your waist. Make sure you finish the exercise with your baby pulled well into your pelvis, otherwise you may stretch your abdominal muscles unnecessarily and pull your spine forward.

THE PELVIC FLOOR

Although the pelvic floor is pierced by three openings, two of which we can normally control separately, in fact the muscles work as one unit when being exercised. Pelvic floor tightening can be done in any position – but perhaps it's easier to begin while sitting down, knees and feet apart, and with body leaning forward and your elbows resting on your knees.

Pull tight on the ring of muscle round the opening of your back passage (anus) at the same time as you

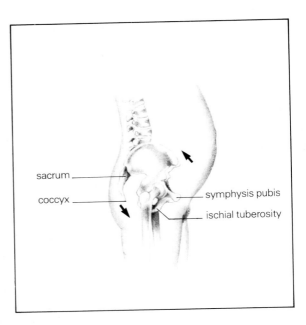

The pelvic tilt involves tipping the bones of the pelvis forward and up while drawing in the abdominal muscles at the same time. Although shown here in the standing position, it can also be done lying, sitting, kneeling, or on all fours.

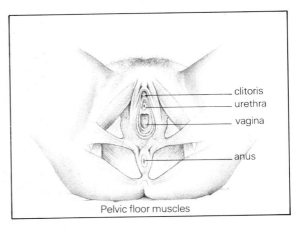

Pelvic floor muscles

The pelvic floor muscles act like a sort of hammock for the pelvic organs, forming a figure of eight around the front and back passages (the urethra and anus) and the vagina. Exercising them as described is extremely beneficial for all women, but especially during pregnancy and after delivery.

try to close the muscle supporting your front passage (urethra) and draw your vagina inwards and up. Hold while you count to four – then relax. Some people find it helps to imagine that the pelvic floor is a lift or elevator which should normally be standing on the ground floor; by tightening and drawing in and up, the lift ascends to the first floor. (Pregnancy and birth take the lift down to the basement!)

A useful test to see if you are exercising your pelvic floor correctly is to try and stop the flow of urine midstream – you will need to be able to do this every time the midwife wants a midstream sample of urine (see p. 20). Another test is to tighten and relax your pelvic floor during lovemaking, to see if your partner notices the difference.

This is the most important female exercise and should be done religiously by women, young and old, pregnant or not, many times every day. It can frequently be the answer to stress incontinence (see p. 55), slight prolapse and can help make sexual intercourse more satisfying for both partners. Being able to relax your pelvic floor can also make an internal examination more comfortable, and may relieve the 'dropping out' sensation which many women feel at the end of their pregnancy.

An awareness of tension or relaxation in the pelvic floor is also invaluable during the second stage of labour and while your baby is actually being born (see p. 88).

RELAXATION

Your body responds to stress (pain, fear or anger) by becoming tense. A typical 'tension posture' involves hunching your shoulders, clenching your fists and gritting your teeth. At the same time your heart beats more rapidly, your breath becomes faster and your body begins to burn up your store of energy as you try to 'run away' from whatever is upsetting you. A certain amount of stress and tension in everyday life is useful, and in fact helps people to perform better; but when the response to events gets out of hand problems begin to arise giving a constant feeling of anxiety which can be exhausting. Relaxation can alter this state, giving you a feeling of ease and calmness.

Pregnancy carries its own stresses. Just being pregnant makes your body work overtime, and the fact that by the end of 40 weeks you are actually carrying an extra ten to twelve kilos in weight increases your fatigue. Worrying about labour and after ('Will the baby be all right? Will *I* be all right?) can increase your stress response.

Antenatal classes are sometimes called 'Relaxation Classes' because it has been recognized for the

Relaxation during pregnancy should not be confined to your preparation classes. In the last weeks, try to find time to put what you have learned into practice, even if it is only for ten minutes a day.

past half century that relaxation can help a woman cope with the normal physiological stress of pregnancy, labour and new parenthood. There are many different techniques for teaching relaxation but the easiest and most logical was devised by a physiotherapist, Laura Mitchell, and is known as 'The Mitchell Method' of physiological relaxation. It is based on the body's response to stress and also on the fact that when one muscle group works, the group that performs the opposite movement has to rest; this is known as 'reciprocal relaxation' and is described in detail in Laura Mitchell's book *Simple Relaxation*.

To deal with the three most common bodily responses to stress (gritted teeth, hunched shoulders and clenched fists) the orders given to your body to change this and to achieve relaxation are:

Jaw: 'Drag your jaw downwards, stop doing it'; now register the comfortable new position in your mind (teeth slightly separated). You have eliminated tension in your jaw muscles.

Shoulders: 'Pull your shoulders towards your feet (making your neck longer), stop pulling' – now register their new position of ease and comfort – your shoulder girdle is no longer in its hunched up position.

Hands: The order is 'Long'; let your hands remain supported on your lap or tummy, then stretch out your fingers and thumbs, stop doing this, and register the new supported position of ease.

Although relaxation is usually taught in a comfortable lying down or sitting position it wouldn't be much use to you if you couldn't use the technique whilst you are standing or walking. Ideally you should practice relaxation in any and every position you can think of; once learned this art can be used every day of your life to help you cope with stress and your tension response; relaxation is not just for labour, it's for living.

BREATHING WITH RELAXATION

The way you breathe can increase your tension response or help you remain calm and relaxed in moments of stress. We've all experienced 'panic breathing' – fast deep gasps, usually accompanied by a dry mouth and pounding heart. Try this little experiment: sitting comfortable, count how many times you breathe out in a minute; probably somewhere between twelve and 25 times. Now slow down your respiration rate by pausing briefly between finishing an outward breath and then letting as much air as you need gently in to your chest; once again count how many times you breathe out. This time it will probably be about half your previous score. This slower, calm, quiet

Positions for relaxation and labour
By practising some of these positions and experimenting with others during pregnancy you can familiarize yourself with different ways to help yourself cope with the pain of labour.

During the first stage many women find that sitting astride a chair with a fairly high back is comfortable (top), resting your head on your arms and with a pillow for support.

Another position that you will probably find more comfortable than lying on your side as the first stage progresses, is to kneel across a bean bag, allowing it to take the whole weight of your abdomen (above left).

Being supported by your partner (above) is helpful and reassuring. Lean against him with your arms round his neck. You can either stand, or kneel on a chair or the end of the bed. Rock backwards and forwards gently during a contraction to help cope with the pain.

Practise squatting during pregnancy to stretch your ligaments and pelvic floor muscles (above), and perhaps to prepare yourself for a more upright position for the first stage. If you aren't used to squatting, start up against a wall with your heels on a book, and progress to unsupported squatting as shown.

During pregnancy, and in the early first stage of labour, it is restful to relax lying down with your head and shoulders supported by two pillows and your abdomen and upper leg supported by more pillows (main photograph).

breathing will actually help you increase your sense of relaxation and control during times of stress; standing in the queue in the Post Office when you're late, dealing with a saucepan that's boiling over on the cooker, comforting a screaming baby when you've tried everything to soothe him, or coping with the contractions of the first stage of labour.

BREATHING IN LABOUR

Some antenatal teachers compare labour contractions to waves on the sea as it gets rougher and rougher, or to mountains getting progressively higher (see p. 82). Your aim is to cope with one contraction at a time; begin each one with a breath out and a command to your whole body (but especially shoulders and jaw) to relax; then breathe comfortably and quietly as you ride your 'wave' or climb your 'mountain', then make your way down the other side. As you breathe out say to yourself 'relax' or 'let go' – each outward breath can increase your sense of relaxation and control and help unwind the tight internal coil of tension.

This slow breathing may be all you need for quite a while in labour, but as the first stage progresses you will probably find that your breathing needs to be slightly shallower and faster at the peak of a contraction. Relax your face and take very gentle sighing breaths through relaxed lips – imagine you're blowing dandelion seeds away one at a time. At the end of each and every contraction, take a deep relaxing breath in, and then out, to make sure there is plenty of oxygen circulating in your body for you and your baby, and also to return you to a relaxed state if you found the contraction a tension-making ordeal.

Until fairly recently all sorts of patterns of breathing were taught for use in labour. Some of these lead to 'over-breathing' (hyperventilation) in the mother and a subsequent decrease in the amount of oxygen reaching her baby. Nowadays we know that labour breathing should be very simple and as near normal breathing as possible. If you begin to feel dizzy and notice tingling or 'pins and needles' in your fingers, hands and face, it could mean that you are 'over-breathing' and have blown out too much carbon dioxide from your body. Immediately cup your hands together, put them over your nose and mouth, keep breathing, and you will be replacing the carbon dioxide.

Occasionally, at the end of the first stage of labour, you may get the urge to push before your midwife feels you are ready; to stop yourself, try saying 'I won't push' out loud. This will keep you breathing and will prevent you holding your breath and bearing down, which could lead to you 'pinching' your cervix between the back of your pubic bones and your baby's head if the cervix isn't yet fully dilated (see p. 88).

Pushing in the second stage of labour may take a while to get right; some people like to hold their breath as they push down; others find it easier to push with a steady breath out. When you are in labour, the best advice is to listen to your midwife. She will tell you exactly how to breathe for pushing, and will also tell you when she wants you to stop pushing and to pant instead.

PRACTISING POSITIONS FOR LABOUR

Many antenatal classes will include some ideas for exercises, relaxation positions and movements to help you cope with labour contractions, which you should use together with breathing and relaxation. If you can get used in pregnancy to positions you may not normally rest in, you will find it easier to use them during labour. It is particularly useful if your partner learns these routines too since he will be able to remind you of the different techniques during labour.

When the uterus works in labour, as well as drawing the cervix over your baby's head, it tries to tip forwards as it contracts. For this reason early first stage contractions can be coped with best by using forward leaning positions. Many couples find it mutually comforting if the mother puts her arms round her partner's neck and leans against him, both rocking together. Many women find it comfortable to sit astride a chair or to lean on a chair seat resting the head on a cushion. Kneeling on all fours often eases backache labour, while gentle or firm massage on the back, abdomen and thighs is very helpful when contractions reach their height.

You may already have discussed positions for delivery with your midwife during antenatal check-ups, and in many classes this subject will also be discussed. Many birth experts now favour an upright position for delivery, either as supported squatting, kneeling, or using a birthing chair or special bed. The most common position is sitting propped upright, with knees apart and your hands hooked behind your thighs for support.

Even if you may not want to adopt a squatting position for delivery, it is worth practising simple squatting on flat feet since it helps to stretch your pelvic ligaments and the pelvic floor muscles, making them more supple for birth. Squatting can be uncomfortable at first if you aren't used to it, so start by practising against a wall with your heels on a book, or wear shoes with low heels. You can gradually progress to unsupported squatting as you become looser.

If you have the opportunity, visit the delivery suite during your pregnancy so that you can familiarize yourself with the layout and the equipment, such as the baby resuscitation trolley.

VISITING THE LABOUR WARD

During most hospital classes there is an opportunity to visit the labour ward where you will have your baby. If you miss this it is worth telephoning the Senior Midwife on the labour ward and asking her if you can come round at another time. If your partner or someone else is going to be with you during labour, it would be helpful if he or she could come with you. The sister will probably give you a time when she expects to be less busy than usual – at the weekend or in the evening, or when a lot of staff are scheduled to be on duty.

WHAT TO LOOK FOR

Many women find it really comforting to lie in the bath while in labour, so find out where the bath is. Others find it helpful to walk around during labour, so have a look and see if this is going to be possible. Many women like to give birth in a position such as standing, squatting, or on a bean bag or birthing chair – ask to see if either of the latter would be available and if they have mattresses to make the floor more comfortable. If this kind of equipment isn't available at your hospital it might be worth bringing your own. Discuss it with the midwives and if they seem put out by your request, ask to see the Senior Midwife or discuss it with the doctor at your next antenatal check. It is very sad nowadays if a hospital cannot cater for a woman's needs in this fairly simple way. It might be a good idea to contact your Community Health Council (address in the phone book) and try to get better facilities in your maternity unit – women will be grateful to you for years.

In the labour ward, discuss pain relief; you might be allowed to try out the entonox mask (gas and air). Ask the midwife to show you the baby resuscitator – this is used quite routinely in many births but might upset you at the time if you don't know what it is for (see p. 102). Get to know the layout of the delivery suite and the individual rooms – remember that one of them will become your room when you are in labour for maybe as long as 24 hours. Think about what you might like to bring to make it more comfortable for yourself and your partner – after all it is going to be one of the most important rooms you have ever spent any time in.

CHAPTER THREE

EARLY PREGNANCY

**Your baby's development in the first twenty weeks
of pregnancy and how it affects your body**

The potential for new life begins when the male sperm fertilizes the femal ovum (see p. 12). It is at this point that the sex and physical characteristics of your new baby are determined, such as the colour of the hair and eyes and the bodily physique when he or she grows to adulthood. All such information is carried in the chromosomes which are made up, in turn, of many thousands of genes which are inherited from our parents, grandparents and so on. Each person's unique chromosome and genetic pattern is repeated in every cell in the body, but when life begins it is just as one cell created from the fusion of the mother's ovum with the father's sperm.

CHROMOSOMES AND GENES

The fertilized egg contains 46 chromosomes – 23 inherited from the mother and 23 from the father. Two of them are the sex chromosomes, of which one is inherited from each parent. The sex chromosome in the ovum is always the same and is known as the X chromosome. In the sperm the sex chromosome can either be X or Y. If the ovum is fertilized by an X-carrying sperm then a baby with XX sex chromosomes will develop; this is the pattern for a girl. If the ovum is fertilized by a Y-carrying sperm then a baby with XY sex chromosomes will result – the pattern for a boy. The

Fetal development in the first twenty weeks
In the first few weeks the embryo is so small that it is shown here several times life-size: at four to five weeks its crown-to-rump length is only about 10mm (³⁄₈in), while at eight to ten weeks it doubles in size to about 20mm (³⁄₄in). At twelve weeks the uterus can be felt just above the pubic bone. At sixteen weeks the fundus (top of the uterus) is about half way to the navel, and by twenty weeks a woman is noticeably pregnant, with the fundus at the level of the navel.

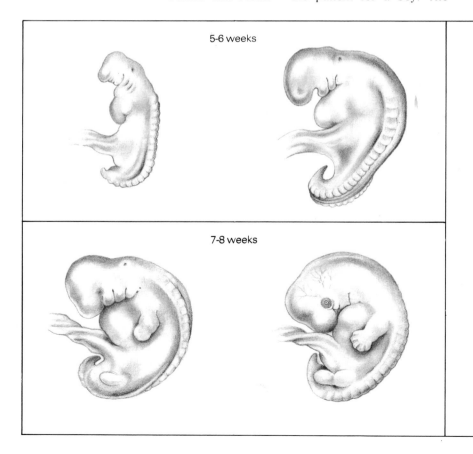

5-6 weeks

7-8 weeks

remaining 44 chromosomes, which are unrelated to the determination of sex, carry the genetic material which decides the outward appearance, the way the body works, and to a certain extent the intelligence and personality.

Since the composition of the genetic material in each sperm and ovum is slightly different, the new life created by their fusion will be unique. You can observe this in your own family. Because you inherit similar genes from your parents and grandparents, there may be quite strong resemblances between you, but no two individuals look exactly the same unless they are identical twins.

TWINS

Identical twins develop when a single sperm has fertilized a single ovum but very early on it has split into two, allowing the development of two babies instead of one, both of whom have exactly the same genetic make up. Non-identical twins develop when two ova have been released at the same time instead of the usual one, and both have been fertilized by two different sperm. The twin babies in this situation are no more alike than sisters or

brothers within the same family; they just happen to develop at the same time and be born on the same day. Identical twins are always the same sex; non-identical twins may or may not be.

DEVELOPMENT OF THE EMBRYO

Once fertilization (the joining of the egg and sperm) has occurred, growth of what is now called the embryo (a word derived from the Greek, meaning 'to grow') now starts to take place. The single cell formed by the union of the ovum and the sperm divides rapidly as it passes along the Fallopian tube, encouraged by the gentle squeezing movements of the tube known as peristalsis. It takes about four days for the embryo to reach the uterus, then it spends a further four days lying free in the cavity preparing its attachment (implantation) into the wall of the uterus which has been specially prepared to receive it by the hormones produced from the ovary, particularly progesterone.

Soon after implantation, the mass of cells now forming the embryo begin to separate into several distinct parts. The outer cells will burrow into the uterine wall, making connections there with blood

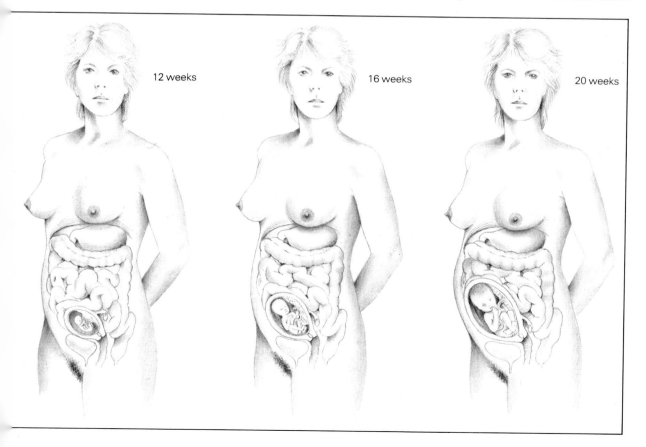

12 weeks   16 weeks   20 weeks

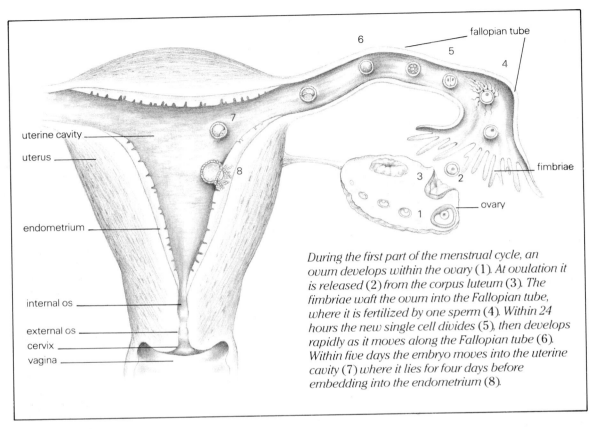

uterine cavity

uterus

endometrium

internal os

external os

cervix

vagina

fallopian tube

fimbriae

ovary

During the first part of the menstrual cycle, an ovum develops within the ovary (1). At ovulation it is released (2) from the corpus luteum (3). The fimbriae waft the ovum into the Fallopian tube, where it is fertilized by one sperm (4). Within 24 hours the new single cell divides (5), then develops rapidly as it moves along the Fallopian tube (6). Within five days the embryo moves into the uterine cavity (7) where it lies for four days before embedding into the endometrium (8).

vessels from the mother's circulation. These cells will eventually form the placenta through which the baby will receive oxygen and nutrition whilst in the uterus. The inner group of cells form themselves into three layers, called the endoderm, mesoderm and ectoderm, from which the baby will develop. The endoderm will be responsible for the formation of the lungs, the stomach and the gut; the mesoderm for the skeleton and its muscles, the heart and circulation, the kidneys and the sexual organs; and the ectoderm for the brain and spinal cord, the face, the eyes, the ears and the skin. All this has happened within two to three weeks of an ovum being fertilized, just about the time when the first period will be missed.

FOUR TO FIVE WEEKS

By week four to five, recognizable structures within the embryo are beginning to form and the blood vessel connections to the placenta via the umbilical cord are becoming established. Once the sixth to eighth week has been reached the uterus has enlarged to the size of a tangerine and the embryo has become curled up and developed a large swelling at one end where the head and brain are being formed. Little protuberances and indentations indicate the sites from which the limbs will grow and the eyes and ears will evolve. The primitive nervous system begins to develop, seen as a ridge of tissue down the length of the embryo, and the amniotic sac now contains a few millilitres of fluid. Also by this time the heart has formed sufficiently to start beating and this can be detected by an ultrasound scan. The length of the baby from crown (top of the head) to rump (bottom) is now about 8-10mm (⅜in).

EIGHT TO TEN WEEKS

Between the eighth and the tenth weeks, the uterus has enlarged to the size of an orange and the baby's face has become more recognizable – the eyes have formed and a mouth and jaw can be seen. The head remains disproportionately large for the size of the body, making up about 50 per cent of the baby's total size at this stage. Around this time it is conventional for this tiny embryonic human to start being called a fetus, a word derived from the Latin meaning 'offspring', which indicates that the developing baby now has recognizable human form. All the internal organs are well on the way to being completely formed and the size is rapidly increasing – by ten weeks, the crown-rump length is approximately 20mm (¾in), a 100 per cent increase in the space of two to three weeks.

TWELVE TO FOURTEEN WEEKS

By the twelfth to fourteenth weeks the baby has developed fully. All the muscles, bones, fingers and toes are in place – as are all the organs, including those of reproduction and the fetus is even moving about the uterus, although these movements are too tiny to be felt by the mother. At this stage the baby's length has reached about 55mm (2¼ in), weighs about 25g (1oz), and the size of the uterus has grown to that of a large grapefruit. It is around this time that the doctor or midwife will be able to feel the uterus when palpating the abdomen – prior to this it has been protected within the confines of the bony pelvis. The placenta is now recognizable as a separate organ.

FOURTEEN TO TWENTY WEEKS

Having completed basic development, from the fourteenth to the twentieth week, the baby now grows rapidly. As the weeks go by, the fetus's appearance becomes more and more like that of the newborn baby with which most of us are familiar. The relationship of the size of the body to the head becomes more proportionate and hair is beginning to appear. Concomitant with the growth of the baby, the uterus also continues to enlarge. By sixteen weeks the top of the womb (the fundus) has reached half way up to the navel (umbilicus) and by twenty weeks the fundus is level with it. At around eighteen to twenty weeks the baby's movements become sufficiently strong for them to be felt as a fluttering sensation. The exact time when movements are first felt does vary and may be a little later or earlier depending on whether this is your first or subsequent baby.

THE IMPORTANCE OF EARLY DEVELOPMENT

From this description of the early development of your baby, you will see that all the organs and vital structures are actually formed by the twelfth week of pregnancy. These first few weeks of life in the uterus are a time of very rapid growth when the baby is at particular risk of damage from harmful outside stimuli such as certain drugs and alcohol which can cross the placenta (see right). Yet you may not even know you are pregnant until several of these early weeks have passed. If you can plan ahead it is best to avoid any known situations which might possibly harm your newly formed baby (see p. 12), but if you have become pregnant accidentally do not worry too much; babies in the womb are remarkably resilient and can withstand many an unfavourable circumstance.

THE PLACENTA

During the second week after conception (about four weeks' of pregnancy in medical terms), the embryo starts to embed in the wall of the uterus. Part of the structure burrows into the soft spongy lining of the womb now called the decidua and forms an implantation cavity. The outer layer of cells of the embryo, called the trophoblast, puts out tiny blood vessels which form links with those of the mother's which supply the uterine wall. These tiny, linking blood vessels form the beginnings of a network which will allow exchange of waste products and nutrients between the baby's and the mother's blood.

Numerous little finger-like projections called villi grow out from the trophoblast in which are contained the blood vessels from the fetus, and these villi form a close relationship with the mother's tissues in the uterine wall. Within a week or two the villi become confined to a circular area around the site of the umbilical cord and their base becomes a layer called the chorion. This circular area forms the definitive placenta and the chorion covers the surface that faces the baby. It is the fact that the chorionic villi are formed from the developing embryo which forms the basis for the test of chorion villus sampling (see p. 28) for the diagnosis of chromosomal or genetic abnormalities in the baby.

The placenta not only functions as the supplier of the baby's oxygen and nourishment and the eliminator of waste products, but it also has a vital role in the production of hormones essential for the maintenance of the pregnancy. These hormones are discussed in more detail later, but in early pregnancy the most important of these is human chorionic gonadotrophin – the hormone which is the basis of most pregnancy testing kits (see p. 16).

The placenta also provides an important barrier to the passage of harmful substances, but unfortunately it does not prevent some getting through, especially drugs such as alcohol and nicotine from smoking. A number of infectious organisms such as rubella (German measles) also pass across quite freely. Fortunately the mother's antibodies which protect her from infection also cross the placenta and so can provide the baby with some passive resistance, especially to some of the most dangerous infections for small babies, such as measles.

The placenta may develop at any site on the walls

of the uterine cavity. Its commonest location is on the posterior (back) wall, followed by the anterior (front) wall and the sides of the uterus. Rarely the placenta forms in the lower part of the uterus next to or covering the cervix. This can give rise to problems later in pregnancy (see p. 62).

THE AMNIOTIC FLUID

Very early in intrauterine life when the embryo is forming its inner and outer layers, a hollow cavity appears between them. This is the amniotic cavity and is lined by a thin membrane called the amnion. Clear fluid collects in this space and there is a net increase of about 5ml (a teaspoonful) per day until at full term (40 weeks) there is a volume of about one litre (2 pints). The fluid originates from several sources. Some of it is made by the amnion itself and some seeps through from the mother's circulation, but quite a large proportion comes from the baby's urine. This is particularly the case in later pregnancy when the urine output may be as much as 0.5 litre (1 pint) per day. Fluid is also removed from the amniotic cavity by absorption back into the mother's bloodstream and as a result of swallowing by the baby.

The functions of the amniotic fluid are to keep the baby at an even temperature, to cushion against injury, to provide a space in which the baby can move easily, and to provide fluid to drink. Just before or during labour the amniotic sac usually bursts and the fluid drains out of the vagina, a process often referred to as the 'waters breaking'.

The amniotic fluid also contains cells and other substances shed from the baby's mouth, nose and skin and these can be very useful for making the antenatal diagnosis of abnormalities involving disorders of chromosomes, or cellular enzymes, and for confirming the diagnosis of spina bifida when the screening blood test suggests this. In the latter situation a protein (alpha feto-protein or AFP) which is present in all babies, leaks through the area of the baby's back which is uncovered by skin and is found in abnormally large quantities in the amniotic fluid. Amniocentesis is used to test for such abnormalities (see p. 27) and is performed at about sixteen weeks of pregnancy when the uterus is easily accessible and there is plenty of fluid.

HORMONES IN EARLY PREGNANCY

Hormones are substances secreted by various organs in the body which are transported in the blood and produce their effects at distant sites. As we have already seen, the sex hormones oestrogen, progesterone and testosterone, secreted by the

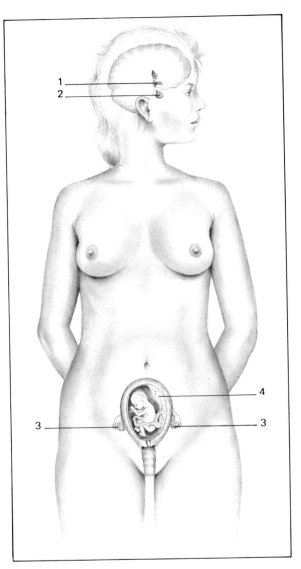

Hormonal activity of reproduction and pregnancy
1 *Hypothalamus (controls the pituitary gland)*
2 *Pituitary gland (secretes LH, FSH and prolactin)*
3 *Ovary (corpus luteum – secretes progesterone and oestrogen at start of pregnancy)* 4 *Placenta (secretes HCG at start of pregnancy, then progesterone and oestrogen in the form of oestriol)*

ovary and testis, play a fundamental role in sexual function and reproduction. Hormones also have a vital role in the implantation and maintenance of the pregnancy itself and in the preparation of the body to meet the increasing demands of the growing baby. Later in this chapter reference is made to the many profound physical changes that take place in women's bodies in anticipation of these demands – these are brought about mainly by the influence of three important hormones, oestrogen and progesterone, which are present in pregnancy, and human chorionic gonadotrophin.

Human chorionic gonadotrophin (or HCG for short) is a special hormone produced by the developing placenta almost from the moment of implantation, and its role is to maintain the function of the corpus luteum in the ovary (see p.10). At this time the corpus luteum is actively involved in producing the oestrogen and progesterone which maintain the endometrium (lining of the uterus) in a suitable state to nourish and sustain the developing baby. It continues to do this until the placenta is mature enough to take over this function at about twelve to fourteen weeks.

During pregnancy the levels of oestrogen and progesterone rise steadily until just before labour starts. As well as their effects on maintaining the pregnancy, they produce many changes elsewhere in the body. Oestrogen, for example, is very important in preparing the breasts for the production of milk and progesterone relaxes smooth muscle in all parts of the body including that in the uterus, dampening down its activity and inhibiting premature delivery. Because these hormones are produced by the placenta, their measurement is sometimes used as a check on how well the placenta is working but since the amount of hormone produced can be very variable even in healthy pregnancies, this sort of test does have its limitations.

The hormone HCG does not have the same pattern of production as oestrogen and progesterone, since its most important role is in the early stages of pregnancy. It reaches peak levels about eight weeks after the last period and then falls to much lower levels by the end of the first twelve weeks. This hormone can be detected in the blood from very early on, often as soon as the time of the first missed period and is a very accurate method of diagnosing pregnancy. Blood testing at this early stage is only performed if there is a special medical indication. Sophisticated immunological tests for HCG in the urine have also recently become available, whereby it is possible to diagnose pregnancy within a few days of the missed period and several of such kits are commercially available, although rather expensive. The standard pregnancy tests are however less sensitive and do not give a positive result until five or six weeks.

The mechanism of the test is rather complicated but practically it consists of mixing a small amount of urine – preferably the first passed in the day since this will contain the greatest concentration of hormone – with some specially prepared re-agents,

and observing what happens. The result is entirely dependent on the amount of hormone present in the specimen tested so if it is negative and yet you definitely think you are pregnant, it may be you have done the test too early, before there is sufficient HCG present. A repeat test a week or so later will give a more reliable reading.

PHYSICAL CHANGES IN EARLY PREGNANCY

To accommodate the changing needs of mother and developing baby, major changes take place which affect almost every system in your body. Many of these alterations start in early pregnancy, and some may reach their full development during this period, thus anticipating the demands the baby will make. Some of these changes are likely to pass unnoticed, but others are more obvious.

BLOOD CIRCULATION AND HEART RATE

The increased blood circulation required to service the pregnancy produces a mild degree of apparent anaemia in early pregnancy, and there are also changes in lung and kidney function, but these are not obvious to most people. However, you may be well aware of your increased heart rate, and the increased blood flow through your hands and feet, which tends to make them warm and moist. This may also make you less tolerant to heat – pregnant women often find they need to wear less clothes in cold weather and are often flinging windows open when others would prefer them shut!

WATER RETENTION AND URINE

The body's handling of fluids is also altered in pregnancy, with large amounts being retained. In early pregnancy the readjustment to this new state is the probable explanation for the frequent need to pass urine (frequency of micturition) noticed by so many women at this time. In later pregnancy water retention may be noticed as slight puffiness, particularly round the ankles (see p. 70).

THE EFFECT OF HORMONES

The hormone progesterone, present in high levels from early pregnancy onwards, causes relaxation of smooth muscle. This produces a variety of effects, contributing to the development of haemorrhoids (piles) and varicose veins, heartburn and constipation. The thyroid gland in the neck becomes enlarged and the general rate at which your body works (metabolism) increases.

Under the influence of the hormones oestrogen

and progesterone, the uterus and cervix become soft, and because of an increase in the local blood supply, the cervix takes on a bluish appearance. Similar changes occur in the vagina and you will notice an increase in normal secretions in this area. However, if these secretions are smelly, accompanied by soreness or itching, or are bloodstained, you should see your doctor at once (see p. 62).

THE BREASTS

The breasts also undergo marked changes from a very early stage; in fact for some women, this may be their first inkling of pregnancy since breast tenderness, tingling and enlargement often precede the first missed period. These changes in the breast are also the result of hormonal stimulation, in particular oestrogen, causing proliferation of the milk producing tissue which continues throughout pregnancy (see p. 149). However the acute feeling of discomfort experienced in early pregnancy does diminish after the first three months.

THE SKIN

Another physical change you may notice is an alteration in the pigmentation (colouring) in your skin. Pregnancy induces extra production of melanocyte stimulating hormone (MSH) from the pituitary gland in the brain. This hormone activates cells called melanocytes to produce the pigment melanin – the same pigment that develops with a suntan. In pregnancy the pigmentation is localized to specific areas, and you will notice it particularly around the nipples, along your cheek bones (chloasma) and along a vertical line from your umbilicus (navel) to your pubic bone – the so-called linea nigra.

You may also notice the development of small red spots, particularly on your upper body and face, which are formed by tiny spreading blood vessels visible just under the skin. These are called spider naevi and are caused by the high level of circulating oestrogen. Both these and the pigmentation fade once the pregnancy is over, but the darkening of the nipples and the linea nigra never disappear completely, although the latter is scarely noticeable when you are not pregnant.

FATIGUE

These profound physical changes which take over almost from the moment of conception are also responsible for the feelings of intense fatigue, faintness and weariness so often experienced in early pregnancy. It seems a curious paradox that just when you feel you would like to celebrate your potential parenthood your body feels exhausted – but you can be reassured these symptoms are only temporary and by the third or fourth month you will feel much better.

Try to rest when you feel tired – either sleep on a bed or sofa for a while, or just drop your head on your arms at a desk or table. If you notice a tendency to feel faint, try not to stand or sit in one position without moving for too long, and get up slowly and steadily rather than suddenly. If you feel faint, just lie down or drop your head between your knees for a minute or two until you feel better.

If you are working and you want to keep the pregnancy quiet for a while, bear in mind that fainting is likely to alert people to the fact that something is amiss. To prevent unnecessary alarm, it might be worth taking someone into your confidence so that he or she can reassure your colleagues that all is well until such time as you want your pregnancy to be common knowledge.

MINOR PROBLEMS OF EARLY PREGNANCY

Although they are so important to the well-being of the baby, the physical and hormonal changes of early pregnancy can and do produce some unwelcome effects in you, the mother. Some of these have already been indicated – increased vaginal secretions, for instance, or breast tenderness. Others are more inconvenient and irritating, but there are ways you can minimize their effect, and they need not worry you, provided you are reassured about the cause. If you have any anxieties that all may not be normal, it is best to consult your doctor or midwife. It is also helpful to know that most do pass within the first twelve to fourteen weeks.

NAUSEA AND VOMITING

Perhaps the most common disorders of early pregnancy are nausea and vomiting. It is estimated that feelings of nausea will be noticed by three-quarters of all pregnant women, and although the symptoms tend to be worst around the middle of the first twelve weeks, in one in ten they start before the first period has even been missed. As with breast tenderness, feelings of nausea may be one of the earliest indications that you are pregnant.

The common belief that this sickness is confined to the morning is not true for most sufferers and the more usual pattern is for symptoms to persist throughout the day. Fortunately these feelings do not last throughout pregnancy and in nine out of ten women they will have settled and virtually disappeared by fourteen to sixteen weeks.

The reason why women should so commonly feel sick at this time is not known. It was once believed to be related to the hormone HCG, but this is no longer thought to be the case. It is almost certainly related to hormonal changes of some kind, however, and is seen much more commonly in pregnancies where excess hormones are being produced, such as twins (see p. 65). In later pregnancy sickness may be associated with heartburn (see p. 53) but this symptom is uncommon in the early weeks.

There are various ways which have been suggested to help you cope with nausea and vomiting, including eating small amounts often rather than two or three large meals each day; avoiding foods and smells that upset you; getting plenty of fresh air and avoiding stuffy atmospheres; wearing loose fitting clothes; and having a dry biscuit or toast before getting up in the morning. It is worth trying each of these until you find something that works for you.

If you feel very ill or are vomiting so much that nothing is staying down then you should see your doctor. You may be developing a serious complication of pregnancy called hyperemesis which will need special management. For less severe cases however it is nowadays very unusual for your doctor to advise medication, as the risks to the baby may far outweigh the benefits to you.

EXCESSIVE SALIVATION

For some women, nausea and vomiting is not as much of a problem as excessive production of saliva. This can happen to such an extent that it is difficult to keep pace with swallowing. Again the reason for this is not known but it tends to disappear in the later part of pregnancy in the same way as sickness. Keeping a good supply of paper tissues handy to spit into will help avoid embarassment until the problem fades.

FOOD CRAVINGS AND TASTE ALTERATIONS

Sometimes in pregnancy you may experience other symptoms related to eating and drinking. Cravings for particular sorts of food (pica) are very common, and may even extend to other things which would not normally be part of your diet, such as coal or wood! These cravings are not usually dangerous unless they prevent you from eating a healthy diet or contain some harmful substances, in which case you need to seek professional advice.

Another common complaint of pregnant women is a metallic taste in the mouth which can persist throughout pregnancy and alter your enjoyment of

particular foods. The reason for these phenomena are not known but may have something to do with meeting the nutritional needs of the baby.

CONSTIPATION AND HAEMORRHOIDS

Another irritating feature of early pregnancy is a tendency to constipation – this is caused by progesterone, which relaxes the smooth muscle of the bowel wall, slowing down the normal elimination of faeces. Unfortunately, it is likely to last all through pregnancy but may be helped by altering your diet so that it contains plenty of fibre, fruit and vegetables. Constipation, like nausea and vomiting, may be made worse by iron tablets and if this seems to be a problem it is worth discussing with your doctor as to whether these are really necessary or if an alternative type could be prescribed.

Straining to open your bowels, particularly if you are constipated, will also encourage the development of haemorrhoids. These are varicose veins of the anus (back passage) which occur commonly in pregnancy because of the congestion caused by the pressure of the enlarging uterus. If the haemorrhoids cause a lot of problems, such as bleeding, itching or discomfort then your doctor can prescribe something for them. Always consult your doctor rather than buying a preparation over the counter at the chemist, since it is important that you use one that is safe during pregnancy.

VARICOSE VEINS

Pressure from the uterus can also cause congestion in the veins of the legs and those around the vulva, an effect that is exacerbated by the relaxant effect of progesterone. For some women this will lead to the development of varicose veins which may result in the legs becoming swollen and uncomfortable, particularly by the end of the day. Support tights and elevation of the legs in the evening will offer some relief. The symptoms tend to get worse as pregnancy progresses, but there is a marked improvement after delivery.

VAGINAL DISCHARGE AND BLEEDING

An extra amount of normal discharge is common in pregnancy as already mentioned, but pregnancy does predispose to certain infections, particularly candida (thrush). In this condition you would notice some itching and irritation as well as a cheesy sort of discharge. Candida can be easily treated by the use of pessaries and will not harm your baby in any way.

Bleeding from the vagina should never be considered as a normal part of pregnancy and if noticed you should consult your doctor as soon as possible. Occasionally slight spotting may occur at the time when a period would have been due, but other causes for the bleeding, such as the start of a miscarriage, would need to be excluded (see p. 58). So-called 'withdrawal bleeding' may be due to insufficient hormonal support in early pregnancy so it, too, must be taken seriously.

KEEPING HEALTHY IN EARLY PREGNANCY

A great deal of the advice which is offered in early pregnancy is a natural extension of that discussed in the pre-pregnancy section (see p. 12). It is very important to review your lifestyle and dietary habits in order to minimize the risk of harm to your baby and to maintain your own good health.

SMOKING AND ALCOHOL

Medically there is no doubt that your baby stands a better chance of being healthy and well nourished if you do not smoke during pregnancy. You may well 'go off' cigarettes at this time anyway because of feelings of nausea, which may make it easier for you to establish the initial break. In the same way many develop a distaste for alcohol and if you can give it up completely then you are minimizing the risk of harm. The evidence about the effects of alcohol in small amounts however is far less clear than for smoking and so you need not feel guilty if you enjoy an occasional drink once or twice a week, but heavy drinking should be avoided.

DRUGS, MEDICATION AND X-RAYS

It is best to avoid all medication in early pregnancy. Most drugs do cross the placenta and potentially could affect the baby, which is developing very rapidly at this stage and is therefore particularly vulnerable. Having said this, most drugs will not harm your baby and if you need any medication, let your doctor know you are pregnant so that a safe preparation can be prescribed. If you have inadvertently taken tablets or medicines and you are anxious about possible effects then it is wise to consult your doctor.

It is wise to be cautious about exposure to other potentially harmful agents, particularly X-rays. If for any reason it is suggested that you should have an X-ray and you think you might be pregnant tell the doctor or the radiographer that this is the case. Some hospitals will not perform X-rays on any woman of childbearing age unless she is in the first ten days of her menstrual cycle.

HAZARDS AT WORK

It is also worth checking whether there are any hazards associated with your place of work – this should be done before pregnancy if at all possible. Particular note should be made of work with chemicals, toxic metals and radiation. Publicity has recently been given to the possible harmful effects of working with VDUs (visual display units) but there is no medical evidence to support this. If you are a nurse or a teacher or work in any profession which takes you into contact with small children, then it is especially important to make sure you have checked your immunity to rubella *before* you get pregnant (see p. 13).

DIET AND WEIGHT

The same guidelines for diet that were given in Chapter 1 for pre-pregnancy fitness apply during pregnancy itself (see p. 13). In particular, this is not a time to diet – it is just as important to put on enough weight as not to put on too much. Don't 'eat for two', but eat sensibly and include lots of high-fibre foods like wholemeal bread, beans and fresh vegetables, which will have the added benefit of helping avoid problems with constipation.

The average weight gain during pregnancy is about 12.5kg (28lb). You do not usually put on much weight in the first twelve weeks or so, especially if you are suffering from nausea, but after that a gain of about 500g (1lb) per week is about right. You will probably notice your shape changing (apart from the obvious protuberance in front!) as fat is laid down to help milk production after the birth (see p. 149). This fat is often distributed round the hip bones, buttocks and thighs. Breastfeeding uses it up quite rapidly and many women find they are actually thinner after breastfeeding for a few months than they were before they were pregnant.

EXERCISE IN PREGNANCY

On the positive side pregnancy is not an illness, and this is a time to enjoy life and prepare for your new baby. If you are used to being active and taking regular exercise there is no need to stop. Athletes, dancers and women who are used to regular exercise can usually continue to 'work out' during pregnancy, as long as you don't push yourself to maintain your pre-pregnancy standard. Warm up before vigorous exercise (which shouldn't be attempted in hot, humid weather or if you yourself have a temperature), and a period of declining activity is advisable to cool off afterwards. Bouncy, jerky movements should be avoided – including

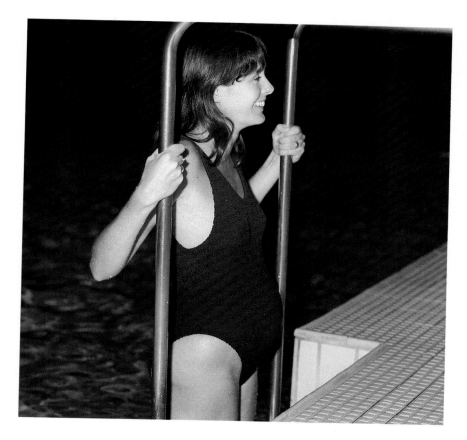

If all is going normally, swimming is an excellent way to keep your body fit and healthy throughout your pregnancy.

jogging – and dangerous sports such as horse riding and skiing should not be attempted. Stretching exercises and positions should be gentle and joints shouldn't be forced or overstretched – due to the action of progesterone, all the ligaments of the body have softened and relaxed; they can easily be damaged by over-enthusiastic exercise.

Many women who don't normally exercise, decide that they would like to do something during their pregnancy to improve their fitness, suppleness, strength and endurance. Yoga and swimming are two particularly safe and suitable forms of exercise and can be continued up until the very late stages. Special classes for pregnant women are commonly available. It may be wise to consult your doctor first, however, and if you embark on yoga for the first time, make sure your instructor is qualified and understands the needs of pregnant women.

SEXUAL INTERCOURSE

Having sexual intercourse during pregnancy is very much a personal decision, but there is no reason why you should not continue with this until late in pregnancy provided everything is normal. Sex during the first few months may be inhibited not by your physical shape but by how you feel. Intermittent nausea and extreme tiredness are not the best of sexual stimulants for many women, and some men may also be anxious in case deep penetration harms the baby. This is quite definitely not the case in the majority of pregnancies.

If you have any worries, or really feel that the physical discomforts of pregnancy are getting in the way of your sex life, talk to your doctor about it, but more especially discuss it with each other. Remember that there are other ways apart from conventional intercourse that you can use to achieve sexual satisfaction. Sometimes the conventional positions adopted for intercourse become too difficult, particularly as pregnancy advances and alternative ways of love-making may need to be explored.

If you have had problems with miscarriages or premature deliveries in the past, or have had complications in your current pregnancy, then these may be reasons why you should avoid intercourse. Again you should be guided by your doctor on this matter. If you are advised to avoid penetrative sexual intercourse for any of the reasons already mentioned, do remember that the seven or eight months involved is not really a long time when the safety of a much-wanted baby is at stake.

CHAPTER FOUR

LATER PREGNANCY

Your baby's development from twenty weeks to full term and its effect on your body

The second half of pregnancy, from 20 to 40 weeks, is the time when the growth of the fetus is outwardly noticeable and when the baby develops the necessary maturity of body and organs to be able to thrive in the world outside the uterus after birth.

LANDMARKS OF FETAL DEVELOPMENT

As we have already seen, between sixteen and 20 weeks, growth of the fetus is very rapid. The head becomes more proportional to the body length and movements can be felt by the mother. It is during this period that detailed growth and differentiation of the parts of the body take place. Measurement of

the fetus is usually taken as the 'crown-rump length', in other words the 'sitting' length of the baby, from the top of the head to the seat. If you have an ultrasound to measure your baby's growth rate it may be this measurement, along with the diameter of the head, that the ultrasonographer will be plotting on the visual display unit. The rate of growth is most between the twenty-eighth and thirty-sixth week (see the table, opposite).

TWENTY TO TWENTY-FOUR WEEKS

At 20 weeks, the vernix caseosa (the cheesy covering which protects the baby in the uterus)

Fetal development from 24 weeks to full term
From 24 weeks the size of the growing baby and uterus has its most direct effect on the mother's body. At 24 weeks the baby is fully formed but very thin. At 28 weeks upward pressure on the stomach can cause indigestion and heartburn. By 32 weeks the baby is beginning to lay down body fat. At 36 weeks the size of the uterus can cause breathlessness as it presses on the diaphragm, but by 40 weeks this may ease as the baby drops deeper into the pelvis, putting pressure on the bladder and groin instead.

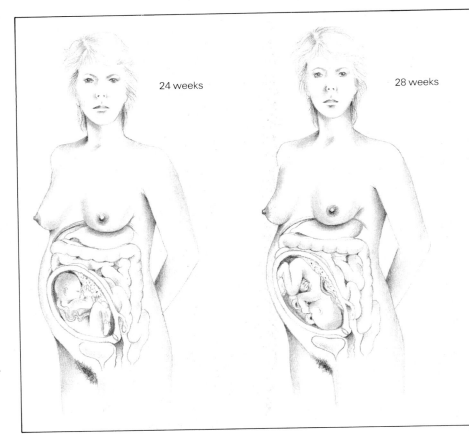

24 weeks

28 weeks

FETAL GROWTH FROM 16 TO 40 WEEKS		
Weeks (after last period)	Size cm. C-R length	Weight g
16	16	110
20	19	315
24	23	620
28	36	1050
32	42	1700
36	46	2500
40	50	3400

collects on the skin. Body hair (lanugo) is present and the nose develops. From 20 weeks the organs are fully developed and simply grow thereafter. By 24 weeks, the fingernails have grown and the head and body become proportional in size. The nostrils open. The fetus moves freely in the amniotic fluid, which is recycled every three hours via the fetus's mouth, kidneys and urethra. Parts of the fetus, especially the head, can be felt when the abdomen is felt (palpated), and the fetal heart can be heard with the help of a portable ultrasound at 20 weeks, and with a fetal stethoscope about two weeks later.

TWENTY-FOUR TO TWENTY-EIGHT WEEKS

At 24 weeks, the fetus overtakes the placenta in weight, but the placenta continue to increase in efficiency. Hearing is well developed and creases and fingerprints develop on the hands and feet. At 28 weeks, the age at which babies are said to be legally viable if born prematurely (see below), the eyes are open and eyebrows and eyelashes have grown. At this stage the skin is wrinkled and quite red. The lungs are not fully developed, but if born at this stage the baby would be able to breathe with difficulty, cry weakly and move his limbs. The enlargement of the abdomen becomes obvious and appears high; the fetus is often in a breech position and movements are vigorous.

TWENTY-EIGHT TO THIRTY-TWO WEEKS

The baby is very skinny at 28 weeks, but by 32 weeks body fat has started to collect and the body begins to fill out, beginning to grow slightly faster than the head. The skin is smoother, the fingernails reach the finger tips, and in boys, the testes usually descend from the groin into the scrotum.

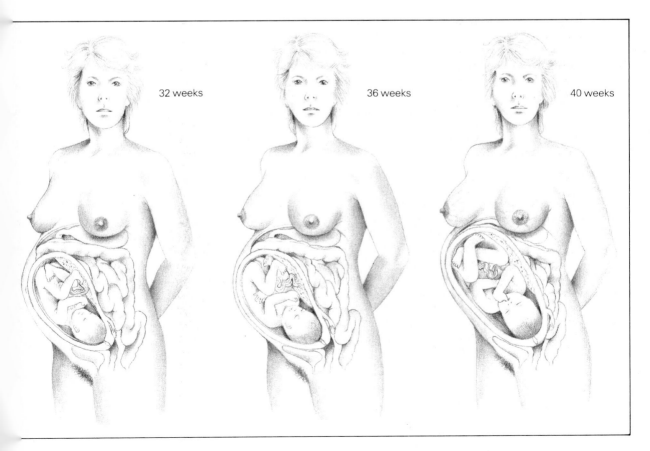

32 weeks   36 weeks   40 weeks

THIRTY-TWO TO THIRTY-SIX WEEKS

THIRTY-TWO TO THIRTY-SIX WEEKS

By 36 weeks the lanugo hair which is so characteristic of preterm babies is beginning to disappear, while the hair on the head thickens. The development of the brain, kidneys, lungs and gastrointestinal tract is now completed after growing progressively from 24 weeks. About 90 per cent of fetuses will have turned to the cephalic (head down) position.

THIRTY-SIX TO FORTY WEEKS

Although the fundus (top of the uterus) will have reached its maximum height by about 36 weeks and be pressing against the diaphragm, the head may engage in the pelvis during the last two or three weeks of pregnancy, especially in primigravidae (women having their first babies). Engagement tends to make the weight of the uterus drop, relieving such problems as heartburn and breathlessness. At 38 weeks, the fetus's mammary glands protrude, the finger nails grow beyond the finger tips and the soft, immature bones are beginning to ossify. The suck and swallow reflexes have developed. The placenta reaches its maximum efficiency at about 38 weeks, maintaining the fetus satisfactorily for another two weeks, after which it ages rapidly. At 40 weeks (term), the baby will be able to breathe without artificial aids, all the reflexes will be fully developed and the lanugo usually has disappeared except on the shoulders. The baby is ready to be born.

FETAL VIABILITY

When a baby is capable of surviving outside the mother's uterus, it is termed viable. Legal viability is at present put at 28 weeks in Britain, but with rapidly increasing paediatric expertise, babies of less gestation, as little as 24 weeks, can with adequate support survive and develop normally. The immature lung is the problem, so such an early baby would have to be nursed in intensive care surroundings with mechanical aids to breathing (see p. 116).

The correct definition of a premature baby is, incidentally, taken irrespective of weight (unlike previously when under 2500g (5lb) was the weight limit, and is a baby born before 37 weeks. Maturity and viability are obviously two very different things.

PHYSICAL CHANGES AND PROBLEMS

Between 20 and 40 weeks the growth of the uterus starts to put pressure on the other organs of your body, and although you will probably feel well, from 20 weeks onwards you are likely to experience some minor discomforts. Consult your doctor or midwife if you are at all worried, however.

WEIGHT GAIN

This may distress some figure and weight conscious women but is both inevitable and desirable as the uterus and its contents grow. As has already been mentioned, the average weight in pregnancy is 12.5kg (28lb), most of which goes on in between 20 and 30 weeks, but during this time a weight gain of under 500g (1lb) per week is desirable. But there is no more reason for being concerned about excessive weight gain than that it is difficult to lose it after pregnancy. Excessive weight gain has not got the profound medical significance which doctors used to believe it had.

Greater weight gain may be associated with oedema – swelling of hands and feet caused by the retention of fluid – and although this is commonly seen in otherwise normal pregnancies, it may be associated with pre-eclampsia. It then becomes of significance (see p. 70).

Static weight or even loss of weight may occur where the baby is growing unsatisfactorily – 'intra-uterine growth retardation'. Here again the mother's weight is a useful piece of monitoring information, which is why it is part of the routine assessment at each antenatal clinic visit.

STRETCH MARKS

Stretch marks (striae gravidarum) are scar-like marks on the skin of the abdomen and sometimes the upper thighs. They are often a rather unsightly red or purple when they first appear, later becoming white. They do not always occur in pregnancy, but when they do they leave permanent marks, although these are not as pronounced as during pregnancy itself. Unfortunately oils, lanolins and other preparations rubbed into the skin do not prevent them.

VEIN DISTENSION

All the surface veins of the body become more prominent as pregnancy progresses. Veins can often be clearly seen under the skin of the abdomen and over the breasts. Actual varicose veins are not uncommon and are most often seen in the legs; as a result of the weight and compressing effect of the growing uterus on the major draining veins of the pelvis, the more peripheral blood vessels become engorged.

Support tights can be of considerable help in minimizing the discomfort of varicose veins but they

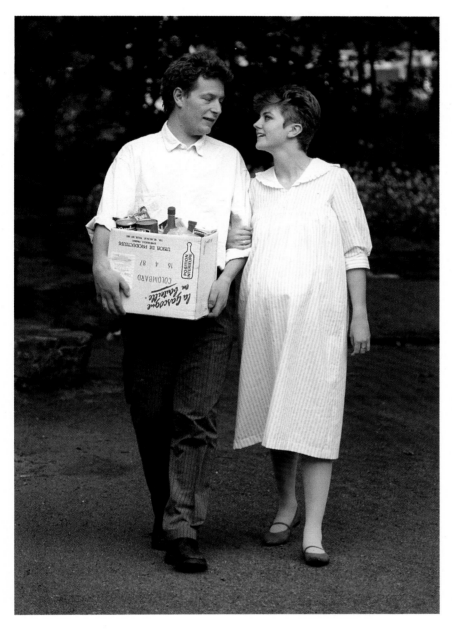

Later pregnancy is a time for gentle exercise and lots of rest. Try to take maternity leave or give up work at least eight weeks before the due date, and it helps if fathers can share the heavier chores.

will not cure or prevent them. If the varicosity is very severe, they can be injected, but as the weight of the pregnancy continues to exert its pressure from above, the varicosities may, unfortunately, return. Surgeons would be very reluctant to operate on varicose veins during pregnancy for the same reason. However, there is no reason why you should not seek treatment once the baby is born.

Varicose veins can emerge on the vulva and cause quite a lot of heaviness and discomfort. Because of their awkward site they are difficult to treat. Sometimes raising the buttocks on a pillow

when resting in bed during the day can give a measure of relief. They tend to disappear quickly after pregnancy.

Haemorrhoids – varicose veins in the rectum – are discussed, along with the often accompanying problem of constipation on page 45.

OEDEMA

Oedema means swelling, and in pregnancy usually involves the hands, feet and lower legs. Sometimes you may notice your face getting puffy. It need not indicate that anything is going wrong – as has already been mentioned it can happen in a perfectly normal pregnancy. Rings may become tight and may have to be removed for the duration of the pregnancy. The longer you are on your feet, the more swollen your feet may become, especially in hot weather. However, since oedema is also a prominent feature of pre-eclampsia, it is looked for routinely at antenatal checks especially in the second half of pregnancy.

There is no specific treatment for oedema, although resting with your feet up as often as possible helps to relieve it in the legs, ankles and feet. 'Water tablets' (diuretics), used in other circumstances to help the kidneys to secrete more fluid, are not advisable in pregnancy because of their possible adverse effect on the fetus. It is not necessary to reduce your intake of fluids by drinking less, and salt reduction is now also known to make no difference.

NOSE BLEEDS

Vascularity – the number and dilatation of the blood vessels – increases in pregnancy, and the blood vessels of the nasal septum (the fleshy structure inside the nose which divides the nostril cavities) are no exception. Nose bleeds (epistaxis) are very common among pregnant women, occurring to a greater or lesser extent – some women never experience them, others have them frequently.

Nose bleeds can be alarming, but are normally stopped by the usual simple measures such as pressure on the bridge of the nose (see p. 278). Contrary to belief, they are not associated with hypertension (high blood pressure) in pregnancy, nor will they produce anaemia unless they are very frequent and very heavy.

ANAEMIA

This is a common problem in pregnancy and particularly in communities where nutrition is poor and there is little if any antenatal care. Physiological or 'natural' anaemia occurs as a result of the normal changes of pregnancy. The red blood cells become 'diluted' and it is normal for the haemoglobin to fall in the middle third of pregnancy. (Haemoglobin is a pigment of the red blood cells and its measurement is used to tell whether someone is anaemic or not). Routine checking of haemoglobin is carried out at the booking clinic and again at 30 to 32 weeks and at 36 to 38 weeks (see p. 22).

Iron deficiency anaemia is the most common form of anaemia in pregnant women, which may be due to a diet deficient in iron adding to the physiological changes already mentioned. Foods containing iron are liver, other meats, fish and most green vegetables, so you should study your diet during pregnancy with this in mind. Most obstetricians will give an iron supplement to pregnant women. Unfortunately iron tablets occasionally have a constipating effect, so that including plenty of fibre in your diet is an important 'back up' to the avoidance of anaemia.

There are also two vitamins involved in anaemia – folic acid and Vitamin B12. Folate deficiency is more common in Asia, but the practice of giving a small folate supplement with iron has made it uncommon in pregnant women in the West. Vitamin B12 deficiency is not common among younger women, unless they are vegans who eat no animal products at all. It is therefore not seen so often in pregnancy.

If you are anaemic you will feel much more tired during your pregnancy, and will be more prone to infections such as urinary infections. It has been suggested that severe anaemia may have an influence on the onset of premature labour. Obviously the effect of any bleeding will be more profound if you are anaemic than if you have a good level of haemoglobin. It is therefore important that anaemia should be detected and treated adequately during pregnancy and before labour.

HEADACHES

Many women seem to have a particular propensity for headaches when they are pregnant. This again may be a hormonal effect, but the actual mechanism is not entirely clear. Analgesics in the form of paracetamol, for example, are safe in pregnancy, but if you are experiencing headaches frequently so that you need repeated doses of pain relief, you should seek the help of your doctor.

The severe headache of imminent eclampsia (see p. 71) is something which every obstetrician is aware of and it may provide a valuable warning sign. Fortunately it is rare.

SCIATICA

Some women experience pain and tingling down the leg due to pressure on the sciatic nerve during pregnancy, although it is usually not more than an annoying discomfort. It may also be associated with the pelvic joint pains described above. It seems to be due to direct pressure of the baby's head on the mother's sciatic nerve, and although there is no specific cure, the discomfort is relieved as the baby's head moves downwards. Rest, heat and analgesics may give some relief.

FAINTING

Fainting is not at all an uncommon phenomenon during pregnancy. In literature, a woman is traditionally recognized as being pregnant by becoming faint in crowded places! Standing too long with the blood pooling in the legs is likely to make you feel faint while you are pregnant, so try to avoid it.

About ten per cent of pregnant women experience a condition known as the 'supine hypotension syndrome'. In this situation, they may feel faint or even lose consciousness for a few moments while lying flat on the back. If the blood pressure was taken at this time, it would be found to be low. The effect is due to the pregnant uterus pressing on the major blood vessels of the abdomen (the aorta and the inferior vena cava) which run behind the uterus.

Try to avoid lying flat on your back for too long during late pregnancy. However, if you do feel faint in this position, roll over on to your side to relieve the pressure on the blood vessels, so that your blood pressure can rise again, and the feeling of faintness will pass.

HEARTBURN AND NAUSEA

Nausea is a common problem in early pregnancy (see p. 44), which usually clears as pregnancy advances. Occasionally, however, it returns, accompanied by vomiting, in the last few weeks of pregnancy. When this happens it is often associated with 'heartburn' (which has nothing to do with the heart), which usually precedes the vomiting.

The unpleasant burning sensation of heartburn occurs when acid from the stomach is regurgitated into the oesophagus (the tube connecting the mouth to the stomach). It is once again a result of hormone action which causes laxity of the stomach sphincter – the tight muscle which blocks the contents of the stomach off from the oesophagus. During pregnancy it takes longer to empty your stomach after eating, which contributes to the problem.

If you suffer from heartburn, take small, frequent and bland meals, avoiding highly spiced or fatty foods, and use an antacid recommended by your midwife or doctor. The problem is often worse at night but can be helped if you sleep well propped up with pillows.

FATIGUE

As pregnancy progresses and your size increases, it is natural that you should feel more tired than usual. Where there are other young children to look after, or if you are working, it is not surprising that you should tire more easily, and if you are anaemic, the situation will be made worse.

It isn't advisable to work right up until the last minute during pregnancy, unless there are good facilities for rest at your place of work and you don't have to travel far to get there. Take advantage of your rights to maternity leave and pay if available (see pp. 294-295), so that you can leave work well before the baby is due.

Resting for an hour or so in the middle of the day whenever possible, and going to bed early at night will help. If you have young children try to persuade them to play quietly with you when you rest with your feet up, or take your rest when your child is having a nap – don't be tempted to use this time to catch up with the chores. If you are found to be anaemic, a good nourishing diet perhaps supplemented with iron tablets will help.

VAGINAL DISCHARGE

Glands in the cervix normally secrete mucus to keep the area moist. During pregnancy these natural secretions increase, so you will notice more vaginal discharge. This should not be a problem, although the dampness can cause irritation, so attention to personal hygiene and wearing briefs made of cotton rather than an artificial fibre can help avoid this. If soreness or irritation persists, you should consult the doctor who will see if you have an infection in the area, (see p. 56).

STRESS INCONTINENCE

Many women who are pregnant experience a slight leakage of urine when they cough, sneeze, laugh or do exercises. This leakage of urine is known as stress incontinence, and during pregnancy it is very common because of the pressure of the uterus on the bladder, and the general laxity of the pelvic floor muscles due to the action of progesterone. Pelvic floor exercises done regularly from the start of pregnancy can help to control this rather embarrassing problem. However, if you do suffer from it, you will probably continue to do so for a little while after the birth as the pelvic floor muscles are extremely stretched. Pelvic floor exercises begun immediately after the birth will strengthen the muscles and the problem should disappear within a few weeks (see p. 140).

INSOMNIA

Difficulty in sleeping can be quite distressing in later pregnancy, when the sheer discomfort of your heavy uterus makes it difficult to settle down

These positions can help relieve sacro-iliac and low back pain.

1 **Pelvic twist:** *Lie flat on your back on the floor. Bend the knee on your painful side, twist that foot round the calf of the opposite leg, then roll your pelvis away from the pain, keeping your shoulders flat on the floor. Gently rock your pelvis back and forth, then carefully return to your starting position.*

2 **Leg up:** *Lie flat on your back on the floor, bend the leg on your painful side right up, taking the knee towards your shoulder and holding it there with your hand. With your other hand, grasp your foot and draw it towards your opposite groin. Gently pull and release your knee and foot several times before carefully putting your leg down.*

To get up after either of these exercises, bend your knees up high, roll on to your side (keeping your knees pressed tightly together), and push yourself up with your hands.

comfortably in bed at night. Your natural worries and apprehensions play a part, and it doesn't help if you find you need to get up to go to the lavatory several times during the night as well.

Simple measures do help: avoiding drinking late at night so you are less likely to need to pass urine; not eating too late; not drinking stimulating fluids like coffee; using extra pillows to give more comfort and minimize the problem of heartburn (see earlier), and practising the relaxation technique described on page 33 or recommended by your antenatal class instructor.

If you are really becoming exhausted from lack of sleep, discuss it with your doctor, who may be able to prescribe mild sleeping tablets to help reintroduce the 'habit' of sleep.

JOINT PAINS

Aches and pains in pregnancy are common; this is not at all surprising when one considers the rate and extent of growth of the uterus. Joints may suffer simply because of the action of the hormone progesterone which loosens the ligaments which hold them normally in a position of stability. The particular joints affected in this way are the sacro-iliac joints, the lumbo-sacral joint which is the joint between the last lumbar vertebra and the sacrum, and the pubic symphysis in front. In the much rarer, more extreme form of involvement of the pelvic joints – pelvic arthropathy – the woman may be totally incapacitated and hospitalization required.

It is difficult to do much to relieve sacro-iliac and lower back pain apart from heat treatment in the form of hot baths and compresses, and simple analgesia. You can help to avoid back trouble by being careful about your posture – try not to allow yourself to lean back to compensate for the weight of the baby in front – and if you need to lift something heavy from a low position, always bend the knees and use the strong muscles of the thighs rather than bending from the waist. When getting up from the floor or the bed, always roll over on to your side and push yourself up with your hands and arms (see the illustrations opposite).

If you do suffer from severe lumbo-sacral or sacro-iliac pain, seek the help of the obstetric physiotherapist in your hospital – the midwife at the antenatal clinic will tell you how to get in touch with her. She may be able to help with manipulation and heat treatment, and can give you a special supporting corset to wear during your pregnancy. In the meantime the positions given in the illustrations opposite can be very effective in relieving this type of pain. Although the effect of progesterone on the ligaments continues for some weeks after the birth,

and you should continue to be careful about posture and lifting, the problem does resolve with the end of pregnancy.

CRAMP

Muscle cramps, especially of the feet and legs, are another troublesome discomfort of late pregnancy. Their actual cause is not known and there is no evidence that extra calcium will help. Since cramp often seems to occur when stretching the legs with the toes pointed down, a simple trick to avoid cramp is always to stretch with your toes pointing up, so that your feet are at right angles to your shins.

If a spasm of cramp wakes you at night, it can be nipped in the bud by pulling your feet up so that the Achilles tendon above your heel and your calf muscles are well stretched. Follow this with some deep massage and vigorous foot pumping and you should escape the painful bruised feeling that bad calf or in-step cramp can leave behind.

SKIN IRRITATION

Spots, acne, soreness in the folds of the groin or the arm pits may develop – but all these fade after pregnancy. Skin rashes are common, although once more the cause is not known. The rashes frequently involve the abdomen and the back. Treating the itching caused by the rash with a mild lotion such as calamine is all that is possible. If you suffer from this type of rash, you should avoid using perfume, talcum powder and other cosmetic body or bath preparations as they make the rash worse. It is best not to use 'biological' washing powders for your clothes, as well. If you are suffering from a more widespread rash, then your doctor might want to look for a specific allergy.

In some severe cases of skin irritation (not always, incidentally, associated with a rash), anti-histamine tablets may be required, but their use during pregnancy must be supervised by the doctor.

CARPAL TUNNEL SYNDROME

The main nerves supplying the fingers and hand pass under a fibrous sheath at the wrist known as the carpal tunnel. This can become swollen during late pregnancy, causing a severe 'pins and needles' discomfort in your fingers, and even numbness and clumsiness of the hand. It is often worse at night.

If you suffer from carpal tunnel syndrome, your doctor may suggest splinting the hand and wrist, which can bring some relief. Sometimes it may be suggested that the sheath is injected with cortisone, but this isn't used frequently during pregnancy because of the high chance of the syndrome recurring. However, it does get better once pregnancy is over, so surgery is not required.

MATERNAL INFECTIONS

There are, needless to say, a very large number of infections which may occur during pregnancy. These are usually coincidental to pregnancy, but every mother who develops an infection of one kind or another is naturally concerned as to whether it will have an effect on her pregnancy.

GENITAL TRACT INFECTIONS

There are two main types of vaginal infection; 'thrush' (Candida albicans or monilia) is discussed on page 45, and is very common throughout pregnancy. The pregnancy is not affected either by the condition or by the treatment for it. Another infection is Trichomonas vaginalis, which produces a thin, yellow, smelly discharge and soreness rather than _itching. Treatment is by tablets containing metronidazole (Flagyl). This drug is better avoided in the first three months of pregnancy but thereafter is safe. In both forms of local vaginal infection both the mother and her partner must be treated.

A common organism found in the vagina is the 'Group B' streptococcus. Its presence is not usually associated with excess discharge, so you may be unaware of its presence. However, as it can cause infection in the newborn baby, it is common practice now in many maternity units to take a vaginal swab and send it to the laboratory to check for the organism's presence as a routine in late pregnancy. If it is found, a course of safe antibiotics is given before labour so that the way is clear, so speak, for the baby during delivery.

Sexually transmitted diseases such as gonorrhoea may also occur in pregnancy. Fortunately this is almost always responsive to treatment by the penicillin group of antibiotics.

Herpes is a problem which has come into prominence in recent years. Genital herpes is common and treatment less than satisfactory. The baby may become affected if he passes through a herpes-infected birth canal, so if the virus is found, then delivery by Caesarean section is advisable.

URINARY TRACT INFECTIONS

These are not uncommon in pregnancy. The effect of the hormone changes in pregnancy means that the tissues of the kidneys and ureters (the tubes that lead from the kidneys to the bladder) expand and become lax, and urine tends to 'pool' in the area,

rendering it more liable to infection.

Routine checking of urine at the booking clinic and at other antenatal check-ups, by sending it for culture in the laboratory, will screen for excess numbers of organisms. If such are found, even if you don't have any symptoms, a course of antibiotics will be given. As in all such situations, the antibiotics used are chosen specifically for their safety in pregnancy. Some antibiotics used for urinary tract infections are suspect, so if you think you have an infection early in pregnancy, make sure you tell your doctor (if you haven't already) that you think you may be pregnant.

A full blown urinary tract infection may bring pain, fever, frequency of passing urine and the risk of premature labour. Here again laboratory testing will indicate which antibiotic to use. In such a case, you must be followed up after pregnancy to make sure the infection is completely eradicated and to check the function of the kidneys.

GENERALIZED INFECTIONS

Quite apart from pregnancy, a mother may develop any infection anywhere in the body – skin, eyes, chest and so on. The same overall rules apply in pregnancy – locate the organism causing the infection, test its sensitivity to antibiotics in the laboratory and treat using of course an antibiotic with no known adverse effects on the baby.

The group of infections which worry mothers most of course, because of their possible effect on the baby, are the common infectious diseases, such as measles, mumps, chicken pox or rubella (German measles). In all these illnesses, if a high fever develops in early pregnancy, then there may be an increased possibility of miscarriage. Mumps has no proven effect; polio virus and measles may give an increased chance of miscarriage or preterm delivery; and chicken pox is rarely associated with serious effects in pregnancy.

Rubella is the problem which is now well identified (see p. 13). If the mother develops rubella in the first three months of pregnancy then fetal abnormalities can develop in as high a proportion as 20 per cent. The abnormalities affect eyes (blindness), ears (deafness), brain, heart or limbs, Termination of pregnancy is clearly justifiable in these circumstances. Between thirteen and sixteen weeks the risk is down to four per cent, and thereafter to one per cent or less.

Laboratory testing of a blood sample will tell you whether you are protected if you come into contact with the disease or, if there is no sign of protection, repeat testing will indicate whether significant infection has recently occurred. You and your

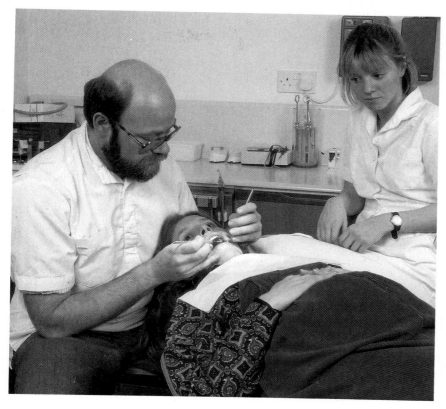

Dental care during pregnancy is important since the increase in the volume of your blood supply can lead to bleeding and gum disease. In the UK dental care is free during pregnancy and for one year after the birth, so it makes sense to have regular check-ups at this time.

partner can then be counselled accordingly, depending when in pregnancy this occurs.

If you aren't immune you will be offered rubella vaccination after pregnancy. You should use careful contraception to avoid pregnancy for three months after the vaccination (see p. 143).

KEEPING HEALTHY IN LATE PREGNANCY

The minor discomforts of pregnancy, and the extra burden of the growing baby, inevitably limit your movements somewhat during later pregnancy. In any case, you will probably find that you are becoming more 'home-based' by choice since your thoughts will be focused on preparing for the birth.

There aren't any special rules about keeping healthy in later pregnancy. A sensible diet, eating little and often if you suffer from indigestion or heartburn, and resting as much as possible have already been discussed. It is useful to keep as active as possible within limits – walking and swimming are good forms of exercise.

Sexual intercourse may be continued as long as you feel like it, although there may be physical restraints in the last weeks. Deep penetration may become difficult, but it won't harm the baby unless you have been specifically advised to avoid it.

DENTAL CARE

It is advisable to ensure that your teeth are in good condition during pregnancy. In Britain, dental care is free for the duration of your pregnancy and for one year after the baby's birth so it is worth taking advantage of this concession.

The gums become spongy with the extra blood supply during pregnancy, which may enhance any existing gum infections. Dental hygiene and advice on the care of your teeth and gums become particularly important so you should be sure to visit your dentist regularly at this time.

TRAVEL DURING PREGNANCY

Travelling long distances can be rather uncomfortable during late pregnancy, and a car journey may have to be planned to accommodate more stops than usual. Take a cushion to tuck into the small of your back to avoid backache. Air travel is not advisable in late pregnancy – many airlines are reluctant to take pregnant women after 32 weeks or so. If it is necessary for you to travel by air after about this stage of pregnancy, you should check with the airline beforehand and let them know that you are pregnant.

PROBLEM PREGNANCIES

A reassuring guide to unexpected or unusual medical
conditions that may arise during your pregnancy

Most pregnancies proceed without any problems at all beyond the minor discomforts and irritations that have already been described in the previous chapter. However, some do not, and it is because they can occur unexpectedly that regular antenatal check-ups are so important. Midwives and obstetricians are on the look-out for problems which even the mother may not suspect, and will do all they can to help your pregnancy proceed to a successful conclusion – that is, the birth of a healthy baby.

MISCARRIAGE

It is unfortunate that a chapter on problem pregnancies has to start with a description of miscarriage, which implies the loss of a pregnancy, but most of these do occur in the first trimester. Fortunately, however, though it is distressing, a miscarriage does not usually mean that you will not have a normal, full-term pregnancy next time.

When a pregnancy does not continue for its full time and is lost before the twenty-eighth week, it is described popularly as a miscarriage, although the medical term is 'spontaneous abortion'. This can occasionally cause confusion, since the word 'abortion' is also popularly used to mean the surgical termination of pregnancy. Medically this is actually called an induced abortion, but to avoid confusion doctors and midwives prefer to call it a termination of pregnancy or TOP.

EARLY MISCARRIAGE

By far the commonest time for miscarriages to occur is in the first three months, and it is thought that perhaps as many as one in four or five pregnancies end in this way, although many women may not even have realized they were pregnant. The reasons for this very high wastage are not fully understood, but when one considers the complex mechanisms of fertilization and implantation discussed in Chapter 3, it is perhaps not so surprising that all pregnancies are not successful.

Sometimes there is a problem with the chromosome make up of the embryo – not every ovum and sperm are perfectly manufactured – and sometimes there is a problem with the implantation of the embryo into the wall of the uterus. In such cases the pregnancy will fail to develop and eventually will be rejected by the uterus. Miscarriages at this stage are not caused by physical injury, despite the belief of popular novelists, nor are they usually precipitated by sexual intercourse.

The symptoms associated with a miscarriage can vary but in the typical situation you would have noticed all the usual signs of pregnancy – a missed period or two, feelings of nausea, breast tenderness and possibly even a positive pregnancy test – and then you would notice vaginal bleeding and cramp-like pains in your lower abdomen.

If the bleeding is very slight and the pain mild or non-existent then this may not be too serious and the pregnancy may well continue normally – this is what is known medically as a threatened abortion or miscarriage. However, it is something that can only be diagnosed by your doctor, so if you have any vaginal bleeding, however little, you should seek professional advice. An ultrasound scan may be necessary to confirm the viability of the pregnancy. If this is normal then you need not worry about the future, the bleeding will not have harmed the baby.

If you experience much heavier bleeding (this can sometimes be very profuse and make you feel weak and faint), with moderate to severe stomach cramps, then it is most likely that you are miscarrying – you may even pass small pieces of tissue, which are portions of the placenta. This is a medical emergency and you will probably need immediate admission to hospital for a minor operation to evacuate the uterus and make sure it is empty, otherwise further bleeding or infection may result. This operation is often referred to as a 'scrape of the womb' or a 'D&C' (dilatation and curettage) and usually involves an overnight stay in hospital.

You will probably be very keen to know why you have lost the baby, but it is often difficult to be any more specific than the reasons stated above, and examination of the products of conception is usually unhelpful. At this stage of pregnancy it is sadly not possible to tell very much about the baby,

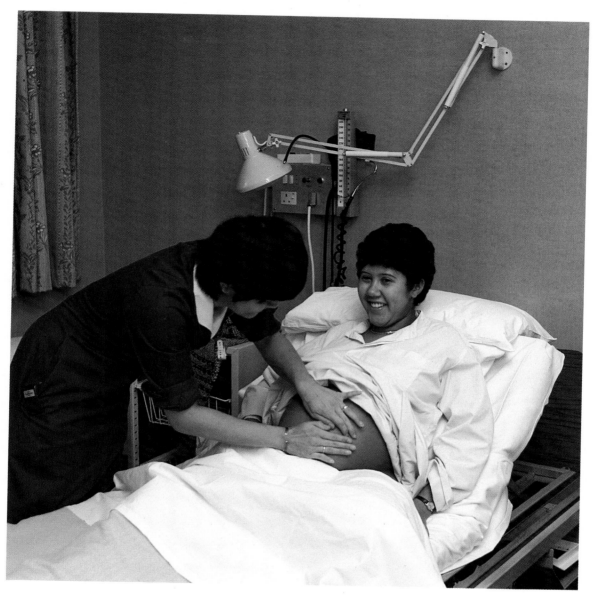

Not all pregnancies run smoothly, but if you have to spend time in the antenatal ward, you know that it is best for both you and your baby.

which is so small it is usually not identified.

Occasionally a pregnancy can cease to continue but will not be miscarried in the way described above. Instead the products are retained in the uterus without further development. This situation is known medically as a missed abortion or miscarriage. The only symptoms here may be a disappearance of the feelings of pregnancy and a little vaginal bleeding or brown discharge. Diagnosis can be made conclusively by ultrasound and

if confirmed then the uterus needs to be evacuated as above.

Having a miscarriage does not mean you will be unable to have children and it is only when a couple have had three miscarriages on the run that special medical investigations are thought to be necessary. Even in that circumstance there is a 40-50 per cent chance of a successful pregnancy in the future. Losing a pregnancy even at this early stage can cause considerable grief but support and help can be provided if you need it (see pp. 297-299). Your doctor will be happy to discuss with you any special precautions for the next pregnancy and how long you should wait before trying again.

LATE MISCARRIAGE

In much rarer circumstances pregnancies can be miscarried in the second three months. Again there can be several explanations for this, some of which, such as premature separation of the placenta and intrauterine death are covered elsewhere.

Miscarriage at this time can also be caused by what is known as cervical incompetence. In this situation the cervix (neck of the womb) is weak and opens up without warning usually around 20 weeks, allowing the contents of the uterus to pass through – resulting in a very rapid miscarriage, sometimes associated with spontaneous rupture of the membranes. Cervical incompetence may be something you are born with, but is more usually associated with cervical damage following surgery or vaginal termination of pregnancy.

If your obstetrician thinks from your medical history that you may have this problem it may be recommended that you have a stitch (known as a Shirodkar or McDonald's suture) placed around the cervix to close it. This is performed under anaesthesia about fourteen weeks into the pregnancy. The stitch is removed again around the thirty-eighth week or when labour starts if this is sooner. You do not need an anaesthetic to have it removed.

ECTOPIC PREGNANCY

Sometimes a pregnancy never gets as far as implanting in the uterus and embeds itself somewhere along the way. Usually this is in the Fallopian tube, and is more likely to happen if the tubes have been damaged by infection or surgery or if there is an intrauterine device preventing implantation in the womb. Symptoms of pregnancy start but the pregnancy cannot develop for long in this environment and so after only a few weeks will be passed out of the tube or rupture through its wall. When this happens there is usually severe pain on that side of the abdomen with a small amount of vaginal bleeding. Severe haemorrhage may occur internally leading to fainting and collapse.

An ectopic pregnancy is a serious medical emergency and will need to be dealt with in hospital. If you think you could have this condition contact your doctor immediately. If examination and further tests confirm the diagnosis then an abdominal operation will be required to remove the pregnancy and usually the damaged tube with it.

Having an ectopic pregnancy does not necessarily mean you cannot conceive again. Your chances will depend on the cause of the ectopic pregnancy and the state of your remaining Fallopian tube.

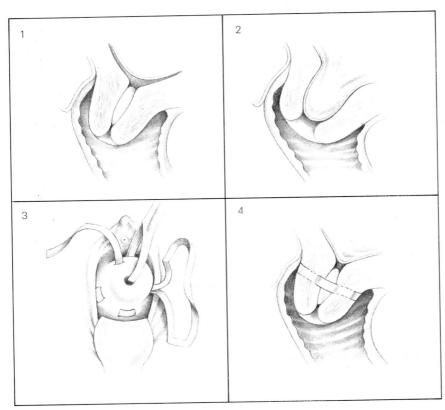

Incompetent cervix
1 In the normal cervix, the cervical os (canal) is tightly closed and sealed with a plug of mucus during pregnancy.
2 In cervical incompetence, the cervix opens, allowing the membranes and amniotic fluid to bulge through the cervical canal, eventually leading to miscarriage.
3 An incompetent cervix can be closed surgically at about fourteen weeks using a 'purse string' suture.
4 The suture shown in cross-section. It holds the cervix closed, preventing the membranes from bulging through. It is removed at about 38 weeks of pregnancy.

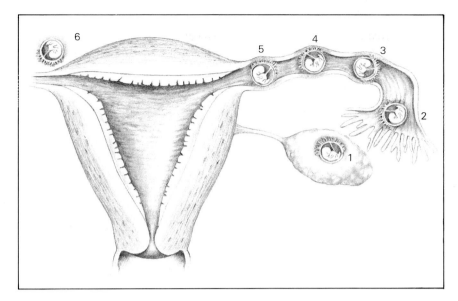

An ectopic pregnancy is one where the embryo does not reach the uterus but embeds itself elsewhere. This is usually somewhere in the Fallopian tube (2-5), but more rarely the embryo embeds in the ovary (1) or outside the uterus within the abdominal cavity (6). An ectopic pregnancy usually fails and has to be removed surgically.

THE RISK OF PREMATURE LABOUR

Arguably the problem of prematurity exercises the minds of obstetrician and paediatrician more than any other single problem in obstetrics. The aim of every obstetrician and midwife is to give to the mother and father a healthy mature baby undamaged by pregnancy or delivery. Prematurity is a threat to this aim.

A premature labour is one that starts after the twenty-eighth week of pregnancy. Before that it would constitute a miscarriage if the fetus is born dead, although in practice many babies born nowadays as early as 24 weeks of gestation can survive with the support of an up-to-date neonatal intensive care unit (see p. 116). In most cases, the basic cause of the onset of premature labour, or premature rupture of the membranes, is not known, but certain background factors, listed in the table right, are however, well defined, and should alert your obstetrician so that extra monitoring of your pregnancy can be arranged if you are at risk.

To stop premature labour in its tracks would seem the obvious thing to do, but that is not always possible. Certain drugs are available which act to inhibit the uterus from contracting. They can be given initially by intravenous drip and subsequently in tablet form, but these cannot be used under all circumstances, such as when there has been an antepartum haemorrhage, and they are not without some unpleasant side-effects to the mother, such as dizziness, faintness and rapid pulse. However this is a small price to pay for improving the prospects for the baby.

Although this treatment can be administered for several weeks in some cases, the most important function for these drugs is in delaying labour for 24 for 48 hours. This is to enable the mother to be given steroid injections which can help to improve the baby's lung maturity, by apparently increasing lung surfactant (see p. 118).

ALLOWING PREMATURE LABOUR TO PROCEED

In some circumstances it may be sensible to allow a premature labour to proceed, especially if there is an neonatal intensive care unit in the hospital or nearby (see p. 116). If the membranes have ruptured it may not be advisable to attempt long-term inhibition of labour because of the risk of infection. If the cervix is already dilated more than four

---

FACTORS ASSOCIATED WITH PREMATURE LABOUR

☐ Multiple pregnancy

☐ Antepartum haemorrhage

☐ Intrauterine growth retardation (fetus 'small for dates')

☐ Cervical incompetence

☐ Congenital abnormality of the uterus

☐ Diabetes

☐ Excess amniotic liquor

☐ Generalized infections, e.g. kidney infection

☐ Previous history of premature labour

centimetres labour will progress anyway. Labour should be allowed to progress also if the estimated weight of the baby is over 2000g (5lb) or the definite gestational age is more than 34 weeks.

If such a premature labour takes place in a hospital without neonatal intensive care facilities, then urgent transfer of the mother to such a unit has to be arranged, before labour progresses to any extent. A premature labour has to be very carefully managed and this is discussed in Chapter 7.

RECOGNIZING PREMATURE LABOUR

It is often difficult, especially for a first-time mother, to recognize the signs of premature labour. Braxton Hicks contractions (see p. 76) can be quite cramping and regular. However if regular pain is accompanied by hardening of the uterus, a 'show' and certainly if your membranes rupture, you should go to hospital immediately.

If you are in any doubt, telephone the senior midwife on the labour ward for help and advice. Because everyone is so aware of the problems of prematurity, it is more than likely that her advice will be to come to hospital at once for admission, to be rested, observed and monitored by the cardiotocograph which will show exactly what is happening to your uterus and the condition of the baby. This information, plus a clinical examination, will then guide the obstetrician as to what action to take, based on the factors discussed above.

Quite often, a mother may stay in the antenatal ward for some time after a threatened premature labour, and the pregnancy is conserved for as long as possible. Rest is the key, and mothers become very bored in this situation, but there is the compensation of knowing that every day nearer to full term that the baby can be maintained in the uterus increases his chances of survival.

BLEEDING DURING LATER PREGNANCY

When bleeding occurs from the vagina after the twenty-eighth week of pregnancy and before the birth of the baby, it is called 'antepartum haemorrhage'. It is important to realize that the bleeding need not be heavy, in spite of the implications of the word 'haemorrhage'. Blood loss may be quite slight, but you should always treat it seriously and contact your doctor at once, since slight loss can herald a much bigger loss, and the sooner everyone is alerted the better.

There can be several possible sources of antepartum haemorrhage. Sometimes the bleeding may be accompanied by other symptoms, although this is not always the case.

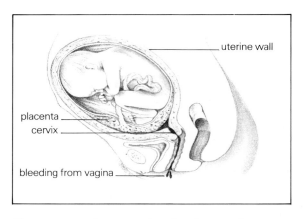

Placenta praevia means that the placenta is very low, partially or wholly covering the exit from the uterus. It is a major cause of painless bleeding during pregnancy.

PLACENTA PRAEVIA

Placenta praevia is a major cause of antepartum haemorrhage – probably accounting for between 20 and 40 per cent of all cases. Placenta praevia – which literally translates as 'placenta first' – means that instead of being positioned somewhere towards the top of the uterine wall, the placenta is partly or completely attached to the lower segment of the uterus. This usually results in part or all of its mass covering the area of the internal os of the cervix. The internal os is a tight ring of muscle at the top of the cervix. It is gradually pulled up into the lower uterine segment as pregnancy progresses and during labour will become part of the lower uterine segment as the whole cervix is dilated (see p. 76).

Depending on how low is the site of the placenta, the condition is classified into four types, ranging from type 1, where it does not quite reach the opening of the uterus, to the 'complete' type 4, where the placenta totally covers the cervix. Placenta praevia is frequently diagnosed at early scanning of the pregnancy. Often no bleeding results; this is because as the lower segment of the uterus is formed as the uterus grows, the placental site is 'pulled up' away from the cervix. What appears as a low-lying placenta at sixteen to eighteen weeks may be seen on a repeat scan at 30 to 32 weeks to be a normally situated placenta.

Placenta praevia is thought to occur in about half a per cent of all pregnancies. The cause of such an abnormal site for the placenta is not known, but in a multiple pregnancy (twins, for example), it is more common simply because a larger placenta, or even two placentae may be involved, thereby covering a larger area of the uterine wall.

The features of a placenta praevia are quite typical. You may experience a sudden painless loss of blood which is very often slight at first. If it recurs, which it is likely to do, and if there is a major degree of placenta praevia, the bleeding may become heavy. When you are examined, the doctor may well find that the baby is lying transversely or obliquely across the uterus, simply because the placenta is preventing the head from getting into the lower segment of the uterus.

Bleeding occurs as the internal os region of the cervix is pulled up into the lower segment of the uterus during pregnancy. The placenta becomes dislodged from its site and a tiny area is exposed, and it is surprising how much bleeding can come from such a small area. However, unless the quantity of blood loss is such as to affect you adversely (with a sudden drop of blood pressure and rapid pulse – in other words, the onset of 'shock'), the fetus remains undisturbed. Although you may be alarmed by the amount of blood you lose, you can be reassured that your baby will be quite safe, in contrast to other causes of antepartum haemorrhage. However, once placenta praevia has been diagnosed, the well-being of the fetus will be checked by electronic monitoring to get a trace of the fetal heart rate (see p. 81).

Bleeding from a placenta praevia tends to occur quite late in pregnancy: 60 per cent occurs after the thirty-sixth week. As a result, it is a golden rule among obstetricians never to give a mother with bleeding in later pregnancy an internal examination. If you suffer from bleeding at this time, your doctor will suspect placenta praevia and will be anxious not to touch the low lying placenta, thus precipitating further bleeding. Instead, you will be given an abdominal examination, looking first for areas of tenderness (see placental abruption, overleaf), and for the lie of the baby – transverse or oblique, or perhaps longitudinal but with an unusually high presenting part (head or breech). You will be given an ultrasound scan as well which can accurately detect the position of both the placenta and the baby.

TREATING PLACENTA PRAEVIA

If you experience slight bleeding, and your doctor suspects placenta praevia, you will be referred without delay to the hospital where you are booked to have your baby, or to the nearest large maternity unit if you had been planning a home delivery. If the bleeding is heavy, the maternity 'flying squad' will probably be called out. The obstetrician in the team will check your health and the baby's heart rate, and will put an intravenous 'drip' into your arm to maintain fluids. The doctor may also take a blood sample to double-check for cross-matching in case of more severe haemorrhage and the need for blood transfusion. You will then be transferred to hospital by ambulance.

Once in hospital a more detailed history will be taken and your notes will be checked. You will also be asked some relevant questions: Have you had a scan earlier in pregnancy? Was there pain when you bled? How much have you lost – a cupful, a milk bottle-full? What were you doing when it started? For example, sexual intercourse with deep penetration could precipitate bleeding from a placenta praevia of major degree.

Your pulse rate, blood pressure and temperature will be checked, and you will be given an abdominal examination. The fetal heart rate will also be checked again. You will almost certainly be given an ultrasound scan at this stage to check the site of the placenta.

Although you won't be given an internal examination, the doctor may decide to pass a speculum into your vagina – this is an instrument which will allow examination of the cervix, which is commonly used for taking cervical smears. A polyp of the cervix may be the cause of a small bleed especially if it was disturbed during intercourse, so it is worth having a look at the appearance and condition of the cervix to rule this out. (A polyp is a small 'tag' of tissue, full of blood vessels, which bleeds readily to touch. It is harmless and can be removed by a simple operation after pregnancy.)

The treatment in hospital following the initial investigation once again depends on how severe the bleeding is, and what stage the pregnancy has reached. If the bleeding is severe, a maternal shock has to be corrected by blood transfusion or equivalent treatment and the baby must be delivered at once regardless of maturity. Severe bleeding usually means that there is a major degree of placenta praevia which would prevent a vaginal delivery, so for the sake of speed an emergency Caesarean section would be carried out (see p. 96).

In mild bleeding, however, the object would be to conserve the pregnancy. You are admitted to hospital for observation, but nothing further would be done until an ultrasound scan confirms the degree of placenta praevia. If the placenta is found to be very low an elective Caesarean section will be arranged. This is because in a major degree of placenta praevia bleeding is likely to recur and the position of the placenta would again prevent a vaginal delivery. 'Elective' simply means that a convenient date and time will be pre-arranged and these will be determined particularly by the maturity of your pregnancy. Your doctor will try to wait until

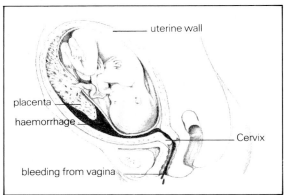

Placental abruption means that part of the placenta becomes detached from the uterine wall and bleeding occurs behind it, associated with pain. The

abruption may be 'revealed' (above) with vaginal bleeding, or 'concealed' (left), where the blood collects at the placental site but does not escape.

you are at least 37 weeks pregnant, so you may have to stay in hospital for several weeks.

If the diagnosis is in any doubt or the degree of placenta praevia appears to be minimal then your doctor might want to carry out a vaginal examination first, although this is rarely necessary nowadays with the sophistication of ultrasound scanning techniques. However if it is thought necessary, a vaginal examination will be done under general anaesthetic with everything prepared for an immediate Caesarean section, in case the doctor 'hits oil' and precipitates bleeding during the examination. However this examination is only done if it seems possible that the placenta is *not* praevia and therefore vaginal delivery could be allowed.

THE RISK TO MOTHER AND BABY

It must be emphasised that the risk to mother and baby from placenta praevia are nowadays very slight, provided that warning signs are acted upon at once. Even if bleeding is severe, the maternal blood pressure can be maintained by adequate transfusion and adequate facilities can be made ready for an emergency Caesarean delivery.

Placenta praevia is not a problem that need necessarily recur in a subsequent pregnancy. If you have to have a Caesarean because of this problem, there is no reason why you should not have a vaginal delivery next time, if all else is normal.

PLACENTAL ABRUPTION

One of the commonest causes of vaginal bleeding after the twenty-eighth week of pregnancy is abruption of the placenta, or abruptio placentae, to give it its classical title. Another rather old fashioned name

is accidental haemorrhage. Placental abruption needs swift treatment, since it is potentially dangerous to the health of both mother and baby.

In placental abruption, the placenta is situated normally in the uterus, in the upper segment, and either on the front or back wall or across the top (the fundus). The bleeding occurs behind the placenta, shearing it off from its attachment to the uterus. This may be slight, or it may extend to a much greater degree, even occasionally lifting the placenta off its attachment to the uterine wall altogether. Placental abruption occurs in as many as two per cent of all pregnancies and is thought to account for 60 per cent of all cases of antepartum haemorrhage.

Like placenta praevia, the actual reason for a placental abruption is not known, but there are several recognized associated factors. For example, it is more common in women who have had several children, and it may complicate a pregnancy already complicated by high blood pressure. Trauma – in the form of some accidental external damage – plays a small part, but it can follow a blow on the stomach, such as experienced in a car accident, for example.

The fundamental difference between the antepartum bleeding associated with placental abruption, as opposed to that experienced in placenta praevia, is pain. The amount of visible bleeding is usually slight, but the amount of bleeding behind the disrupted placenta can be quite considerable and pain results from the tension produced by the trapped blood.

Pain may also be accompanied by tenderness and irritability of the uterus, and indeed labour may ensue. Finally, and most importantly, the oxygen supply to the fetus is interrupted to some extent, fetal distress may result and prompt action may be required on behalf of the baby. Apart from these serious problems, the situation may be complicated by maternal shock caused by loss of blood, failure of her blood to clot in severe cases, and temporary kidney failure, also in severe cases.

TREATING PLACENTAL ABRUPTION

When you are initially examined by your doctor, placental abruption will probably be diagnosed if you have had bleeding with associated pain; if your uterus is generally rather hard, tender and irritable or has an area of marked tenderness on examination; and especially if the fetal heart rate is fast or slow or showing 'dips' in association with the activity of the uterus. You will be admitted immediately into hospital in the same way as described for placenta praevia, above, but how you are treated subsequently depends on the severity of the abruption. You will probably be given an ultrasound scan which may show evidence of a blood clot behind an area of uterus. However, in major degrees of abruption there will be no time for scanning.

In a mild case of placental abruption before 37 weeks of pregnancy, where there was only slight blood loss, with no distress of the baby and the mother's condition is good, you would be scanned to confirm the diagnosis and then advised to rest in bed in hospital. Yours and your baby's condition would be monitored carefully to try and conserve the pregnancy as long as possible. If the abruption occurs after 37 weeks, then your membranes would be ruptured and labour induced (see p. 87). Rupturing the membranes appears to 'clamp down' the uterus on the bleeding spot, preventing further extension of the abruption. Obviously the baby's condition would be closely monitored during the ensuing labour.

Moderate placental abruption might consist of more loss of blood – say 500-1000ml (1-2 pints) – although not all would be visible and measurable, a raised pulse and lowered blood pressure, much pain, a very irritable, tender uterus and probably evidence of fetal distress.

Here the baby would have to be delivered urgently and an emergency Caesarean section is required. Your condition would have to be corrected by blood transfusion and special steps taken to correct the inability of your blood to clot (if this has happened) and to preserve kidney function.

Severe abruption is a rare but extremely important obstetric emergency. The mother would be profoundly shocked, her uterus tense and very tender, and unfortunately the baby, who has had his life-line cut, does not usually survive. In such a life-threatening situation, the labour would be induced as soon as possible, with adequate transfusion and close monitoring of the mother.

OTHER REASONS FOR BLEEDING

It has already been mentioned that a polyp of the cervix may cause a small loss of blood, which, after 28 weeks, must be classified as antepartum haemorrhage, although it is not serious. Other rare local conditions causing bleeding may be severe inflammation of the vagina due to infection, a cervical ectropian (cervical erosion), which sometimes occurs during pregnancy, or even more rarely, cervical cancer. All these conditions would be borne in mind by the obstetrician when examining the mother through a speculum in the vagina, following a small antepartum haemorrhage.

Apart from the extremely rare case of invasive cervical cancer, no active treatment would be given to any of these local conditions during pregnancy. Your doctor would probably arrange for an ultrasound scan to be done as well to make quite sure that a low lying placenta was not after all the cause of the bleeding, and the local condition simply coincidence.

Quite a large number of women are admitted into hospital with a slight bleed which has to be classified as of 'unknown cause'. A scan excludes placenta praevia, there is no evidence of placental abruption and no local condition can be found.

Even so most obstetricians would prefer to regard such cases as probably mild abruptions, and although the treatment would be to conserve the pregnancy, they would want to monitor mother and baby, probably with a few days in hospital, for the rest of the pregnancy.

MULTIPLE PREGNANCIES

A multiple pregnancy of course means more than one baby in a pregnancy – twins, most commonly (1 in 80 pregnancies), triplets less commonly (1 in 80×80), and still less commonly, quadruplets or more.

It seems a pity that the topic has to be put into a chapter entitled 'problem' pregnancies. It would be nice to think that the mother with twins would not look on her pregnancy as a problem, but rather as an exciting, if challenging, prospect. Hopefully the description and explanation which follows will help to emphasise the latter rather than the former.

We talk about twins simply because that is the most common form of multiple pregnancy. Any additional points on triplets (or more) will be made where relevant.

TYPES OF TWINS

Twins are described as binovular (non-identical) or uniovular (identical), which means that they either develop from two separate eggs or from the one fertilized egg dividing into two at an early stage. In binovular twins each fetus is separate, with a separate placenta and two sets of membranes (amnion and chorion). In uniovular twins there is a single placenta and one chorion but each fetus usually has a separate amniotic sac. Uniovular twins are always the same sex, but binovular twins may not be. Binovular twins are no more alike than any other brothers or sisters from the same family. The proportion of binovular to uniovular twins is approximately 60:40. At birth it is sometimes quite difficult to tell whether twins are identical or not, but parents obviously want to know this. The placenta has to be examined by a pathologist, but even so, the diagnosis might have to be confirmed by a special blood test.

DIAGNOSING MULTIPLE PREGNANCY

How do we recognize if you are going to have twins? First of all your uterus would be bigger than would be expected for the calculated dates. As the pregnancy grows there seems to be an excess of fetal parts when your abdomen is examined and often two heads can clearly be felt. If there is a family history of twins (it is an hereditary trait) then

In many twin pregnancies, both babies adopt a cephalic (head down) presentation. These twins have a separate placenta and amnion (inner membrane) but share a single chorion (outer membrane).

the diagnosis seems highly likely.

Confirmation of the diagnosis will nowadays be made by ultrasound scan; it is then that a 'head count' shows whether there are two or more babies present. In the absence of ultrasound a single X-ray picture will also give the diagnosis, but this cannot be done until quite late in pregnancy to avoid damaging the fetus (or fetuses). An ultrasound picture can diagnose the situation as early as eight weeks of pregnancy.

PROBLEMS IN A TWIN PREGNANCY

Increased nausea may be experienced in early pregnancy, and may lead to actual vomiting, often well into the second trimester. Ask your doctor's advice if this becomes incapacitating. In later pregnancy all the minor discomforts of pregnancy may be exaggerated – haemorrhoids, varicose veins, ankle swelling, heartburn and so on – all made more troublesome as a result of the extra size of the uterus. There is more amniotic fluid – especially with uniovular twins – and the uterus considerably distended, so it is not surprising that these discomforts appear. This is especially so in triplets or quadruplets where the uterus can become enormously distended. When the babies begin to move, you may find it very uncomfortable and they may make sleeping difficult. Use extra pillows to take the pressure off your abdomen, and don't be

WHY DO TWINS OCCUR?	
As is so often the case the reason for twinning is not really known, but several associated factors are recognized which are listed below.	
Family history	There is a strong familial tendency to twins
Older age groups	The chances of twins increase over the age of 35
High parity	The more babies a woman has the more likely she is to have twins
Racial factors	Twinning is more common in Africa and Asia (except the Far East) than in Western countries
Fertility drugs	Nowadays this is a recognized 'risk' factor in twin pregnancies (or more). The use of fertility drugs has certainly increased the chances of a multiple pregnancy simply by increasing the number of eggs available for fertilization.

Another common twin presentation is for one baby to be cephalic, the other breech. As shown here, most non-identical twins have separate amnions, chorions and placenta.

If one twin is smaller than the other, the baby may be forced to adopt a transverse lie. The safest form of delivery for these babies would probably be by Caesarean section.

afraid to ask your doctor for a mild sedative. Try to avoid sleeping on your back as this may cause faintness. If you are working, you should expect to give up at least twelve weeks before the expected date of delivery.

Other problems are associated with multiple pregnancies. Pre-eclampsia (see p. 70) is one, anaemia is another (see p. 52) and the bigger placental area in a twin pregnancy may mean the chance of a placenta praevia (see above). The onset of premature labour is a risk that is recognized and steps will be taken to avoid it.

Premature labour is a direct result of the over-distension of the uterus.

ANTENATAL CARE FOR THE TWIN MOTHER

Bearing these points in mind it makes sense to take special care of you antenatally to minimize your discomfort and make sure the pregnancy continues for as long as possible.

Once twins (or more) have been diagnosed, you will be advised to have all your antenatal check-ups at the hospital and your progress will be closely monitored by the senior members of the obstetric team. If you are found to be anaemic, you will be given iron tablets to correct this, and it is important to pay particular attention to maintaining a good balanced diet.

Your blood pressure will be closely monitored, and you will be advised to take extra rest. A twin

pregnancy is very tiring and you will probably need to give up work earlier than most pregnant women. Indeed some obstetricians will recommend that you are admitted to hospital for a period of rest between, say, 26 and 32 weeks.

The babies' growth will be maintained by regular ultrasound scanning. Twin babies tend to be individually smaller and one may be much smaller than the other, so that it is valuable to watch their growth in the uterus. The babies commonly lie in one of the positions illustrated, which can make a difference to the way labour is managed, and many twins are eventually delivered by Caesarean section. Twin births are discussed in Chapter 7, but need not necessarily be problematic.

THE PHYSICALLY-HANDICAPPED MOTHER

We see many more handicapped mothers nowadays in the antenatal clinic. There are probably two reasons for this. One is that advances in medical care are such that women, born disabled, are helped to lead a much more complete life including in many instances marriage and child bearing. The other is that road accidents are increasing, leading to 'acquired' handicap and these women may, with care, go on to bear children.

There are many types of handicap, from deafness or blindness which may cause a problem of adjustment when caring for the newborn baby, to major handicaps such as paraplegia.

PARAPLEGIA (PARALYSIS)

This severe disability may have been present since birth or it may have been acquired through trauma – a motor traffic accident for example. It is of the utmost importance that you get thorough pre-pregnancy counselling if you are in this position, so that together, the doctor, you and your partner can map out a picture of how things will be during pregnancy and particularly how you are going to cope after the birth of the baby.

Associated medical conditions such as kidney problems have to be assessed, as well as how much extra nursing care you yourself require as a result of your disability (such as impaired bowel and bladder control). Then everyone must consider the help you will have with the new baby from your family, friends, social services or voluntary organizations.

If you have become paraplegic as the result of a road accident it is obviously necessary to check the size and shape of your pelvis in case it was significantly damaged at the time of the accident. There is no reason why such a paraplegic mother should not have a vaginal delivery but if any pelvic abnormality exists then Caesarean section will be necessary. In any case help with forceps is likely to be required in the second stage of labour since you will not have the power to push and deliver the baby yourself (see p. 92).

Help with the care of the baby afterwards is essential but paraplegic mothers are quick to adapt, and devise methods to overcome their disability.

MULTIPLE SCLEROSIS

The cause of this neurological disease is still unknown. Cruelly, it tends to manifest itself in women in their late twenties or early thirties, when they may already have started a family, or are just starting to plan for it. In its more advanced stages multiple sclerosis causes paraplegia, so careful counselling before pregnancy is essential. There is some evidence, for example, that there is an hereditary element in the disease and this fact alone may deter many such couples from contemplating pregnancy. However, many MS sufferers have fairly mild symptoms and feel able to contemplate childbirth for the sake of their partners', and their own, fulfilment.

Pregnancy seems to have no effect on the long term outlook for the patient with multiple sclerosis but unfortunately the patient who is already pregnant before the disease reveals itself, seems to develop a greater degree of disability.

Pregnancy and labour may be normal but again delivery may have to be by forceps.

PELVIC DEFORMITIES

These may result from accident or disease or to be present from birth. Basically the degree of deformity must be assessed by x-ray so that a decision can be made as to whether a vaginal delivery is possible or whether a Caesarean section will be required. If there is any real doubt then, for the safety of the baby, the latter course will be chosen.

EXISTING MEDICAL PROBLEMS

If you already suffer from an existing medical condition, such as heart disease or diabetes, it does not necessarily mean you should not have a baby. However, it is clear that your pregnancy is not going to be as straightforward as that of someone who doesn't suffer from any of these conditions, and you can expect to have more medical monitoring and more intervention during your delivery for the safety and health of yourself and your baby.

HEART DISEASE

We do not see severe heart disease nearly so often nowadays. This is because congenital (developmental) heart conditions are detected early in life and with the advanced techniques of cardiac surgery now available, are corrected well before childbearing age. Rheumatic heart disease is also much less common nowadays.

However, women do still suffer from heart disease, and also have babies. Occasionally, the problem may not be discovered until the woman is pregnant, so it is essential that the doctor examining a pregnant woman in the booking clinic listens carefully to her heart. If an abnormality is discovered then the opinion of a heart specialist is sought; in fact it is crucial to the success of the care of a pregnant woman with a heart problem that her case is shared between obstetrician and heart specialist.

During pregnancy, adequate rest is essential, and may involve a stay in the antenatal ward for observation at any time during pregnancy, but especially in later pregnancy – if the condition is severe enough to warrant it. It is important, of course, to avoid anaemia and to treat any infections promptly. If dental treatment is required it must be covered by antibiotics.

DIABETES MELLITUS

Although pregnancy worsens a diabetic's condition and is equally dangerous for mother and baby, this somewhat alarming statement does not mean that a diabetic woman should not undertake a pregnancy. What it does mean, however, is that the care of a diabetic pregnant woman must be in the hands of experts – preferably a combined team (as for the cardiac mother), in this case a diabetologist and obstetrician – and that the control of her diabetes must be as strict as possible.

DIAGNOSIS

If you are already diabetic when you become pregnant, you will be well aware of the management of your own condition. Occasionally however pregnancy induces a condition known as gestational diabetes, in which the ability of the body to handle sugar becomes abnormal only during a pregnancy. There are particular signs which may point to this possibility, such as previous large babies (over 4.2 kg or 9lb); an unexplained stillbirth; a family history of diabetes; obesity; and repeated appearance of sugar in the urine during pregnancy.

One of the changes that takes place in the function of the body during pregnancy allows the kidneys to spill sugar over into the urine. But when this occurs repeatedly in a pregnancy, further investigation must be carried out. This consists of a glucose tolerance test. First of all you will have a sample of blood taken when you have had nothing to eat for a certain length of time, and your blood sugar level will be measured. You then drink 50g (2oz) of glucose in solution and further blood sugars are measured half hourly for the next 2½ hours. A normal glucose tolerance 'curve' is shown at the top of the graph on this page; a diabetic one in the centre and one which suggests gestational (pregnancy only) diabetes at the bottom.

PROBLEMS OF DIABETES IN PREGNANCY

During pregnancy, it is important that you control the diabetes very strictly because pregnancy does make it worse, bringing with it other complications. Before diabetes was properly understood and controlled, the picture for diabetic mothers and their babies was a rather depressing one. They were likely to suffer distension from excessive liquor and pre-eclampsia (with high blood pressure) was often associated with it. The diabetic mother was also more prone to various infections. Diabetes could cause the baby to grow very large in the uterus, with consequent difficulty in labour and with delivery.

Diabetes also brought with it an increased chance of abnormalities in the baby, and the likelihood of premature labour was increased. If the baby was very large he or she might suffer the trauma of a

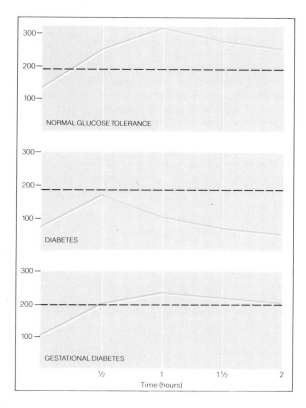

Glucose tolerance curves. **Top:** *In a normal pregnant woman.* **Centre:** *In a previously diagnosed diabetic.* **Above:** *In a woman with gestational diabetes (diabetes of pregnancy).*

difficult delivery. There was also a higher risk of stillbirth if the mother's diabetes was not controlled, and in the neonatal period, babies of diabetic mothers often suffered respiratory difficulties, low blood sugar, and infections. But these risks are minimized nowadays by strict control of the diabetes. With increasing understanding of the implications of diabetes on the pregnancy – and vice versa – and increased expertise in the control of diabetes the outlook for the diabetic mother and her baby is nowadays greatly improved and almost all diabetic women can plan two or three pregnancies confidently provided they are prepared to cooperate with the strict medical supervision which is required for the sake of mother and baby.

THE MOTHER WITH DIABETES

If your diabetes is already being treated, your obstetrician will work closely with your physician throughout pregnancy. Your diet will be controlled at 1500-2400 calories per day with 150-250g (6-8oz) of carbohydrate and 100g (4oz) of protein.

If you were using oral agents for the treatment of your diabetes this will be changed to insulin by injection so as to maintain stricter control over blood sugar levels, and you may be admitted to hospital as often as necessary to supervise that control. However, you may be taught to monitor your own blood sugar at home, especially if the diabetes has only appeared in pregnancy.

In many centres you can phone the hospital diabetic unit and discuss these results directly to assess any alteration of insulin requirements. If diabetes is only seen as a potential threat, only your diet need be controlled, but your pregnancy will be strictly monitored.

Nowadays there should be no need for intervention in a normal vaginal delivery unless there are complicating features such as hypertension or fetal distress, when a Caesarean section would be carried out. Needless to say, great care in the control of blood sugars during labour, delivery and in the puerperium must be maintained.

HYPERTENSION AND PRE-ECLAMPSIA

First of all a definition. The left side of the heart (the left ventricle) pumps blood through the arteries and smaller vessels of the circulation and the blood returns to the right side of the heart via the veins. There is a higher 'head' of pressure stemming from the left ventricle than from the right, which means that the flow of blood will be maintained. This is known as the arterial blood pressure or simply the blood pressure, and it varies between 120 and 80mm mercury above atmospheric pressure.

At the beginning of pregnancy the level measured represents your non-pregnant level. This is one reason why it is important to be seen by a doctor as early as possible. However, in the middle third of pregnancy (the second trimester) the blood pressure drops slightly.

High blood pressure or hypertension can be a problem in pregnancy and can have all the potential for disaster. But if it is recognized and managed with skill and care, both mother and baby should emerge from the pregnancy fit and well.

To simplify what is quite a difficult and complex subject, women suffering from hypertension in pregnancy can be considered in two groups. In the first group, there is pre-existing hypertension, that is a significantly high level of blood pressure (more than 140/90) known to be present before pregnancy begins or, as so often happens, discovered early in pregnancy (before 20 weeks). This is one of the reasons why it is so important for a mother to start antenatal check-ups early in pregnancy for the blood pressure reading recorded at the booking clinic represents her non-pregnant level of blood pressure (see p. 21).

The second groups suffer from a condition peculiar to pregnancy called pre-eclampsia (also known as pregnancy-induced hypertension). No one yet knows the cause of this condition, which is characterized typically by a rise in blood pressure, swelling of hands and legs (oedema), and the appearance (in the more severe forms) of protein in the urine.

CAUSES OF HYPERTENSION

There may be no known cause for pre-existing hypertension (in this case called essential hypertension), or the raised blood pressure may be due to other conditions such as kidney diseases, diabetes or other rarer conditions.

Although as has already been mentioned, the cause of pre-eclampsia is unknown, there are several associated background factors which make it easier to identify the woman at risk. These include a first pregnancy or a pregnancy following one which was severely affected; women with a family history of hypertension especially involving pregnancies; women who are hypertensive before pregnancy (referred to as 'superimposed pre-eclampsia'); women with diabetes or kidney diseases; multiple pregnancies; and poor socio-economic backgrounds. It is interesting to note that for some reason the incidence of pre-eclampsia in women who smoke is lower, but for smokers who do develop the condition, the outlook for the baby is not at all hopeful.

PROBLEMS WITH HYPERTENSION AND PRE-ECLAMPSIA

There is no doubt that if hypertension is at all marked and certainly if there is pre-eclampsia, a pregnancy does not fare so well. The mother may be at risk of kidney problems and in severe uncontrolled cases, there is the chance of eclampsia developing (see later).

So far as the baby is concerned, the environment within the uterus in either of these conditions is not at all favourable. The placenta functions less well and the baby grows more slowly than one would expect for the dates, leading to a 'small for dates' or 'growth retarded' baby (see p. 72). In severe cases, abruption of the placenta may occur with associated heavy bleeding (see earlier) and death of the baby is an increased risk.

Essential or pre-existing hypertension may get worse as pregnancy progresses. If you are already having treatment for the condition, the dosage of the drug used may need to be increased, or you may need to start treatment for the first time in pregnancy. So far as pre-eclampsia is concerned, left alone the condition almost always deteriorates as pregnancy progresses.

TREATING HYPERTENSION AND PRE-ECLAMPSIA

It is obvious that hypertension in pregnancy is taken very seriously indeed. The problem is that there are no symptoms to help you realize that an important situation has arisen. This is especially true of pre-eclampsia where you may have known nothing of hypertension previously, and feel perfectly well. It is therefore often difficult to accept the restrictions suddenly placed on you by the doctors – the need for extra rest, for example, and even the need to come into hospital for closer observation of your blood pressure.

However it is important to take your midwife or doctor seriously if she informs you that your blood pressure has risen to an unacceptably high level, compared to your pre-pregnancy level. In point of fact, pre-existing hypertension of a mild degree may not require any treatment. The only important feature of management is to keep a very close eye on you, so you will be seen more frequently for antenatal checks and may be admitted to hospital, if necessary, to monitor for either deterioration of the blood pressure or for the appearance of pre-eclampsia.

More severe degrees of hypertension however, will require drug therapy. The drugs will be chosen for their safety in pregnancy and again in liaison with a physician specializing in this area. Close monitoring will be of great importance. The aim of your care if suffering from hypertension will be to keep your blood pressure at acceptable levels, compatible with your safety and the healthy growth of the baby. This will be done until the baby is mature enough to be born – ideally at term, but often at 36 to 38 weeks.

There is no cure for pre-eclampsia, either, except to deliver the baby, so the aim is to control your blood pressure, monitor fetal well-being and to step in and deliver the baby preferably when he is mature and conditions are favourable for induction of labour (at around 38 weeks).

If the environment for the baby within the uterus is clearly no longer ideal (shown by worsening blood pressure levels, increasing protein in the urine, and evidence of fetal distress shown on a heart-rate tracing), the situation calls for prompt action. It may arise well before term, sometimes as early as 26 to 28 weeks, and certainly before 38 weeks, so Caesarean section may be necessary and the baby may need special care.

ECLAMPSIA

Eclampsia is also associated with high blood pressure and is a very serious condition which only affects pregnant women. It can occur antenatally, as early as 26 to 28 weeks in rare cases, and it also occurs during labour or in the immediate puerperium (up to 48 hours after the birth). Eclampsia is typified by convulsive fits which occasionally happen out of the blue, but mostly in women already suffering from pre-eclampsia (see above). Although much rarer than pre-eclampsia, eclampsia poses a very high risk for the mother, and equally for the baby if it occurs before the birth.

Eclamptic fits are like the convulsive fits of epilepsy and are handled in the same way. First of all the fit is treated. The airways are cleared to ensure that the patient has a good supply of oxygen, then a sedative such as diazepam is given intravenously to control the convulsions, as well as a hypotensive drug to lower the blood pressure.

During the eclampsia the mother runs the risk of kidney failure, brain haemorrhage and an associated condition called 'disseminated vascular coagulation' (DIC). In this the blood fails to clot and the risk of uncontrollable haemorrhage develops, unless the situation is recognized and treated.

If eclampsia occurs during labour, the birth is speeded up, and unless labour is already far advanced an emergency Caesarean section will be required. Both mother and baby will need intensive care for some days after the event.

EPILEPSY

Epilepsy is a common condition and many women who are epileptics have children. Pregnancy may cause an increase in the number of fits but this is by no means always the case and often epileptic women remain in the same state of control as before pregnancy.

Provided that control of fits is good, pregnancy does not present many problems. However, severe, repeated fitting, known as 'status epilepticus' can be disastrous for both mother and baby unless treated promptly and adequately.

Some drugs used to control epilepsy are thought to cause developmental abnormalities in the fetus (teratogenic) so these are best avoided. But others – such as carbamazepine – appear to be safe and can be used in pregnancy.

Frequent monitoring of the drugs used is essential in order to maintain just enough in the blood to control fitting. The levels seem to fall more quickly in pregnancy so that adjustment of dosage may be required from time to time.

RHESUS ISO-IMMUNIZATION

The problem of rhesus iso-immunization is described and its effect on the baby discussed on pages 22 and 122. The conditions is now rare, thanks to the 'Anti-D' injection which can be given to rhesus negative mothers, but even so, occasional cases do slip through. If a mother is found to have antibodies present in her bloodstream which would in effect be attacking her baby's red blood cells, then careful supervision of her pregnancy preferably in a specialized rhesus clinic is essential if her baby is not to be severely affected.

If you are found to have antibodies, a careful history is taken at booking of previous pregnancies, miscarriages and so on, and both yours and your partner's blood is checked. After this, the level of antibodies in your blood is measured every month or more often if necessary.

It may be necessary to carry out repeated amniocentesis to sample the liquor and measure its bilirubin content. The amount of this substance indicates the rate at which fetal red blood cells are being broken down, and therefore the degree to which a baby is affected. A severely affected fetus may be given an intrauterine transfusion of a small amount of rhesus negative blood direct into the abdominal cavity under ultrasound control to allow the fetus to remain in the uterus until mature enough to be born. Even so, early induction of labour – or even delivery by Caesarean section – may be necessary, and the affected baby will require special neonatal care (see p. 122).

THROMBO-EMBOLISM

The risk of deep vein thrombosis (clotting) is something of which the public is well aware because of the publicized connection with the contraceptive pill. It usually occurs in the leg, and may be associated with pain. It is equally well known that a piece of clot may occasionally break off and travel to the lung, with fatal results. Such an event is tragic in any age group, but in a young mother is profoundly so. There are factors which predispose some women to this problem. The older mother is at greater risk, as is one who has had several children. Obesity is a factor, and so is long confinement to bed, for instance, following surgery. Knowing this, doctors are on the look-out for 'at risk' women and take precautions – early mobilization after surgery, special 'pressure' stockings to wear in bed, dietary restriction to reduce weight and so on.

The treatment for deep vein thrombosis is with anti-coagulant drugs. It is a fairly rare occurrence in pregnancy but when it happens anti-coagulant

tablets would have to be replaced by injections of a drug called heparin; mothers can be taught to administer this to themselves. Treatment would almost certainly have to be continued for a minimum of six weeks after delivery.

Pulmonary embolus – that is, when a piece of clot lodges in the lung – may follow a deep vein thrombosis or may occur out of the blue. It causes chest pain, breathlessness and a little blood may be coughed up. Confirmation of the diagnosis is made on X-ray or by a lung scan, and the treatment – which is urgent – is with anti-coagulants.

THYROID DISEASE

Occasionally a woman who is already on treatment for an over-active thyroid gland falls pregnant. Treatment must be continued during pregnancy and careful supervision and regulation of these drugs maintained throughout. Sometimes the problem is an underactive thyroid and the same principle of treatment applies.

Breastfeeding may or may not be allowed depending on the drugs being used and in all cases the baby must be tested for over or under-activity of his thyroid.

PROBLEMS OF FETAL GROWTH

Fetal growth can cause concern during pregnancy, either because the fetus is too small or too big. Of course there is a wide range of normal birth weights (see graph opposite), but babies born below the 10th percentile are classified as small for gestational age (small for dates) and above the 90th percentile, large for dates.

Small babies may be premature (born early but an appropriate weight for their period of gestation) or simply small (but mature) or small for their dates – sometimes called 'growth retarded'. This last situation has been increasingly recognized in recent years and requires expert care if the outcome of pregnancy is to be successful.

CAUSES OF GROWTH RETARDATION

The actual cause is obscure but several background factors are recognized. One of the most important is poor placental function – and this happens where high blood pressure, pre-eclampsia, kidney disease or diabetes exist in the mother. It may occur following partial placental abruption and possibly in prolonged pregnancy (beyond 42 weeks).

Twins and higher multiples are often smaller than average – this is not surprising since they have less room and the other may have fewer resources, but

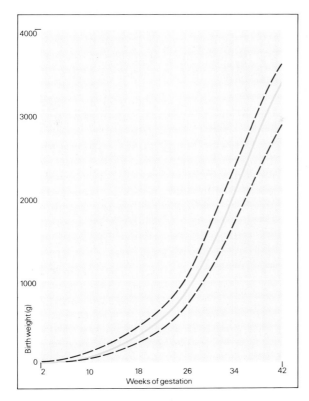

The range of normal fetal birth weights according to the weeks of gestation. Weights below the lower centile may indicate a 'small for dates' baby.

occasionally one baby may be considerably smaller than the others.

Another rare cause may be due to infection, for example by rubella (German measles), and chromosome abnormalities may be associated with small-for-dates babies. Poor maternal nutrition is a contributing factor. but more importantly, smoking has a highly significant relationship to the incidence of growth retardation in pregnancy. It has been proved conclusively that mothers who smoke during pregnancy have smaller babies than those who do not. Smoking constricts the blood vessels and restricts the passage of blood carrying oxygen and nutrients to the baby.

DISCOVERING GROWTH RETARDATION

Suspicions are aroused that the baby may not be growing well when the uterus appears to be small for the dates. Measuring in centimetres from the pubic bone (pubis symphysis) to the top of the uterus (the fundus) gives a fair estimate of the duration of pregnancy. If the gestational age has been confirmed by early ultrasound scan and a discrepancy develops between it and the symphysis-fundal measurement, then the doctor will suspect growth retardation.

Repeated scanning (every two weeks) will show a discrepancy between the measurement of the head (nature seems to watch over the brain, and the head measurement grows), and the circumference of the abdomen (which grows poorly). Meanwhile, other simple clinical features become apparent. The mother's weight, for instance, remains static or even drops; the measurement of her girth likewise.

Growth retardation may arise in the absence of other complications but not infrequently a mother may have high blood pressure, which would alert the doctor to the possibility of a growth retarded baby. Dealing with the problem in this situation can be difficult, as a decision has to be made as to when the environment within the uterus is actually *less* favourable to the baby than the environment in a special care baby unit would be. The mother and baby have to be monitored by frequent visits (weekly or even more often) to the antenatal clinic, for routine weighing, examination and clinical assessment of the growth of the baby, and by frequent scanning (every fortnight is a useful interval).

Many doctors would want to monitor the baby's health daily or two or three times a week by repeated cardiotocograms – tracings of the baby's heart beat pattern. This is a bit like phoning in to the fetus to ask how he is, and getting a beat-by-beat reply!

The mother would also be monitored by other tests which indicate how well the placenta is functioning. This is done by measuring levels of the hormone oestriol, for example, in the mother's blood or urine. These tests tend not to be as useful nowadays in the face of our ability to 'phone in' and get an immediate answer from the baby, but are still used by some doctors as a method of 'tracking' the function of the placenta.

When it is obvious that the baby has, in a sense, outgrown his placenta – or has simply stopped growing – then delivery is the only answer. Induction of labour may be the choice under favourable circumstances, especially if the mother has had a previous baby, the cervix is ripe, and there is no immediate fetal distress. But if the baby seems to be seriously affected, then Caesarean section will be chosen as the safest method of delivery.

The care of a mother carrying a baby which is growth retarded must be intensive, so it is often sensible and necessary that care is provided within the hospital, so that moment by moment supervision can be offered. Resting can help to increase oxygen flow to the baby. In other cases it will be sufficient to see the mother twice a week, say, in the antenatal

The normal position for a baby at term. The lie is longitudinal, the presentation is cephalic (head down) with occiput anterior (the baby facing the mother's back).

Some abnormal positions which may lead to difficulty at the delivery. 1 Breech presentation 2 Oblique lie 3 Transverse lie due to placenta praevia 4 Occiput posterior (face to pubes).

clinic and to attach her to the electronic fetal monitor (cardiotocogram) at those times to assess directly the well-being of the baby.

THE LARGE-FOR-DATES BABY

The opposite problem is the 'large for dates' baby. As we have seen this means that the birth weight exceeds the 90th percentile for the gestational age. The background to such a situation may simply be inheritance – the parents may both be big. It has already been mentioned that diabetes causes larger-than-average babies, but it is as well to remember that the 'dates' may be wrong – women are quite often unsure of the date of their last menstrual period – and that the size of the baby may seem big but is actually appropriate for the true dates.

The management of a diabetic mother's pregnancy has already been described. In other situations if the baby seems unduly large (and this is confirmed on ultrasound scan) then Caesarean section may have to be carried out or, if there is a possibility of a vaginal delivery, a trial of labour will be conducted. This means that the doctor will allow labour to proceed to see if the baby can be delivered. The progress of labour is watched very carefully, and the well-being of both mother and baby are monitored. If there seems to be a difficulty, the doctor can then be ready to intervene with Caesarean section, if necessary.

ABNORMAL LIE

By about 36 weeks the lie of the baby has become stabilized within the uterus and is normally longitudinal (straight up and down) most commonly with the head presenting. In certain abnormal circumstances the position of the baby in relation to the uterus may be oblique, or even directly transverse. If a baby's lie is oblique on one examination, then changes on a subsequent examination to transverse, it is described as an 'unstable lie'.

CAUSES OF ABNORMAL LIE

There are several causes for unstable, oblique or transverse lies. A uterus which has borne several babies becomes 'floppy', loses tone and the maintenance of a longitudinal lie is more difficult. Excess liquor may allow the baby to 'float round' even to a late stage in pregnancy. This may be caused by such conditions as diabetes, rhesus iso-immunization, or some abnormality of the baby.

It is quite common for at least one of the babies in a multiple pregnancy to lie abnormally, because of space problems in the uterus. Similarly a low lying placenta 'blocks' the way for the baby to take up his normal longitudinal lie, while a pelvic brim of small size has the same effect of 'blocking' the baby. Finally, and rarely, abnormalities of the shape of the uterus may restrict the way the baby lies.

DIAGNOSIS

The midwife or doctor will discover an abnormal lie on palpating the abdomen. If necessary it will be confirmed by ultrasound scan or X-ray. The reason will be looked for at the same time, scanning to locate the placenta, or X-ray to measure the pelvis, and so on. One of the fundamental points must be to re-check the dates and the maturity of the baby – after all, although a 36 week baby may be expected to have stabilized the lie, a 32 week one may not have, so the doctor will want to make sure that he or she is not dealing with 'wrong dates'.

DEALING WITH AN ABNORMAL LIE

If an oblique or transverse lie is found between 32 and 35 weeks, then it can be left but you will be seen frequently to monitor the baby's position. After 36 weeks, the cause must be looked for as above.

By 38 weeks, you would be safer in hospital in case the membranes should rupture. This is more likely in this situation, as neither the head nor the breech are positioned to 'plug' the lower segment. As a result the membranes bulge against the internal os of the cervix and may rupture early, allowing the cord or an arm to prolapse.

If this happens, an emergency Caesarean Section may be required to rescue the baby.

If labour begins and the lie can be converted into a longitudinal one and maintained there by enhancing the contractions with an intravenous infusion of syntocinon (see p. 86), then a vaginal delivery may be possible, but obviously a close watch has to be maintained to ensure that the lie does not revert to oblique or even transverse.

THE ANTENATAL WARD

In the previous pages, the possibility of hospitalization during a difficult pregnancy has frequently been mentioned. It is of interest to know that the first antenatal bed was established in the United Kingdom in 1901 for the purpose of studying the abnormalities of pregnancy. At that time high blood pressure was at the head of the list of problems.

Nowadays antenatal wards with many beds are established in every maternity unit. There are of course many reasons for admission to these wards. Some of these have already been mentioned, such as hypertension and pre-eclampsia, or where the baby is growing poorly – 'light for dates'. Simple surgical procedures, like inserting a Shirodkar suture for cervical incompetence, are dealt with through the antenatal ward, and where there has been a previous history of premature labour, a mother may be admitted to hospital for rest and observation round about the time of the previous onset of premature labour. Antepartum haemorrhage, for whatever reason, may require a stay in hospital, and women suffering from diabetes or some cases of rhesus iso-immunization may be hospitalized. An acute urinary tract infection may need treatment in hospital, as indeed, may many other abnormal situations in the pregnancy.

Fundamentally admission to the antenatal ward will be for observation of both mother and baby more frequently and more closely than is possible in a single, even weekly, visit to the antenatal clinic. It is often said that a mother is being admitted 'for rest'. It must be admitted that the amount of rest you can obtain in a busy antenatal ward which in many units is shared with postnatal mothers – and their babies! – is somewhat limited, although for a tired mother with other children at home it does offer rest and care. But in the main the reason for admission is for intensive monitoring of both mother and baby.

ON THE WARD

What can you expect in the antenatal ward? First, and perhaps most important of all, visiting times are usually very generous. There are usually periods of rest when visitors are not admitted, but otherwise partners, parents and families are allowed to come and go fairly freely.

It could be that you may have to face admission to hospital for an extended period of time – up to six or eight weeks for example. If you are admitted for a period of rest however, if both yours and your baby's condition seem stable, you may be allowed to go home for weekends to break the monotony and boost your morale. It is essential however that your partner or someone else reliable is also at home and able to look after you. On Monday you would return to hospital so that close monitoring of your condition can start again. Some units have established a day ward where mothers suffering from hypertension for example, or with a growth retarded baby, can come and spend the day resting, having their blood pressure taken and the baby's heart monitored at intervals, returning home in the evening.

There is no doubt that where other young children are involved, considerable distress and disruption to a family unit can occur if the mother has to come in to hospital for an extended period. This is where grandparents, family and friends can play such an important supportive role. The Social Services can be alerted where necessary too and every help will be given to the mother so that she can rest in hospital with some peace of mind.

CHAPTER SIX

LABOUR AND BIRTH

A moment-by-moment guide for both parents to the
progress of labour and normal birth of your baby

Labour is the name given to the process during which the uterus contracts repeatedly, the cervix opens and is pulled up over the baby's head. The baby and placenta are then expelled through the vagina. Labour is divided into three stages: during the first stage the uterine muscles thin the cervix, then pull it up and open so that the baby's head can pass through. The second stage pushes the baby down the birth canal and out through the vagina, and the third stage consists of the expulsion of the placenta and membranes, often called the after-birth.

WHAT HAPPENS DURING LABOUR

The uterus is a large muscular bag closed at the bottom by the cervix, the ring of muscle which normally dips into the vagina. Throughout your pregnancy the muscle contracts regularly with painless Braxton Hicks contractions (so-called after the doctor who first observed them). As you approach full term you may be able to feel these contractions quite strongly as the uterine wall hardens. They are quite often mistaken for actual labour pains (see p. 78). Braxton Hicks contractions do not usually have an effect on your cervix during the first and second trimesters. As you approach term your cervix will have softened due to the action of progesterone and as labour begins the muscle fibres of the uterus shorten, pulling the cervix up into the lower uterine segment.

THE FIRST STAGE

At first the cervix is simply being thinned (effaced) and during this time the contractions are often not particularly noticeable. In second and subsequent labours, many women are not aware of this process at all and may only realize they are in labour when the cervix is already dilating. Once the cervix is fully effaced it begins to dilate (open) and the uterine contractions become more efficient. The cervix dilates slowly at first, then dilatation becomes quicker and quicker, in response to stronger, longer and more frequent contractions.

The cervix has to dilate to about 10cm (4in) in diameter to allow the baby's head to pass through. You may hear your midwife or doctor refer to your cervix being two or four centimetres dilated during internal examinations in labour; once it is five centimetres dilated it is referred to as half dilated and the midwife would feel a rim of cervix all round the baby's head. At three-quarters dilated the cervix can only be felt at the front and sides of the baby's head, and the last part of the cervix to be taken up is the front edge. When the cervix is fully dilated labour enters the second stage. The membranes usually rupture by the end of the first stage, if they had not done so before labour really started.

THE SECOND STAGE

While the cervix has been dilating the baby's head comes lower and lower inside your pelvis. During the second stage, the muscular effort is expulsive; in other words it is pushing your baby down through the vagina (the birth canal). The skin inside the vagina is normally folded and crinkly; as the baby's head descends, the vaginal walls stretch and become smooth to allow the baby to pass through. As the baby's head descends it rotates so that it is facing the back as it emerges. It then rotates to allow the shoulders and body to be born.

THE THIRD STAGE

The third stage of labour often passes without mothers really taking much notice. After a pause of five to ten minutes the uterus contracts to expel the placenta and membranes; alternatively you may be given an injection to speed the contraction and the midwife will gently ease the afterbirth out by pulling on the cord. The midwife or doctor will check to make sure that the placenta has come away cleanly.

HOW LABOUR STARTS

Labour starts in different ways, but remember that with the first baby labour may take longer than you expect. Most first labours last at least twelve hours

The normal birth

1 *During the first stage of labour, the uterine contractions gradually thin and open the cervix.* 2 *Towards the end of the first stage, the cervix is almost dilated, and the membranes usually have ruptured.* 3 *In the second stage, the cervix is fully dilated and the uterus produces strong, expulsive contractions.* 4 *The baby's head rotates to face the back and presses against the* perineum, *stretching the tissues as it emerges through the vagina. This is known as crowning.* 5 *Once the head has been delivered, the baby rotates again to the side, gently guided by the midwife, to allow the shoulders, then the body, to emerge.* 6 *The third stage is the delivery of the placenta and membranes. The midwife presses one hand on the abdomen to keep the uterus in place, and gently pulls the cord with the other.*

from start to finish and sometimes longer. There are women who have their first babies in an hour or two but they are extremely rare. Women are often surprised by just how long and tedious labour can be.

A couple of days before labour starts, many women experience a bout of diarrhoea, and many others have a 'show' as the plug of mucus that has been keeping the cervix closed and protecting the uterus from infection comes away. This plug of mucus is gelatinous in texture and may be slightly blood-stained. It comes away painlessly, often when you go to the toilet. These are signs that labour may be approaching, but they may occur several days before anything concrete happens – or they may not happen at all.

FALSE ALARMS

Some people experience quite strong contractions for a few hours, which then cease, and others think that the strong Braxton Hicks contractions of late pregnancy are in fact the onset of labour. This can be very disappointing after the long weeks and months of pregnancy, and partners and friends may have to find things for the mother to do to keep her mind off it! Stress incontinence (a small gush of urine on sneezing or coughing) can also sometimes lead mothers to think their waters may have broken. The temptation in this situation, especially if you are at full term or even later, is to go to hospital or call the midwife. But it can be very embarrasing to have told your parents and neighbours that you are off to hospital only to come home again after a false alarm.

If this happens to you don't worry too much – it can even happen to pregnant midwives! The midwives in the labour ward are very sympathetic about false alarms – if you turn up they will probably monitor you for a while to make sure that you really aren't in labour, and maybe suggest you stay overnight if there is a bed. If you are having the baby at home it isn't so bad, as your midwife can come to you to check and reassure you either way.

COPING WITH EARLY FIRST STAGE

When your labour really starts you will have painful contractions of the uterus, which often feel like period pains, or stomach cramps, or back-ache; they come regularly so that you can time them – perhaps every ten or fifteen minutes; and they don't go away. The pains become stronger and stronger and the space between them gets shorter. Some women can actually feel the cervix being pulled open as the baby's head pushes down against it and the uterine muscle pulls it up.

It is much more comfortable during this early stage to be at home. You have all the things around you that you like; you can do what you like – watch television, have light food and drink, arrange for other children to be looked after, call your partner if he is at work, go for a walk in the park or to the local shops. You can check that you have everything packed and ready for the hospital as well.

During this early stage of labour it is sensible to keep your bladder as empty as possible by passing urine every hour and a half or so.

WHEN TO GO TO HOSPITAL OR CALL THE MIDWIFE

There will come a time when the uterine contractions are very painful and strong and seem to be coming very quickly – every five minutes or even less. The pain comes in waves, of about 30 seconds duration to start with, rising to 90 seconds or even two minutes towards the end of first stage. At this point you will probably need to stop what you are doing and try to relax through the pain – many women find it helpful to vocalize in some way at the height of the contraction. At this stage however there are still spaces in between the contractions when you can rest and relax.

Now is the time to go to hospital, either by calling an ambulance (dial 999) or by getting your partner or a friend to drive you there. Do not try to drive yourself. Call the labour ward before you leave, so they can collect your notes if you do not keep them yourself, and prepare a room for you.

If you are having your baby at home this is also the time to call your midwife and doctor, although many community and independent midwives like to be informed right at the beginning of labour, even if they do not come to you straight away. You will have to ask your midwife what she prefers.

IF YOUR MEMBRANES RUPTURE

If your membranes rupture, shown by a gush of warm, clear fluid from your vagina, then you should call your midwife or go to the hospital straight away. This can happen quite unexpectedly, even though you have not felt any contractions at all. It means that the membranes have ruptured and that the amniotic fluid has escaped.

It is important to be examined straight away if this happens. In very rare cases the umbilical cord can drop down (prolapse) in front of the baby's head when the waters gush out. The cord could be pinched by the pressure of the head, depriving the baby of oxygen. Although it is almost impossible for prolapse to happen when the baby's head is deep in

WHAT YOU WILL NEED IN HOSPITAL

2-3 nightdresses	Front fastening nightdresses in light material are best, particularly if you are going to breastfeed.	Magazines and books	To read in the postnatal ward.
Nursing bras	You will need at least two, and possibly one a larger size to support you during the engorged stage two or three days after the birth.	Writing things	To write letters to your family and friends. Some people like to record a 'labour and birth diary'.
Breast pads	One box, to protect your clothes from milk leakage.	A natural sponge	To wipe your face – it is also nice to suck cold water from when your mouth is dry.
Cotton pants	These can be more comfortable than belts to wear with sanitary pads.	Something to wear during labour	It is more comforting to wear your own dressing gown, nightdress or comfortable maternity dress during labour than a hospital gown. Many people prefer to wear nothing when it comes to giving birth.
Maternity strength sanitary pads	Take at least two packets.	Change for the telephone	There will be coin boxes in the hospital so that you can contact your family and friends after the birth. A reverse charge call will probably be accepted however by anxious grandparents!
Towels	Most hospitals are quite short of linen and will expect you to bring your own towels.	A photo or picture	Something to look at during labour – a beautiful scented flower would do as well.
Toilet articles	A sponge bag containing soap, talc and other articles for washing and bathing, plus toothbrush and paste.	A camera	For pictures of baby and parents immediately after the birth.
Pillows and pillowslips	Two or three of your own pillows are more homely than hospital pillows which tend to be covered with polythene and are therefore very hot.	Honey	Many women find spoonfuls of honey nourishing and easy to digest during labour.
A dark-coloured flannel	To have over your face during labour to exclude light.	Sandwiches and a flask of coffee or tea	For your partner or birth assistant – it can be a long time before he can get to the canteen, and anyway he might miss something!
Sweets	To suck during labour; pastilles are nice and comforting and provide a little sugar to keep your blood sugar level up. Mints sometimes help to keep your mouth fresh and help avoid nausea.	Baby clothes	If the hospital is short of linen it might be prudent to bring a couple of nighties for your baby's use.
Cassette player or radio	To listen to during labour.	Salt	Ordinary cooking salt is soothing and healing in the bath, and many hospitals run short in busy postnatal wards.

the pelvis (known as engaged), it is important to have it checked. Most first babies' heads are engaged before labour starts, but the heads of second and subsequent babies may not engage until you are in labour, so if the waters break a few days early the danger of cord prolapse is greater. The membranes also protect the baby from infection through the vagina, which, though unlikely, could occur if labour has not started after about 48 hours. However, for most women labour will start within 24 hours of their waters breaking.

If the amniotic fluid is green, and it can be as dark as cooked spinach, it means that there is meconium present in it. Meconium is the contents of the fetal bowel, and a baby who is distressed in the uterus may open the bowels, passing meconium into the amniotic fluid. This is very serious and you should go to hospital at once, even if your waters have only leaked a little.

If you think your waters are leaking a little when your baby is due, it is worth being assessed by a midwife. Often when the waters are just leaking slightly the small hole in your membranes will heal over and the leaking will stop. If your waters leak

In order to assess the progress of your labour when you arrive at the hospital, your midwife may ask you where you can feel the pains, how long they last and how frequently they are occurring.

and it is still several weeks before your baby is due, then you should always go to hospital or call your midwife (see p. 61).

WHAT HAPPENS IN HOSPITAL

When you go to hospital you will go straight to the labour ward, no matter what time of day or night it is. The baby's father is always welcome – nowadays in Britain more than 90 per cent of fathers witness the birth of their babies, and it is often remembered by them as one of the most exciting and moving events of their lives. It is also extremely helpful and supportive for the mother to have her partner or someone else close to her throughout labour, especially in hospital, where a long labour may mean a change of midwife at some stage.

The initial procedures may vary a little from unit to unit, but what follows is typical. Your community or independent midwife will probably follow much the same procedures when she comes to you for a home delivery. In the hospital, a midwife will be assigned to you and you will be shown into one of the rooms. Some hospitals allow you to labour and give birth in the same room, others will move you into a special delivery room for second stage.

The midwife will ask you what is happening and why you felt it was time to come (or to call her, if you are at home). She will want to know if the

ELECTRONIC MONITORING

Most large maternity units will suggest monitoring you electronically for a period of about twenty minutes in early labour, using a machine called a cardiotocogram. Small pads strapped to your abdomen pick up the baby's heart beat by ultrasound and measure the strength of your contractions onto a continuous graph.

waters have broken, how much the baby is moving, how you are feeling in yourself and what each contraction feels like and how long it lasts. She will then check your general health – your temperature, pulse and blood pressure will all be measured. She will ask you to give a specimen of urine for testing. She may time your contractions and will feel your abdomen to check which way the baby is lying and whether the baby's head is engaged. She may also listen to the baby's heart with a little ear trumpet known as a Pinard's stethoscope.

The midwife will then do an internal examination. She will be feeling for your cervix to work out whether you are in established labour and how far advanced it is. She will also be feeling for the baby's head to see how low down it is lying and how deep inside the pelvis it is. If your baby is breech (see p. 98) she will be checking to see how far down the baby's bottom is and whether any limbs are descending first.

Some units suggest that mothers spend about 20 minutes being electronically monitored, which gives a very accurate picture on a moving graph of the strength and timing of your contractions and their effect on the baby's heart beat. When you have settled in and before contractions have become too painful the midwife may ask you if you would mind doing this. Straightforward monitoring is done by strapping electrodes round your abdomen with belts. This can be quite uncomfortable if you have to lie on the bed so ask if possible to be monitored while sitting in a chair. You will feel more in control of the situation if you can keep upright during labour and the ability to keep moving can be a great help in coping with contractions (see p. 82).

Some modern units may have remote control monitors available which feed the information being picked up by the electrodes into a small apparatus rather like a personal stereo, which you wear on a strap round your neck. This then transmits the data to a larger, fixed unit which prints out the graph. It still entails a certain amount of paraphernalia, but is much easier to cope with as you are able to move around.

If the midwife or obstetrician suggests that you should be monitored throughout your labour, it is

Towards the end of first stage, when the contractions are at their height, you may feel the need for quiet, dim lights, and the reassurance of your partner's presence to support you.

worth asking whether this is really necessary. The technology is very sophisticated and the medical staff are often very interested in the information that is being recorded. However, monitoring is restricting, which makes it difficult for you to cope with the pain of labour in the way that suits you best. Monitoring should not really be necessary throughout labour unless there are signs of fetal distress, your contractions are found to be abnormal (irregular or weak), or if you are having an epidural anaesthetic. These situations are discussed later and in the next chapter. Monitoring is sometimes also used if you are being induced or your labour is being accelerated, or if you have an existing medical condition which means that your own and your baby's condition need to be closely watched throughout labour.

If you are at all anxious about electronic monitoring, it might be wise to talk about it during one of your antenatal check-ups towards the end of your pregnancy and have your wishes written into your notes. Alternatively your partner or birth assistant could discuss the situation with the midwife for you in the labour ward so that you can concentrate on the contractions.

COPING WITH LATER FIRST STAGE

Once monitoring has been completed, it is a good idea to try to keep moving, walking about, leaning on whatever is handy during each contraction. The positions discussed on page 35 may be helpful. Some women find it very comforting to lie in a bath of warm to hot water, others just want to lounge on the bed, or on a bean-bag. Others find kneeling on all fours is comforting, or perhaps leaning on a chair seat supported by cushions. Only you can decide at the time what is right for you, which is why it is so important to have available all the different mats, surfaces and other equipment in the labour ward.

As labour progresses, you will need to pass urine frequently in order to keep your bladder empty so that it does not impede the baby's progress through your pelvis. Drink refreshing and nourishing drinks, and keep yourself fresh with a flannel or soft sponge wiped over your face from time to time. Cologne can be refreshing too. You can keep your spirits up by thinking that each contraction is one less to be had, each contraction is one nearer to being able to see and hold your baby. Like any other long, muscular effort, such as running a marathon or climbing a mountain, labour is an endurance test; it goes on for a long time and takes a lot of energy and dogged determination. You just need to keep at it and realize that this is really only a short time in the whole of your life, and that millions of women would be envious of you at that moment. It is particularly helpful if your partner can be encouraging you in this way, too.

As the contractions become stronger and closer together – lasting for up to two minutes and with what seems no pause between them, you will become more and more self-absorbed, going deeper and deeper inside yourself. You won't want to chat to the midwife or your partner, and you may find you are irritated by interruptions such as the midwife wanting to see what is happening to the baby, because you will just want to concentrate on what is happening inside your body.

Perhaps the best way of coping with the contractions of labour is to relax and surrender to their sensation. They are very painful, but you may be able to cope with the pain if you can just let yourself be carried along with it. The body releases natural analgesics (endorphins) to deaden pain when it is relaxed and allowed to do what it needs to do.

THE TRANSITIONAL PHASE

There comes a point when time becomes irrelevant, the contractions are really strong and close and you try every method to get comfortable: standing, leaning against your partner, lying in the bath, lying on the bed, leaning forward on to a work surface or a chair, wriggling your hips, rocking, crawling, walking about. Nothing seems to help – and at this point many women have a crisis: 'I can't bear it any longer, I've had enough, I want to go home, when will it stop, give me an epidural, anything!'

Midwives are very used to seeing women reach this point in labour, which is known as the transitional phase. It means that very soon your cervix will be fully dilated and you will be ready to push your baby out. Your midwife will try to distract you – she may send you off to the lavatory to pass urine, for instance, and just going for a little walk to the lavatory may make you feel more on top of things again.

PAIN RELIEF

The midwife will probably examine you internally at this point to see how far your cervix is dilated. If you still have quite a while to go she may suggest that now is the time for you to try some analgesia (pain relief) if you haven't done so already. It is up to you – many women can go through labour without any analgesics, but different people have different pain thresholds, and if your labour is very long and you are getting very fed up you may feel that you would like something to help the pain. The important thing is not feel that you are a failure if you accept some pain relief, nor to feel that you are being forced into having it if you don't want it. It is your choice.

PETHIDINE

Pethidine is given as an injection into your thigh or buttock. It is a strong analgesic and also seems to help your cervix to relax and dilate more quickly. If you have pethidine you will have to stay on the bed unless the dose is very small as it makes you feel very sleepy. Most midwives mix another drug called phenergan in with the pethidine to stop you feeling sick. However this drug also has the side-effect of making you forget your labour, so if you don't want this to happen you might want to suggest that phenergan isn't added to your pethidine injection.

Some women find pethidine very helpful as it gives them a little 'time out' when they can doze between contractions – although the pain isn't completely deadened, the drug seems to help women to detach themselves from it. Other women, however, complain that they just feel drunk and out of control, and that it doesn't really help the pain at all. It is a difficult decision to make, especially if you don't know how it is going to affect you.

Pethidine passes across the placenta and can make the baby very sleepy and slow to breathe after the birth. The baby may need to be given an antidote by injection after the birth, which fortunately works very quickly.

ENTONOX ('GAS AND AIR')

Entonox is a gas consisting of half oxygen and half nitrous oxide. The nitrous oxide is analgesic and helps the pain, while the oxygen increases the supply to the baby and keeps you feeling fresh. Entonox is preferred as an analgesic by many women, because it is breathed in through a small face mask or mouthpiece which you can hold yourself and use when you need it.

It takes about four deep breaths of the gas before the analgesic begins to take effect. The apparatus makes a loud swooshing noise each time you breathe in the gas, which is a useful distraction as well. The idea is to breathe in the entonox as the contraction begins so that the analgesic effect is greatest when the pain is at its height.

One of the simplest forms of pain relief during labour is the inhalation of entonox (a mixture of nitrous oxide and oxygen), which can be self-administered through a mask held firmly over the mouth and nose.

In hospital entonox may be brought to you in a cylinder or may be piped directly through a nozzle in the wall. At home, your midwife will bring a cylinder of entonox with her for your use. Entonox doesn't restrict you completely – you can either lie on the bed, sit in a chair or stand to breathe it in, but you are of course constricted by how far the tube will stretch.

EPIDURAL ANAESTHESIA

An epidural anaesthetic (or block) consists of a quantity of local anaesthetic injected into the epidural space in your spinal column, which deadens all sensation in your lower trunk. Before you have it you will need to sign a form giving your consent. This is a reasonable request on behalf of the hospital authorities, as administering an epidural is a skilled procedure which like all such procedures does involve a tiny element of risk. However if you are asked at any point to sign a permission form for 'any procedures necessary for childbirth' it is worth thinking twice about it. These forms are very questionable and probably have no legal validity at all: you can't sign your rights away for a whole period of time, each procedure should be negotiated separately. If you are faced with one of these forms you can either sign it and realize that it is not valid, or not sign it at all.

To administer the anaesthetic, a very fine tube (catheter) is passed through a needle into the epidural space around the spinal cord. The needle is then removed. The anaesthetic drug is injected through the catheter, and all subsequent 'top-up'

injections are given down the plastic tube which is secured to your back with sticky tape. You will be asked by the anaesthetist to curl into a tight ball so that your chin is right down on your chest – this position separates the bones (vertebrae) of your spine. The anaesthetist will then numb the skin of your back with an injection of local anaesthetic before inserting the needle and catheter carefully between the third and fourth lumbar vertebrae.

One dose lasts about two hours and it can be topped up as labour progresses. The catheter is inserted in the lumbar region just above the point where the nerves connected to the uterus enter the spinal cord, anaesthetizing you below that point, but you remain awake and alert throughout labour and usually require no other form of pain relief.

If you have an epidural you will need to have an intravenous drip put into your arm. This introduces sterilized water plus glucose and salts to keep you fresh. Your baby's heart will also need to be monitored continuously with the electronic fetal monitor, and as there is sometimes a tendency for a woman's blood pressure to drop during an epidural this will be monitored regularly as well.

Obviously all this equipment is going to mean that you will be confined to the bed for most of your labour, which can be very boring. Occasionally epidurals don't work very well, or only partly anaesthetize you, which can be very trying. There is also a higher incidence of forceps deliveries associated with epidurals because the anaesthetic has a very relaxing effect on your pelvic floor which can mean that the baby's head does not rotate into a good position for birth.

*Transcutaneous nerve stimulation (TNS) is a
relatively new form of pain relief during labour. A
hand-operated stimulator activates the nerves that
lead to the uterus to produce natural pain-relieving
substances called endorphins.*

TRANSCUTANEOUS NERVE STIMULATION (TNS)

TNS is an analgesic technique that is often used in
the treatment of acute or chronic pain, and which is
now being more widely used during labour. It is
produced by a small battery-powered electronic
stimulator. Four electrodes (rubber pads) are taped
to your back over the nerve roots which supply the
uterus. The tingly, throbbing 'pins and needles'
sensation can be very soothing during a contraction
and has the effect of blocking some of the pain
messages going to your brain. It also stimulates
your body to produce some of its own pain-relieving
chemicals – endorphins. TNS can be very helpful if
you have back pain in labour – if your pain is in the
front, massaging your abdomen at the same time
can be very soothing.

Many women like this form of pain relief when it
is available; it doesn't restrict you at all, and you
remain in charge of it at all times.

SIMPLE AIDS TO PAIN RELIEF

If you think about how you usually cope with pain
you will find that you already know quite a lot about
analgesia. Some people like to curl up in a ball and
let the pain flow over them. Others like to massage
the hurting part, either with very firm strokes on your
back, or smooth and gentle, almost stroking movements, over your abdomen. Deep massage may be
helpful for back pain; your partner could try
kneading your back with both fists. Some women
feel associated pain in their thighs and find it
helpful to have them massaged deeply.

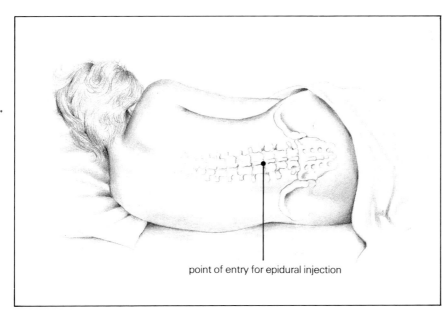

point of entry for epidural injection

*The epidural
anaesthetic is injected
into the epidural space
round the spinal
column through a
small gap between the
third and fourth lumbar
vertebrae (back
bones). When the
catheter is inserted the
mother curls up on her
side with her knees
bent to widen the gap
between the vertebrae
as much as possible.
An epidural anaesthetic
completely numbs the
uterus, lower back and
pelvic floor for about
two hours per injection.*

Heat and cold help pain too – a hot water bottle or an ice pack pressed against the part that hurts, both bring relief in their different ways. Baths have already been mentioned – some women stay in the bath for six or seven hours, just having the water topped up now and then, and women have even given birth in the bath.

Many women like to walk around or lean against a piece of furniture while rotating their hips or rocking gently from side to side. This can also help to rotate the baby into an advantageous position. It is soothing too, if everyone is silent and the room is darkened, or perhaps you could lay a dark flannel over your face for a while.

FATHERS DURING LABOUR

Some men become quite distressed when they see their partners in pain, especially if like many women, you decide you need to vocalize during contractions. It is very good to hear a noise when you are in strong labour, even if it is you who has to provide it. If you feel relaxed and at ease with the midwife you will feel less inhibited about making a noise, and partners need to be warned about this tendency to grumble, moan and groan, so that they realize what a tremendous help it can be to a woman.

However fathers can also play a very supportive role in helping with massage, holding and comforting their partners, giving drinks and wiping brows. A father can also discuss medical procedures with the midwife or doctor when they are suggested, especially if it is something he knows may worry you.

MEDICAL INTERVENTION DURING LABOUR

Throughout the first stage your midwife will be doing regular checks on your health and the condition of the baby in the uterus. In hospital an obstetrician will probably come in to see you from time to time and to ask the midwife how things are progressing. If you are at home your GP might come in at some time during the labour and may try to be there at the birth, although he may not be involved at all, and only visiting after the baby is born.

Every now and then the midwife will take your pulse, your blood pressure and occasionally your temperature. She will listen to the baby's heart during and between contractions with a Pinard's stethoscope or a portable ultrasound, or may ask if you would mind being monitored by the electronic fetal monitor again. It has already been mentioned that continuous monitoring should not be necessary unless there is concern about your baby's health, in which case a clip may be attached to your baby's scalp to monitor the baby directly. If it is felt that your baby needs monitoring in this way, your membranes will probably have been broken already to check for the presence of meconium (see p. 119).

ARTIFICIAL RUPTURE OF THE MEMBRANES (ARM)

Breaking the bag of waters round the baby is known as artificial rupture of the membranes (ARM). It is a completely painless procedure in itself, and is done to speed labour up or to examine the liquor for the presence of meconium (see above) if there are concerns about the health of the baby.

There are several disadvantages in having your membranes ruptured. This action often makes contractions much more painful and thus harder to cope with. It creates a passage for infection to enter the uterus, which means that you will need to give birth within the next 24 to 48 hours. If your labour is not really established and the contractions cease, the risk of having a Caesarean section is increased if your membranes have already been ruptured. However, ARM is a very effective means of speeding up labour if it is dragging on very slowly and you are becoming tired.

ACCELERATION OF LABOUR

If your labour seems to be prolonged, the midwife or doctor may suggest accelerating it artificially. There are good reasons for this. A labour that becomes prolonged (more than about eighteen hours) can lead to infection and dehydration in the mother, and infection and hypoxia (lack of oxygen) for the baby. If your progress is going more slowly than that indicated on a graph of average cervical dilatation (partogram), then the situation may be becoming abnormal and there are probably good grounds for speeding things up.

The first step would be to rupture your membranes, as described above. In most cases the doctor or midwife would wait for up to four hours before intervening further, in the hopes that normal progress of labour can be restored in the ARM alone. However, if nothing much seems to be happening and your contractions are still weak, irregular, or the cervix is not dilating more quickly, then a synthetic hormone called syntocinon will be introduced through a drip into your arm. Syntocinon is modelled on oxytocin, the natural hormone which initiates the contractions of labour.

Syntocinon speeds up contractions and makes them more regular and efficient, but they are more painful than normal contractions and most women need to have an epidural to cope with them. On the other hand, with your midwife and partner support-

To accelerate labour, a fluid drip containing the artificial hormone syntocinon is inserted into your arm, usually through a vein in the back of your hand. It may mean that you are confined to the bed for the rest of your labour, and you may feel more comfortable with an epidural.

ing you through every contraction you may find you can manage with only simple analgestic help, such as entonox (see p. 83).

BACKACHE IN LABOUR

Many women having their first baby, experience a long, trying labour with backache, because the baby is lying with her back against your back (the occipito posterior position), instead of the more usual 'back to abdomen' position (occipito anterior). In this position the baby needs to rotate around to the front of your pelvis in order to be born.

If you experience a backache labour, there are several things you can do. Firstly, it is good to spend as much of your labour as possible on all fours. This relieves your back and is also an excellent position for your helpers to massage your back and to put hot or cold compresses on it. Sometimes you can relieve the boredom of just being on all fours by standing and leaning forward on to a work surface or table top, or even against a high bed. If the labour drags on for a very long time, it is worth considering having syntocinon and an epidural, because the much stronger uterine contractions induced by the drug sometimes manage to rotate the baby into a better position more quickly.

INDUCTION OF LABOUR

Sometimes women go far beyond the date they thought the baby was due. This can be a very frustrating time as a week or maybe two can go by without anything happening. Some obstetricians may suggest an induction of labour when you are ten or fourteen days overdue. After 40 weeks of pregnancy, the placenta can begin to lose its efficiency so your doctor will be checking your baby's health very carefully if your pregnancy extends beyond this length of time. There are other medical reasons for induction at term or even before, however. For instance, if your blood pressure is very high, or if you are diabetic and the doctor does not want the baby to grow any bigger (see p. 71) you would be advised to have an induced labour, or perhaps your baby is not growing fast enough and the doctor feels that he or she would thrive better once born, rather than continuing to full term in the uterus.

An induction of labour means starting it off artificially. Usually you go into hospital the night before the induction, and a pessary will be inserted into your vagina, containing a hormone called prostaglandin which helps to soften and 'ripen' the cervix. This is sometimes enough to start labour off naturally, especially if you have had more than one child.

If labour hasn't begun the next morning, your membranes will be ruptured and you will have a syntocinon drip put into your arm to stimulate your uterus to contract. The contractions which are induced in this way are very painful almost immediately and you may need an epidural to cope with them. The baby's heart rate will also be monitored electronically as this is an unnatural situation, and movement may be restricted as a result. Induced labours can seem to take a very long time because you spend the whole time in hospital,

One of the commonest positions for second stage is to be propped upright on the bed, gripping your thighs for support, and dropping your chin on to your chest as you push with each contraction.

and many induced labours in fact result in Caesarean deliveries.

It is worth bearing all these factors in mind if your doctor suggests induction as a possibility. Sometimes it is worth asking for time to think it over, and unless the doctor can point to a definite indication that labour should proceed as soon as possible, you have more time to allow it to start naturally. Remember that the normal length of a pregnancy can vary from 38 weeks to 42 weeks. Of course, many women who are overdue find the last few weeks of pregnancy very uncomfortable and boring and are only too pleased to be offered an induction.

INTO SECOND STAGE

Imperceptibly the contractions begin to change; they become less frequent, less demanding, and you begin to feel huge pressure on your vagina and rectum as if you need to open your bowels very urgently. Quite involuntarily you will begin to push with the sensation, just as you do when you are opening your bowels.

As soon as you get this feeling, alert your midwife. She may not want you to push just yet until she has done an internal examination to check that your cervix has completely dilated. If there is a rim of cervix left, she will ask you not to push but to gently pant each time a contraction comes on to stop yourself from pushing with it. It can also be very helpful to kneel on all fours with your bottom in

the air and your chin on the ground – the so-called knee-chest position – which takes the pressure of the baby's head off your vagina and rectum and makes it easier to stop pushing.

BIRTH POSITIONS

Once the midwife is certain that the cervix is completely dilated and it is safe for you to push, you can get into position for the birth. Second stage contractions aren't painless – in fact many women find they hurt quite a lot – but the more you push the more numbed you begin to feel and the more excited you are likely to become at the thought of the imminent birth.

The length of second stage varies enormously. For some, it can take an hour or more, while for others a few pushes are enough. Many doctors and midwives are unhappy to allow a mother to go on pushing much longer than an hour and a half, because of the increased risk to the baby and because the mother may become exhausted. In this situation they may suggest helping the birth with forceps or ventouse (see p. 94). A seriously delayed second stage, due to malpresentation or position may result in an emergency Caesarean section (see p. 95). However, the vast majority of births proceed perfectly normally without the need for any medical intervention and most women are able to push their babies out without help.

When you are pushing, you need to have your

The baby's head appears through the bulging perineum (known as crowning), stretching the vagina open. The head is moulded and elongated as it is squeezed through the birth canal.

The head is delivered and the baby begins to breathe. At this point the midwife may insert a tube to suck out excess fluid from the baby's mouth, while the baby rotates and the body emerges.

The cord is clamped and cut and if all is well the baby is wrapped and given immediately to the parents. This is always an emotional moment, even for the midwives who deliver several babies every day of the year!

knees wide apart to ensure that your pelvis is as wide open as possible. Some mothers push their babies out sitting upright on the bed, supported by lots of pillows; others lie down; others squat with support from their partners and midwives or supported on a birthing stool or special bed; others stand with legs bent and apart or lie on their sides with one leg held up. Other women kneel on all fours and push from this position. Once again do what feels right at the time, but it is helpful to know that being upright or on all fours allows gravity to help the baby's descent.

'CROWNING'

The vagina is soft and stretchy due to the action of progesterone and it opens out with the advancing head. On inspection by the midwife, first of all only a small amount of the baby's head is seen. Each time you push, the baby's head descends further and further until it is said to be 'crowning' – pressing against the perineum and stretching it wide apart – as the widest part of the baby's head begins to move through the vaginal opening and the crown of her head becomes visible.

The sensation of stretching can be quite alarming and many women feel they are literally splitting. However the skin becomes so stretched that it is completely numb, and although some women do 'give way' and the skin tears a little, you don't feel it at the time.

EPISIOTOMY

Sometimes the skin around the vagina is quite firm and is impeding the baby's entrance into the world, or the midwife may be worried about the baby's

An episiotomy incision may be postero-lateral (1), J-shaped (2) or median (3), depending on the circumstances when it is needed.

heart beat so may want to speed things up. In this case she or the doctor may ask you if she can perform an episiotomy – a small cut to enlarge the opening of your vagina. Before doing it you will be injected with local anaesthetic to make you completely numb.

An episiotomy has to be stitched after the birth, whereas some 'tears' or superficial grazing may not need to be. There is some evidence to suggest that natural tears heal better than episiotomies although this is disputed. It is very common to be given an episiotomy for a forceps delivery, but if you have an epidural it may not be necessary because of the perineal relaxation caused by the epidural. But in other circumstances, try to make sure you understand the reason for suggesting it, and if you feel strongly that you don't want to have an episiotomy, have this recorded in your notes beforehand.

THE BIRTH

Most babies' heads are facing downwards at birth so if you look down you will see the back of your baby's head emerging. Some women like to touch the baby's head at this point. If you can't see what is going on, the midwife might be able to hold a mirror for you. When the head has emerged the midwife will run her fingers round the baby's neck to make sure the cord isn't tightly round it. Then the baby's head turns to the side so that the first shoulder slips out, followed by the second shoulder, and then with a quick, smooth motion the rest of your baby's body slides out and the midwife will probably lay her immediately on your abdomen while she clamps the cord.

Many midwives use a small, soft plastic tube to suck out any moisture from your baby's mouth and throat at this stage, although not all babies need this. If a baby does still have a mouthful of amniotic fluid or an accumulation of mucus, 'sucking out' can help breathing to be established more easily and quickly. Some babies cry quite lustily at this point; others make little noise at all. This is perfectly all right so long as the baby is breathing normally and 'pinks up' without difficulty (see p. 102).

DELIVERY OF THE PLACENTA

Once the baby is born or just as she is emerging, it is common for you to be given an injection of syntometrine, a substance which helps the uterus to contract strongly. This helps to dislodge the placenta because the part of the uterus wall where it was embedded shrinks down, sloughing the placenta off. Most midwives will have clamped the cord immediately the baby is born so that the

After the birth, when mother, father and baby have all had a chance to relax, there is usually a reviving hot drink to enjoy while you get to know the baby.

syntometrine does not have a chance to get into the baby's circulation. The midwife will then gently pull the placenta out. This process takes about three minutes.

Some women choose not to have syntometrine, preferring to wait for the placenta to come out naturally and for the cord to stop pulsating of its own accord. This means that the time after the baby is born is conducted at a more leisurely pace. It usually takes about 20 minutes for the placenta to be delivered naturally, but can take longer – up to an hour or more. Putting your baby to the breast and letting her suckle can help deliver the placenta and to make the uterus involute more rapidly, so many women do this immediately after the birth (see p. 104).

The other reason that syntometrine injections are given is that doctors believe that it prevents women from bleeding dangerously after the birth. The original studies which indicated the need for this injection were done some time ago when women were less well nourished and had more children, so there may not be the same necessity to use syntometrine today. This is being researched at the moment, but in the meantime doctors and midwives prefer to be on the safe side and give the injection, with your permission.

Occasionally, the baby may need further sucking out or warming. The midwife will take her to the resuscitation table that will already have been prepared in the delivery room, and sometimes a paediatrician will be called in to help, or in some circumstances may be on hand at the birth (see p. 102).

Once the baby is born and the afterbirth delivered, the midwife or doctor will stitch up a tear or episiotomy if necessary. The area will be thoroughly numbed again with local anaesthetic and you will be asked to lift your legs into the lithotomy position, resting them on two slings fixed to the end of the bed for the purpose. Stitching can take up to 30 minutes to complete, but it is important that it is done carefully so that the area heals with as little subsequent discomfort as possible.

You may be offered a cup of tea, and the midwife may offer you a blanket bath, so you can change into a clean nightdress if you need to. If your partner is with you, you will probably be given an opportunity to spend a little time alone together with your baby while the midwife writes up your notes. If all is well with the baby, both of you will be wheeled up to the postnatal ward within an hour or so, and you will be able to get some rest.

THE ASSISTED BIRTH

The types of medical assistance that may be
needed to help with the safe delivery of your baby

A spontaneous delivery, as described in the previous chapter, happens when the mother delivers her baby through the vagina virtually unaided – 'virtually', because, of course, some help is almost always necessary from the midwife, even if it is only to lift the baby out. An assisted delivery, however, is one where the medical staff take over most or all of the work in delivering the baby – with forceps, for example, or by Caesarean section.

A breech delivery, where the baby is born bottom first, is also 'assisted', in that however nearly spontaneous it may be, a doctor is almost always required to bring out the baby's legs and arms, and then to supervise the controlled delivery of the head. Similarly the birth of twins, although usually a perfectly normal delivery, may require the active assistance of the midwife or doctor, and if a mother suffers from some existing medical condition, such as heart disease, she will probably need assistance to avoid exacerbating her condition. It is these situations which are described in this chapter. Stillbirth and perinatal death are also covered, to help parents face this tragic situation.

FORCEPS DELIVERY

Forceps are instruments designed to cradle the baby's head in a rigid metal frame so that the baby can be pulled out of the pelvis without compression on the head. They were first introduced into midwifery practice in England in the seventeenth century, by the Chamberlen family. There is quite a variety of types of forceps, ranging from small, very light ones designed to lift out the baby when it is right down on the floor of the pelvis, to long flat ones (Kielland's forceps) which are designed to rotate the baby's head into the favourable occipito anterior position (face to back) for delivery.

Most mothers are naturally nervous about having to be delivered by forceps but it must be emphasised again that the blades act as a 'cage' to protect your baby's head during the delivery – they do not harm the baby in themselves – and their use is always in the hands of someone fully trained in their application or under close supervision.

THE NEED FOR FORCEPS

There are a number of situations where forceps may be necessary. One of the most common is a prolonged second stage, where the baby's head is not moving down the birth canal in spite of strong pushing by the mother. Alternatively, second stage may need to be curtailed, if the mother has high blood pressure, or there are signs of fetal distress on the electronic monitor (cardiotocogram). It is important also to ensure the controlled delivery of the baby's head in a breech birth.

However, forceps delivery will only be undertaken if certain conditions exist. Normally forceps will not be used to help bring the baby out in a breech birth which is delayed, as the forceps cannot fit round the buttocks. (However, the forceps can be used in the latter part of a normal breech delivery – see later.)

It is clearly most convenient if the baby's head is presenting normally, with the crown of the head (occiput) in front; abnormal presentations, like face or chin are more difficult to manage (see later). The head must also be at or below the ischial spines of the pelvis (see p. 11). If the baby's head was above this level, this used to involve a procedure known as 'high cavity' forceps, but as it is known to be dangerous to the baby it is never undertaken nowadays; in these circumstances an emergency Caesarean section would be performed instead.

Forceps cannot be used either if there is any disproportion between the mother's pelvis and the size of the baby's head. If this turns out to be the reason for a delayed second stage, then once again a Caesarean section would be performed.

Forceps cannot be used if the cervix isn't fully dilated, so the medical staff would wait until this happened, or again may decide that it is safer to perform an emergency Caesarean, depending on

The baby's father is almost always allowed to stay with his partner for an epidural Caesarean, even if the operation is unexpected. Both parents can then see and hold their baby while the mother is being sutured (stitched).

For a forceps assisted delivery, the blades of the forceps are inserted carefully one at a time on each side of the baby's head, then locked together before gentle traction is applied.

For a ventouse assisted delivery, the suction cup is slipped into the vagina sideways, then applied to the top of the baby's head by means of a vacuum. Gentle traction is then applied.

the circumstances. Above all, there must be adequate anaesthesia for the mother. Many forceps deliveries are performed with an epidural in place (indeed the epidural anaesthetic may unfortunately be the reason for the need for forceps); otherwise the perineum is completely numbed with an injection of local anaesthetic.

USING FORCEPS

If you are found to need the help of forceps, the doctor will make sure that a paediatrician is on hand at the birth. The baby may need help in clearing his airways of fluid, and may need oxygen as well, especially if forceps have been required because of fetal distress.

For the delivery, you will be placed in the lithotomy position – with legs bent and held up and open by resting in stirrups on poles fixed to the bed. Your legs and perineum are draped with sterile towels and the whole procedure is carried out like a surgical operation, with full sterile precautions. If you are having an epidural already, the doctor will proceed; otherwise you will be given an injection of local anaesthetic. Once you are completely anaesthetized in the area, your bladder will be emptied by catheter and you may need an episiotomy, if you haven't had one already. Depending on the reasons for needing a forceps delivery, it takes on average three to five minutes to deliver the baby.

As has already been mentioned, a forceps delivery is not dangerous to the baby, especially now that the practice of high forceps delivery has been abandoned. However it is not uncommon for

marks from one or other of the blades to be left on the side of the baby's face. These may look quite worrying, but they fade within a day or two.

VENTOUSE EXTRACTION

The ventouse consists of a metal cup which is placed over the baby's head and attached by a rubber tube to a machine which creates a vacuum. A chain also runs down from the cup; when a vacuum is produced under the cup, an area of the baby's head is sucked into it, giving it a firm grip on the scalp. Traction can be applied via the chain so that the baby's head can gently be pulled down the birth canal.

The ventouse is used in very similar circumstances to forceps, and some obstetricians simply prefer to use it. It can also be used to rotate the head to a more favourable position for delivery, and in theory at least, it can be applied to the baby's head before the cervix is fully dilated.

It is very unlikely to damage the baby in any way, but it does produce a characteristic puffy, rounded area on the baby's head after delivery, known as a 'chignon'. This is the part of the scalp that was sucked into the cup by the vacuum. It is prominent at first, but subsides within a day or two.

CAESAREAN SECTION

The Caesarean section is an historic operation for the delivery of a baby; it is the surgical technique whereby a baby is delivered through an incision in the uterus and lifted out through the abdomen. The present rate of deliveries by Caesarean section averages twelve per cent, including elective and emergency Caesareans.

ELECTIVE AND EMERGENCY CAESAREANS

There are many reasons for delivering a baby in this way, some of which have already been mentioned. Caesareans are usually referred to as 'elective' or 'emergency'. An elective Caesarean is one that is planned antenatally because it is clear that a normal vaginal delivery will not be possible, while an emergency Caesarean is one that has to be performed without prior warning because of some unforeseen circumstances once labour has started, or because the health of mother or baby suddenly deteriorates during late pregnancy.

An elective Caesarean may be planned several weeks in advance, or only a day or two, but you will know exactly when the operation is going to be performed and will be admitted to hospital the day

before. For healthy mothers, there is often the opportunity to have the operation performed under epidural anaesthesia, which means that you will be awake throughout and can see your baby as soon as he is born. Of course, you won't feel any pain and you won't be able to see anything during the operation as the area of the incision will be masked by sterile towels.

Sometimes, your partner may be allowed to come into the operating theatre with you in these circumstances and provided the baby is healthy when delivered, he will be able to hold the baby and talk to you while you are being stitched. It is particularly comforting to have your partner with you while the epidural anaesthetic is being injected and during the time it takes effect. This may be anything from 30 minutes to an hour, and you may become quite apprehensive during this waiting time.

The birth of the baby only takes a few minutes, but the 'tidying up' afterwards can take about 25 minutes. Your own recovery after the operation is

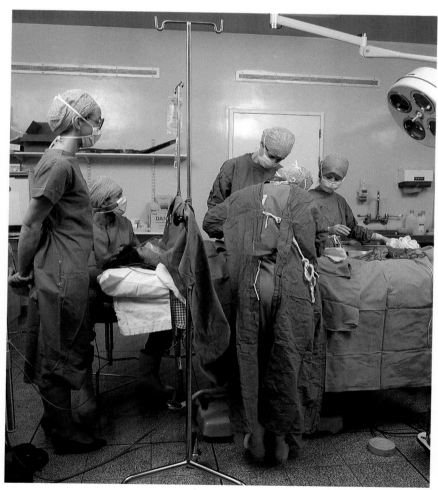

A Caesarean section performed under epidural anaesthetic takes place in an operating theatre, sometimes in the delivery suite, or else in the general hospital operating area. It is performed under full sterile conditions and everyone present, including the baby's father, wears gowns, hats and masks. Towels are carefully draped across the operating table so that the surgical procedures are masked from the parents' view.

usually much more rapid after an epidural Caesarean as you do not have to cope with the trauma of a general anaesthetic.

An emergency Caesarean may be required without warning at any stage of labour. If you are already having epidural anaesthesia it may be possible to perform the operation as described above, with you awake throughout, or there may be time to set up an epidural before the operation is performed. However if speed is essential or there is serious doubt about yours or your baby's health, then a general anaesthetic will be required and you will be fully asleep during the delivery.

REASONS FOR CAESAREAN SECTION

You will need an elective Caesarean if your pelvis is too small or the wrong shape to allow the baby's head to pass through it safely. This is usually discovered during a first labour, which results in an emergency Caesarean, and elective Caesareans would be arranged for subsequent births. Some

Being awake during a Caesarian section can be a nerve-wracking experience, even though the incision is hidden from your view, but it does mean that you can see your baby at the very moment of birth.

obstetricians suggest Caesarean section for breech presentation, although many allow you to go into labour, letting it proceed normally probably under epidural anaesthetic, but being ready to step in if the baby shows signs of getting stuck. If you have had more than one Caesarean section in the past, you will almost certainly have to have a Caesarean for any subsequent babies as the scar tissue can weaken the uterine wall.

An elective Caesarean will be performed also for most cases of placenta praevia, even if the amount of bleeding has been small, partly because the placenta is impeding the baby's exit from the uterus, but also to avoid excessive haemorrhage during the birth. The obstetrician would be unlikely however to allow an epidural anaesthetic in this case. Certain cases of premature delivery would be performed by elective Caesarean too, for instance for triplets.

Depending on the circumstances, a mother with hypertension (high blood pressure) or pre-eclampsia may be delivered by elective Caesarean, or an emergency Caesarean may be required. Severe fetal distress during labour often calls for an emergency Caesarean, and certain cases of placental abruption would mean that the baby should be delivered as soon as possible – again by Caesarean section performed under general anaesthetic.

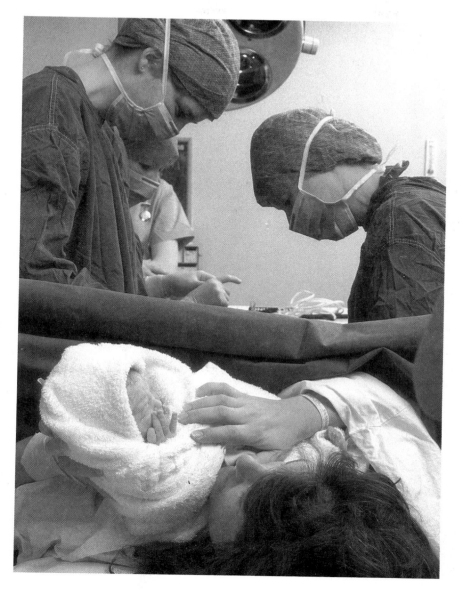

One of the main advantages of a Caesarean section performed under epidural anaesthesia is that if all goes well you can actually hold your baby after the birth. Stitching the uterus and abdominal wall is the longest part of the operation, but it is always masked off from the mother's view by carefully positioned drapes.

THE OPERATION

A Caesarean takes place in an operating theatre under full sterile conditions – it is a major piece of abdominal surgery, like the removal of an appendix or any other internal organ. The classic Caesarean incision used to be a vertical one in the upper part of the uterus, but nowadays the obstetric surgeon usually uses a transverse incision in the lower uterine segment, using the so-called 'bikini' incision through the abdomen for cosmetic reasons.

The skin incision is deepened through the layers of the abdomen to reach the abdominal cavity. The uterus is then opened through its lower part also by a transverse incision. The membranes bulging through the incision are opened and the baby is lifted out – head first if he is presenting that way or, if it is a breech presentation, gently extricated by grasping round the baby's ankles and pulling him from the uterine cavity.

The cord is clamped and divided, the placenta is then extracted and finally the uterus and abdominal wall are sutured (stitched) layer by layer so as to restore the normal anatomy. The entire procedure usually takes about 30 minutes.

Recovery from a Caesarean section is slower than for a spontaneous delivery but nowadays you need only be in hospital for about a week. The discomfort from the abdominal wound makes progress slower, but with better modern techniques of suturing

For a breech delivery, the baby's legs, body and arms are delivered first (above). As the baby's head is the largest part, an episiotomy is usually recommended. Then the midwife lifts the baby's legs and body out of the way to enable the doctor to apply forceps to protect the baby's head during its delivery (above right).

(stitching), even this is less of a problem than it used to be. The wound takes about two to three weeks to heal completely and it is best to arrange for your partner or someone else to help you as much as possible at home until you are fully recovered (see p. 138).

For the future, it is worth knowing that if you have a baby delivered by Caesarean section it does not necessarily mean that every other delivery will have to be the same way, unless the reason for it is a recurring one, such as a small pelvis. It is perfectly possible for your next baby to be delivered vaginally as normal.

BREECH PRESENTATION

A breech presentation is when the baby's buttocks (or breech) is the lowermost part, rather than the head. Most babies will have turned into the cephalic (head down) position by the last few weeks of pregnancy; in four per cent of cases they do not. The baby may have both legs and hips flexed so that he is curled up and only his seat is presenting – this is known as a complete breech. If both legs are extended at the knee, so that the baby's heels are at the level of his ears, it is known as a frank breech; if one or both of the baby's feet are tucked under the buttocks, thereby becoming the presenting part, it is called a footling breech.

If your baby is breech, it may be possible to have a vaginal delivery, but your doctor will want to be

satisfied that certain criteria have been fulfilled before allowing it. Your pelvis must be of adequate size and shape so that there is no delay in the delivery of the baby's head. (As it is the largest part of the baby, but will be delivered last, the head is obviously the most crucial part of the delivery.) The baby himself should not be too big, which would mean of an estimated weight not greater than 3.5kg (7½lb). If he was thought to be bigger then a Caesarean section would probably be suggested instead. Similarly, if there were complicating factors like hypertension, diabetes and so on, then a Caesarean section would again be safer, as it would be for a baby that was small for dates or premature. Some obstetricians think that a complete or footling breech presentation are also more safely delivered by Caesarean, because of the risk of cord prolapse.

EXTERNAL VERSION

It is possible for a breech to be converted to a cephalic presentation by swivelling the baby round in the uterus, a manoeuvre known as 'external cephalic version'. However nowadays few obstetricians would attempt this, and there is no purpose at all in trying it until 34 weeks, since many babies will revert spontaneously to the breech position before then. At the end of the day the number of breech deliveries carried out by an average maternity unit remains much the same whether external version is carried out or not. As it is not without some small risk, of disrupting the placenta, for instance, it is rarely used.

DELIVERING A BREECH BABY

It goes without saying that a full team of doctors and midwives must be present for the breech delivery, and a paediatrician will be present to receive the baby to check and stabilize his condition if necessary. The first stage of a breech labour proceeds more or less as normal, although you are likely to be monitored frequently, if not continuously. You will probably be advised to have an epidural as forceps may be required to help the delivery of the head, and it is useful to have it in place in the event of an emergency Caesarean. An episiotomy is almost always performed for a breech delivery, as the baby's buttocks and body are not as wide as the head and the perineum will not usually be stretched enough to allow the head to pass through without this incision.

In second stage, the baby's buttocks are allowed to deliver as spontaneously as possible, after which the midwife will lift out the legs. Then the shoulders are rotated so the arms can gently be brought down and the head is allowed to descend on to the perineum. This part of the delivery is done quickly, with the fetal heart being monitored continuously. The delivery of the head is then carefully controlled by the attending doctor, either by hand or with the help of forceps.

Some authorities feel that there is no place for a vaginal breech delivery and that Caesarean section should be the method for all such deliveries. But most obstetricians consider that providing the antenatal assessment of both mother and baby is carried out scrupulously there is no reason why a vaginal delivery should not be permitted.

THE BIRTH OF TWINS

Although a twin birth need not necessarily be assisted, very many are because difficulties can arise with the delivery of the second twin. This is usually due to some form of malpresentation (see p. 66), or possibly because of fetal distress, especially if one twin is much smaller than the other, which is frequently the case. Preterm labour is also a likely complication with twins, although steps will be taken to try to prevent it (see p. 61). Naturally a full team of medical experts will be on hand, including paediatricians to look after the two babies. Triplets or higher multiples are always delivered by Caesarean section.

The birth of the first twin is usually straightforward if the presentation is cephalic, and may even be quite trouble-free if breech, since twins are usually smaller than average babies. Reasonably enough, parents of twins want a birth with the minimum of intervention, but if the second twin is to be delivered safely there must be a minimal delay between the two babies.

Once the first twin is delivered your abdomen is examined to check the lie of the second twin, and to correct it if possible. There is often a pause in the contractions, but they usually pick up again quite quickly or can be stimulated with syntocinon in an intravenous drip. The membranes of the second sac are then ruptured, if they haven't already done so.

If the baby's presentation allows it, a vaginal delivery follows, although a breech presentation (which is quite common in the second twin) may require the help of forceps in delivering the head, especially if the baby is small or preterm. If the second baby shows any signs of distress, due perhaps to cord prolapse, he will be delivered immediately with the help of the ventouse extractor (see p. 94) if the head is presenting, by forceps if the head is low enough, or by breech extraction, which simply means the deliberate extraction of the baby from the pelvis by the obstetrician.

Because the uterus is excessively distended by twins, there is an increased risk of haemorrhage following delivery, so special precautions will be taken to avoid it. If you have a drip in place the syntocinon dose will be increased, if not you will be given an injection of syntocinon to speed up the delivery of the afterbirth, and you will be examined to make sure nothing is retained in the uterus.

Twins are tiring to look after the first few weeks and months so it is a good idea to take the opportunity if offered to spend as long as possible in hospital getting used to caring for them. If they are premature, they may anyway have to spend some time in the Special Care Baby Unit (see p. 116).

DELIVERING A PRETERM BABY

The fundamental point to remember about a preterm delivery is that the baby is particularly fragile and immature and great care has to be taken throughout. Whether to allow a vaginal delivery or perform a Caesarean section is a difficult decision.

If labour is progressing fast, which is likely to be the case if you have had children before, then a vaginal delivery is best, but with your baby's heart rate being monitored continuously. Extreme care with the delivery of the head is necessary – it must have a controlled, gentle exit from the birth canal, so a wide episiotomy may be necessary.

If the labour is very premature, or the baby needs to be delivered early because of some problem, such as high blood pressure or placental abruption, then a Caesarean section would be the safest form of delivery, and this is certainly the case with a preterm breech presentation or a multiple pregnancy.

Delivering a preterm baby is a highly skilled operation, requiring a full team of experts. There will also be senior paediatricians and nursing staff from the Special Care Baby Unit present, with mobile incubators at the ready to ensure the baby's survival, especially if he is very immature.

DELIVERIES REQUIRING INTERVENTION

No two labours are the same, and unfortunately, a labour that starts perfectly normally may well require intervention by the medical staff in order to affect a safe delivery. Fetal distress is one such problem – if your baby shows signs fo asphyxia during either first or second stage the doctor or midwife may want to speed up the delivery with syntocinon, help the birth with forceps or ventouse, or it may even necessitate an emergency Caesarean (see above).

DELAY IN LABOUR

A frequent cause of unexpected intervention is delay in the progress of labour. One very important potential reason for this is the occipito posterior position. Here the crown of the baby's head (occiput) is at the back instead of the front, and the baby's face is turned towards your front. Almost inevitably the head is thrown back slightly (deflexed), presenting a longer diameter to the pelvis, so there will be less room for the head to pass through. Not only that: to rotate to the anterior position the baby has to turn 180°, which takes time.

This is probably the most common cause of delay in the first stage of labour, particularly in the first-time (primigravid) mother; not infrequently it leads to a Caesarean delivery. In the second stage, the midwife or doctor may be able to rotate the head by hand, or by using Kielland's forceps.

Other, rarer, reasons for delay are a brow presentation, where the head is markedly deflexed, or a face presentation. In both of these, Caesarean section will be necessary unless, in the case of a face presentation, the chin is already lying to the front, when a spontaneous delivery is possible.

HYPERTENSION AND LABOUR

If you suffer from any pre-existing medical condition, such as diabetes or heart disease, your labour will of course be very closely monitored and you will be given all the help you need to maintain your own well-being and that of your baby (see p.68). The medical staff will be equally vigilant if you are suffering from high blood pressure (hypertension) or pre-eclampsia, which are generally caused by the pregnancy rather than predating it (see p. 70).

An epidural anaesthetic is particularly helpful in lowering the blood pressure, and you may be asked to accept this for the sake of your baby. Your blood pressure may also be controlled during labour, using drugs usually given in an intravenous drip. Equally, monitoring the baby's heart rate throughout labour is imperative, along with frequent, or continuous, recording of your blood pressure level. Naturally, this will be very restricting, but you know that your baby's safety is the over-riding concern.

Provided that your blood pressure remains satisfactory throughout labour and that the baby's condition does not give rise to concern, a spontaneous delivery should be possible. It may, however, be necessary to curtail the second stage of labour, using forceps if any delay occurs.

After the birth and for the first few days of the puerperium (see p. 132), your blood pressure will continue to be measured at frequent intervals, and treatment with drugs will be continued if necessary. If you were found to be hypertensive from the early stages of pregnancy, further investigation as to its cause will be continued postnatally. If you suffered from high blood pressure or pre-eclampsia you should make sure you attend your six-week postnatal check-up at the hospital (see p. 139) so that the implications for future pregnancies and your own health can be discussed and you can be referred back to a specialist physician if necessary.

LOSING YOUR BABY

Sadly not all pregnancies end in the birth of a perfectly formed and healthy baby. For some parents the tragedy will be that their baby is born dead, medically known as stillbirth, for others that the baby will die shortly after birth, a neonatal death. (If the fetus dies before 28 weeks, it is deemed to be a miscarriage, or spontaneous abortion – see page 58).

The period of time around birth and the week which follows it are known as the perinatal period and statistics are collected annually on the numbers of baby deaths during this time. From these we know that over the years the perinatal death rate has been steadily falling and in England and Wales at present it is just under one in a hundred.

THE CAUSE OF DEATH

There are three major reasons why a baby may die at this time. The oxygen supply to the baby in the uterus may be reduced, sometimes because of problems with the placenta or umbilical cord, and the baby may die of asphyxia before it is born or shortly afterwards; the baby may be born with a major physical abnormality which cannot be corrected; or the baby may be born very much too early and die because of his immaturity.

Sometimes it is very difficult to be precise about the exact cause of a baby's death, but should this happen to your pregnancy then it will probably be the most important question you want answered. The doctors attending you will want to help you all they can and may well ask for your permission to perform a post mortem examination. This examination not only gives very important information sometimes on the cause of death, but just as importantly can exclude a number of other problems which may otherwise have been relevant, although it does not always provide the answer.

COPING WITH THE LOSS

If you have the misfortune to lose your baby then the intensity of your feelings and the expression of your grief often make it very difficult for you to take in all that is happening. The medical and nursing staff will also be distressed, so this may not be the best time for lengthy explanations. You will be offered the opportunity to see and hold your baby, perhaps to give him or her a name, and to have some private moments together. Baptism can be arranged if this is your wish. Most units will also take a photograph of the baby which you may like to keep. Do not worry if you cannot accept this when first offered – the hospital retain it in your notes for you.

As with any death there are certain legal formalities which must be dealt with. In the case of a stillbirth, the birth does not need to be registered but a special medical certificate has to be taken to the registrar within 42 days. In the case of a neonatal death, first the birth must be registered and then a death certificate presented to the registrar within five days. The registrar can then issue, in either circumstance, a certificate of burial or cremation. It is now possible to register a first name for your baby, but you have to ask for it if this is your wish.

This is a desperately difficult time for decision-making but you will be faced with one more choice, once the legal formalities have been dealt with, as to whether you would prefer a hospital or private funeral. In the former circumstance the hospital will take all the arrangements off your hands. They usually organize a burial in a local cemetery, which of course you may attend if you so wish. The grave may be a communal one, so arranging a personal memorial may be difficult. If a private funeral is preferred then you can make arrangements with an undertaker according to your own wishes. A member of the hospital staff familiar with the local situation can help here.

You may want to leave hospital quickly, but immediate discharge is not always possible. You can choose whether you would prefer to be in a room to yourself or whether you would welcome the company of other mothers. Quite often it is possible for your partner to stay with you, through the night as well as during the day, and this can be very comforting for you both.

AT HOME WITH THE FAMILY

When you do go home you may find it difficult to talk to your relatives and particularly to other children in your family, who often feel that their thoughts or actions may have had something to do with the baby's death. Meeting other pregnant women or those with young babies may also be difficult. You will be visited by your community midwife and probably by your doctor who can advise you on practical problems such as lactation, and who can put you in touch with local self-help groups, if the hospital have not already done so. Talking to other parents who have had a similar experience can be very consoling and a helpful leaflet called 'The Loss of your Baby' can also be provided by the hospital or can be obtained from the new Health Education Authority (previously the Health Education Council).

THE POSTNATAL CHECK

Before you leave the hospital you will have seen the Consultant who looked after your pregnancy, or a senior member of the team, and an appointment will have been made for you to come back and discuss your case in detail once all the results are available. This could be anytime from two to six weeks from the time of the baby's death and may also be attended by a paediatrician if your baby received special care after birth. It is helpful if you have listed all the questions you would like to ask beforehand. In this interview the doctors should give you as precise an explanation of what happened as is possible and discuss its implications for the future. You may like to ask about the timing of another pregnancy, and any special tests or management that might be advised. If the doctor thinks that specialist genetic or other medical opinions are necessary then these can be arranged. An invitation to return at some time in the future, perhaps when considering another pregnancy, is often offered but do not hesitate to ask for a further appointment if, on reflection, you have further questions. The process of grieving may take a long time to work through and you must not feel guilty about this. Even though you may not have known your baby for very long, his or her loss is no less painful than losing a close relative or friend.

THE NEWBORN BABY

Getting to know your newborn baby during the first few hours and days after the birth

For new parents, the first view of your baby immediately after the birth is often an extremely emotional occasion, especially with your first child. But this emotional feeling is almost always accompanied by a feeling of apprehension about the baby's condition, his apparent fragility, and whether you will be able to look after him properly. And if the birth has been at all difficult or prolonged for the mother, you may not feel particularly drawn to your baby at all and may feel guilty about whether you can ever learn to love him (see p. 137). But a normal newborn baby is an extremely resilient being, and although not designed like a calf or foal to struggle to his feet within minutes of the birth, the newborn baby has instincts and reflexes which are designed to help him survive.

IN THE LABOUR WARD

Most full term babies who are born normally require no special attention at birth and you are likely to be able to touch your baby as he is born and let him lie on your stomach before the cord is cut, after which he will be given to you to hold (see Chapter 6).

If you need a Caesarean section or forceps delivery, if there is any anxiety about the baby's condition or indeed if you are having twins then the midwives will have arranged for a paediatrician to be present at the delivery. You are likely to be so absorbed in the labour that you will probably not notice his arrival. In many instances his presence is merely a precaution and his service is not required. However, you may find that once the cord is cut, instead of being given to you, the baby is taken to the paediatrician who will be waiting by the resuscitation trolley at the side of the room. In the great majority of cases this does not preface a serious problem.

It is very common for babies to have a lot of mucus and fluid in the airways at birth and to require suction to clear them, or to be a little slow to start breathing regularly and to remain a bluish colour. Sometimes this is because they have been a little asphyxiated during the delivery or it is a side effect of analgesics such as pethidine during the labour. In this case the paediatrician might give the baby some extra oxygen for a few minutes or he may even need to help the respiration either with a mask over the baby's face or by inserting a tube into the airways. Usually the baby will be breathing well within a few minutes and remains pink without extra oxygen. The paediatrician will probably remain for another few minutes just to check that all is well before confirming that the baby will be able to go with you to the postnatal ward.

Sometimes the baby is a little slow to breathe in the first few minutes even when there has been no problem identified during the labour. In this case the paediatrician will not have been informed and the midwives, who are specially trained in techniques of resuscitation, will do what is necessary while the paediatrician is called.

Even if there are no particular problems at this time you will find that the staff are most concerned to ensure that your baby does not become cold. Newborn babies are particularly inclined to lose heat because they are wet and naked and have a relatively large surface area. Even if you have been able to deliver the baby on to your own abdomen and he is crying vigorously the staff will be anxious to dry him and wrap him in warm towels and blankets. It is most important that they are able to do this. They will feel, rightly, that they have failed in their duties to your baby if his temperature drops.

THE APGAR SCORE

As soon as the baby is born, the midwife or doctor will be observing his condition closely and assessing it in terms of the Apgar score, so called after the doctor who first described it. Five features – the heart rate, the respiratory rate, colour, activity and response to stimulation – are assigned a score between zero and ten, so that a baby who is pink and very active and responsive will be given a score of ten, while a baby who fails to breathe and is limp, needing resuscitation, will get a low score. The score is usually calculated at the ages of one and five minutes and only later if resuscitative measures are still required. Many babies who have very low

Apgar scores respond very well to resuscitation and may not even require admission to the Special Care Baby Unit (see Chapter 9).

You will probably not even realize that the midwife is calculating the score because she will be doing it by observation while she is busy delivering the afterbirth and attending to you and the baby. When things have quietened down a little later, she will write the scores into your notes. Many professionals are sceptical about the actual usefulness of the Apgar score system, but it is very widely used and remains the most efficient shorthand way of describing the baby's state of health in the minutes immediately after the birth.

WEIGHING AND MEASURING

If you are able to hold the baby immediately after delivery the midwives will probably leave him with you while they tidy everything else up. They will then ask you if they can just borrow the baby for a few minutes to have a quick check that all is well, or they will have a quick look at him during any resuscitation that is required. It is part of the midwife's statutory duty to weigh, measure and to examine the baby at this time to ensure that there are no major congenital abnormalities. While this is being done they will also tend to the umbilical cord which will probably have been left fairly long with a metal clamp on it. A light plastic clamp will be put about an inch from the umbilicus itself and the cord cut just beyond this.

In the majority of maternity units the babies are also given some Vitamin K at this time. This is in order to prevent a rare bleeding illness, known as haemorrhagic disease of the newborn, which very occasionally effects even completely fit full term babies. The Vitamin K may be given by mouth but if the baby is at all preterm or if there has been any problem necessitating Caesarean section or forceps delivery, it may be given by injection into the thigh.

PUTTING THE BABY TO THE BREAST

If you are intending to breastfeed your baby you will probably want to feed him as soon as possible after the birth. You may still be relatively immobile because of an epidural anaesthetic or because of stitching and you will need some help either from your partner or one of the midwifery staff. Most babies are very alert at this time and suck well. As the baby begins to suck you will experience not only the sensation of the 'let down' reflex within the breast (see page 150), but often a fairly strong contraction of the uterus. This arises because oxytocin, the hormone released during suckling, acts upon the uterine muscle as well as on the muscle in the milk ducts in the breast. This contraction helps to deliver the placenta and minimizes bleeding from the uterus.

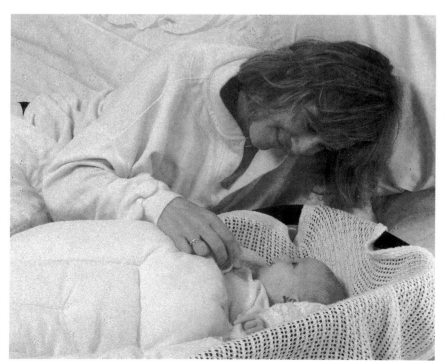

Many parents are surprised by how alert their babies are immediately after the birth, if pain-relieving drugs such as pethidine have not been used and the baby is well. A baby will look fixedly at his parent's face if held about twenty centimetres (eight inches) away, and will seem to look round the room, sometimes remaining wakeful for several hours after delivery.

THE BABY IN THE FIRST FEW HOURS

While the midwives will be keen to dry the baby to prevent his becoming cold they will not go to any great lengths to clean him while you are still on the labour ward, apart from wiping his face, so he is still likely to have odd bits of blood and occasionally meconium, (fetal bowel contents), on him. If the baby is at all early you may find that he has a thick creamy material known as vernix on the skin. There is no hurry to clean away any of these substances, as it is much more important that you and your partner are able to hold and admire your child for as long as possible.

It is often a great surprise to new parents to see how wide-eyed their baby is in the first few hours after delivery, often staring up at his mother or father or gazing around the room and appearing to explore his surroundings. It has been shown that many babies spend the greater part of the first twelve hours after delivery awake and that it is in the second twelve hours that they are more likely to sleep.

Before you leave for the postnatal ward, usually an hour or so after delivery, the midwives will check the baby's temperature and will confirm that the colour is good and that there are no problems with breathing.

It is common, especially after a Caesarean section or forceps delivery, for women to get as far as the postnastal ward without having been able to have a good look at the baby without clothes on. You will have been reassured by the staff in the delivery room that all appears to be well and it is a great excitement to be able to inspect the baby yourself. Sometimes the appearance of the baby is rather a surprise. Newborn babies are often not the red, wrinkled creatures we would be led to believe.

THE HEAD AND HAIR

One of the things that often first strikes the parents is the shape of the head. If you have had an elective Caesarean section or a breech delivery then the head is likely to be round, but if you have had a normal delivery the head will have 'moulded' in order to aid its passage through the birth canal, and may be tall and elongated. If the labour has been long this may be very marked and the appearance further complicated because of swelling of the scalp known as 'caput'. Caput arises because of the pressure on the scalp during contractions, but it resolves rapidly over the first day or so.

The bones of the baby's head are of course mobile and just as they have moved to enable the head to 'mould', so over the next few days they will return to a normal position, the caput will subside and the head will become a normal shape.

To facilitate the moulding of the baby's head during birth, the four bones of the skull are not fused and there are areas at the top and at the back of the head which are covered only with a tough membrane – these are the fontanelles. The posterior fontanelle is usually closed before birth, and if not will have closed within a very short time afterwards. The anterior fontanelle, or 'soft spot', with its characteristic diamond shape, is probably one of the most worrying things for first-time parents – the baby's head seems so vulnerable, especially as you may notice the fontanelle pulsating, particularly when the baby cries. However the membrane is very tough and it does not matter if you touch it, when you are washing the baby's hair for instance. The anterior fontanelle takes quite a long time to close completely – twelve to eighteen months is quite normal.

Occasionally, the baby may have an area of swelling on the head which is caused by bleeding over one of the bones of the skull (cephalhaematoma). There may be more than one of these swellings, which, although not serious, are much slower to resolve than a caput, and may not disappear for several weeks. They can be rather unsightly and as they settle you may notice as you run your finger over them that there is a depression in the centre. This will gradually extend outwards as the collection of blood becomes liquid and disperses. All this can be worrying, but it does not cause any subsequent problems.

Within a few days of birth you may notice a blister or patch of thick white skin appearing centrally on the inside of the lips. This is related to sucking and is quite normal.

The amount of hair on your baby's head at birth does not bear any relation to how thick it will be subsequently. Some babies are born with a great deal of hair; unfortunately most of it usually falls out by about three months of age.

If the baby is preterm there may be some downy hair (lanugo) over the body, especially on the shoulders. This has usually disappeared in white, Afro-Caribbean and oriental babies at full term, but it is normal for Asian babies often to be born with a considerable amount of body hair.

EYES AND EARS

The white of the baby's eyes is often not as clear as in older children and the colour of the eye tends to be a deep blue. True eye colour develops over the first year.

Occasionally little red areas are visible on the

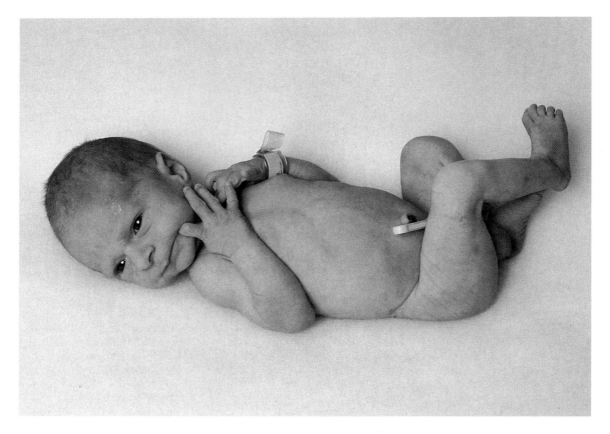

A normal newborn baby, photographed within 24 hours of the birth. The cord clamp is not removed for four or five days, when the remains of the umbilicus has dried to a leathery stump.

white of the eye to either side of the coloured iris. These are small haemorrhages which arise because of the high pressure as the head comes through the birth canal. They will resolve over the first week or so and will not cause any permanent damage.

The ears of the newborn baby are often more striking than in the adult because they are disproportionately large and less likely to be hidden by hair. If your baby is a little early the cartilage inside the ear may not extend right out to the edge at birth and you may find the ears lying forward. Don't worry, they will soon stiffen up so don't feel that you need to coax them back by sticking them down!

THE SKIN

The texture of the skin in the first few days is very variable and you must not be dismayed if your baby doesn't, from the outset, have the peachy skin of the magazine advertisements.

If the baby is a little early the skin is likely to be a pinkish to red colour and to be smooth. If your baby is at term or a bit late you may find that the skin is rather dry at delivery and seems to be peeling off, especially on the fingers. This peeling can be very dramatic, with apparently very dry skin coming off over the whole body in the first few days. The midwives may rub some light oil on to the skin to soften it during this time. It is only a temporary phase and when the peeling has stopped the skin will be softer.

If the delivery is a bit late or if there has been some fetal distress, the baby may have had his bowels open (passed meconium) while still in the uterus. This may result in yellow or brownish staining of the skin and of the umbilical cord, which will gradually disappear over the first few days.

Afro-Caribbean parents are often surprised because their baby's skin is relatively fair at delivery. You will find however, that the pigmentation increases rapidly over the first few days.

Between about the third day and the end of the first week, you may notice small white spots with a red weal around them appearing over your baby's body and sometimes extending over the limbs and face. This characteristic rash, known as toxic erythema or neonatal urticaria, is usually easily distinguished from infected spots. It is not serious and requires no treatment.

Another common and totally innocuous spot is the small cream, pearly spots known as milia, which are present over the nose and cheeks. These are often seen in great numbers during the first few days and sometimes persist for some weeks.

After the second day you may notice your baby's previously normal pink skin becomes yellow because of jaundice. This is very common even in healthy full term babies (see page 121).

BIRTH MARKS

The majority of pigmented birthmarks and the common raised strawberry marks seen on the skin of babies are not present at birth. However, you may notice flat red marks of various shapes and sizes over the eyelids, on the centre of the forehead and at the nape of the neck. These are the well known 'stork marks'. The ones on the face disappear in the first year, while those at the back of the neck tend to persist but are usually well hidden by hair. If present at birth, flat red marks on either side of the face are more likely to persist. The paediatrician will advise you about this.

Another common birth mark is the 'mongolian blue spot'. This is a flat blue-grey mark usually on the buttocks or lower back. They are often small, single marks, but can be multiple and extend over the back. They are particularly common in babies with pigmented skin and become less apparent as the pigmentation of the surrounding skin increases.

THE NAILS

At full term the finger nails are often rather long and they may be stained brown with meconium. This fades within a week or so.

Long nails need cutting (you may find it easier to bite them off, this is a very common practice and totally acceptable). If they are not cut you may find that your baby scratches himself quite badly. Some people suggest putting mitts on a baby when this happens, but they rarely stay on for long. Keeping your baby's nails short is more effective.

THE BREASTS

You may be rather taken aback by the development of your baby's breast tissue which may be marked in either sex, greatly in excess of the breasts of older children. The nipple may be well formed with a well developed pad of breast tissue. In extreme cases you may even notice a slight milky discharge on the nipple. This is because the baby has been exposed to high circulating levels of female hormones whilst in the uterus and the activity in the breast will gradually subside after birth. Sometimes this effect is greater on one side than the other.

THE UMBILICUS

The umbilical cord itself is a clear gelatinous structure through which the umbilical blood vessels which carry blood between the baby and the placenta can be seen. The cord is usually about 1cm (½ in) in diameter but can vary greatly. About 2cm (1 in) of cord will remain at the umbilicus, clamped with a plastic clamp. It dries up very quickly in the few days after birth so that by about the fourth day it looks thin and leathery. The midwife will remove the clamp on the fourth or fifth day, after which the cord stump will drop off within a day or so.

THE GENITALS

Another frequent source of surprise is the prominence of the baby's genitals. Male babies have a well developed scrotum and penis, large in proportion to the size of the body, and Afro-Caribbean and Asian babies will have a pigmented scrotum even if the rest of the skin is still pale.

The labia (lips of the vulva) of female babies often appear to be rather swollen and there is very commonly a mucusy vaginal discharge which may very occasionally be slightly blood-stained. This is another effect of the mother's high hormone levels affecting the baby and diminishes after delivery.

THE LEGS AND FEET

You may be concerned that your baby's legs are abnormal because the thigh, the lower leg and the feet do not seem to be properly aligned, and the lower part of the legs is often bowed inwards. Occasionally of course there is a genuine abnormality but usually these funny postures are purely positional – a newborn baby is naturally curled up – and the midwives or the paediatrician will demonstrate to you that the leg can easily be brought into a normal position. Minor abnormalities of foot position and over-riding toes nearly always correct during the first year as the baby begins to bear weight.

SEEING AND HEARING

As you watch your baby you will see that there is lots of normal movement of all his limbs and you will notice that he is looking around and sometimes seems to be staring in a particular direction, often towards a sunlit window or lamp. It is surprising how many new mothers have been led to believe that their babies will not be able to see straight away but simple observation of the baby's activity will soon dispel this misconception.

If you catch your baby wide awake and not crying and hold him so that your faces are about 25 centimetres (ten inches) apart you may find that he is gazing at you intently, and if you move your head from side to side he may follow you with his eyes. You can play similar games with simple objects such as a brightly coloured ball of about seven centimetres (three inches) diameter. Don't worry if your baby goes cross-eyed at this time. This is very common and is because the baby does not yet have good control over the muscles around the eye which determine the direction in which it is looking.

Formal testing of hearing is complex in the newborn but it is often clear that the baby can hear when he is seen to startle in response to a bang close by, or to quieten in response to a reassuring sound close to him, such as a musical toy, or his parent's voice.

THE POSTNATAL WARD

It is not long since babies on postnatal wards spent most of their time in a side nursery and were only with their mothers at the regular feed times. Now nurseries are largely reserved for bathing babies, and babies remain in a cot at the bedside throughout the day and night. This practice is known as 'rooming in'.

The midwives may suggest that your baby goes to the nursery for the first night so that you are able to sleep. You should only agree to this if you feel quite happy about it and you should discuss plans for night feeds so that the midwives are quite clear as to whether you want to be woken.

After the first night it will almost certainly be assumed that you will have your baby with you and that you will feed him yourself through the night. Even though you may feel tired, this is particularly important if you are breastfeeding as it helps to establish feeding as quickly as possible.

FEEDING

Provided your baby is full term and well grown he will be fed 'on demand', although you may be advised not to let him sleep for more than six hours at any one time until feeding is established.

If you are breastfeeding you will need help with getting the baby on to the breast for the first few feeds (see p. 152). Your milk flow will become established more quickly as you put the baby to the breast each time he cries for the first few days. Don't be worried if you find you are feeding very frequently, even up to about fifteen times a day for a few days; provided that the baby is getting on to the breasts properly they shouldn't become sore.

If the baby cries frequently this is most unlikely to be because you don't have enough milk and there is no need to 'top the baby up' with a bottle after the feed. If the baby cries just put him back on the breast.

If you are bottle feeding you will be provided with pre-packed bottles while you are in hospital. Bottle fed babies will probably demand feeds less frequently than breastfed babies for the first few days. Milk is all they need, clear fluids should not be necessary.

Full term babies are weighed at birth and are then not usually weighed again until the third day. You should expect your baby to have lost some weight at this time. Breastfed babies often lose more than bottle fed babies because they obtain fewer calories in the first few days. This weight loss is absolutely normal and is not going to put your baby at any long term disadvantage: full term babies who have grown well in the uterus will have stores of fat beneath the skin and carbohydrate in the liver which they can use in the first few days, both to help keep themselves warm and to keep their blood sugar at the right level.

Midwives have a rule of thumb by which they calculate the amount of weight loss they consider acceptable (usually up to ten per cent of the birth weight), and they will probably only seek the help of a paediatrician if the loss exceeds this figure or the baby seems otherwise to be unwell. When your baby is next weighed a few days later he will probably be gaining and most babies have re-gained their birth weight by the tenth day.

DAILY CARE

The purpose of keeping you and your baby in hospital for a few days after delivery is not just to ensure your health prior to discharge but also to help you learn how to care for your baby. In many hospitals the baby does not receive a bath until about the third day but you will be shown how to keep the baby clean without resorting to a full scale bath (see p. 169). If the baby is not having a bath the neck area and armpits should be cleaned carefully with cotton wool balls and water or cream. Only water should be used on the face and a clean piece of cotton wool must be used for each of the eyes.

The nappy area is best cleaned with cotton wool balls dipped in tepid water. Always clean in the folds of the groin and upper thigh. Clean a baby girl from the front to back to avoid germs from the anus reaching the vagina. The whole area should then be smeared liberally with a barrier cream, either a zinc and caster oil mixture or petroleum jelly, before the nappy is put on.

Particular attention is paid to the area around the cord (umbilicus) until it has dropped off, usually towards the end of the first week, and its base dried up, usually at about ten days. Various techniques of cord care are available but the most satisfactory and widely used is probably to clean the cord with a small spirit swab and then to powder it with an antimicrobial powder with which you will be provided in hospital. At first the midwife may do this for you, but you will be encouraged to take over as soon as possible.

The cord is inspected carefully every day until it has dried up and dropped off as it is a common site of infection. If the cord, or the area around it, looks inflamed, this may indicate an infection, so ask the advice of your midwife or paediatrician.

THE FIRST BATH

Your baby will probably receive his first bath on about the third day. A midwife or nursery nurse will show you how to bath the baby and then the next day you will probably do it yourself with a member of staff close by in case you are in difficulties. This is when your baby will receive his first hair wash and finally get rid of all those little bits of debris which have been present since delivery.

You have the choice of using a cake of non-scented baby soap and soaping the baby prior to putting him into the water or using a liquid baby wash added to the bath. In terms of cleanliness there is probably nothing to choose between the methods but do remember that once soaped your baby will be very slippery.

Most babies enjoy their bath but some clearly don't until they are a little older. You can keep your baby perfectly clean without a bath so don't feel that you have to perform this ritual daily (see p. 169).

BOWELS

The great majority of babies have their bowels open within the first 24 hours and the remainder before 48 hours. If the bowels are not opened by this time the paediatrician will be informed.

Meconium, which is present in the baby's bowel at birth, is a sticky greenish-black substance often passed in copious amounts on the first day, necessitating a premature first bath! By two or three days the colour of the stool will be lightening, a 'changing stool', so that by four or five days the normal soft yellow stool of the milk fed baby will be passed.

The frequency with which babies have their bowels open and the texture of the stools is very variable and can surprise parents, causing unnecessary anxiety. Breastfed babies stools are very soft, usually light yellow and virtually odourless. Some babies may have dirty nappies with runny stools at every nappy change, while other babies may only open their bowels every two or three days or even once a week! Any of these is perfectly normal – what you need to find out is what is normal for your baby; you should only become concerned if the bowel habit changes or if the baby seems unwell.

Bottle fed babies usually have their bowels open two to four times a day, although it is not uncommon for them to go much more frequently. The stools are usually a yellowish colour and are soft. Occasionally the baby's stools may be green, but provided they are not runny or frequent this is probably normal for your baby. If you have any doubts it is worth showing a little sample of the stool to your midwife or health visitor, once you are at home.

Parents are often distressed because of the tremendous straining and redness of the face which might go on for some time before their baby passes what turns out to be a perfectly ordinary, soft stool. This is absolutely normal behaviour in young babies and you only need to seek guidance if the stool becomes hard (see p. 192).

URINE

Urine is frequently passed at the time of delivery and then not very often during the first 48 hours. Thereafter the baby will have a wet nappy at most feeds. It is most important that you don't leave your baby for too long in a wet nappy as this will lead to a nappy rash (see p. 193).

SLEEPING, WAKING AND CRYING

Babies do not settle straight into a routine from the first day. In fact it is likely that no two days in the first week will be the same. Breastfed babies may feed many times a day in the early weeks and they may sleep for variable lengths of time, ranging between about half an hour and six hours. Similarly the length of time that they are awake varies, some babies commonly lying wide eyed in their cots for prolonged periods. The baby bottle fed on demand is less likely to feed so frequently in the first few days but you will find that the length of time taken between feeds varies.

The practice of 'rooming-in' – having your baby's crib by your bed in the postnatal ward at all times – is now almost universal in modern maternity units. It helps you to get to know your baby more quickly, and means that you can feed your baby whenever he needs it, which helps to establish breastfeeding.

You may find that your baby varies greatly from the one in the adjoining bed in terms of the amount of noise that he makes. Most babies do not really cry very much in the first few days but perhaps your baby will be the exception. Why some cry so much is often difficult to explain. The cause seems to be hunger on some occasions while in many others it can be stopped just by picking the baby up or simply by wrapping him up well in the blanket and tucking it into the cot. In the early days a wet or dirty nappy does not seem to upset the baby. You may worry that your baby is crying because he is unwell but this is unlikely to be the case; quietness and lethargy are much more common signs of problems in the newborn. If your baby does cry a lot at the beginning, it doesn't necessarily mean that he is going to continue in this manner.

VISITING ON THE POSTNATAL WARD

Visiting hours will vary between different hospitals but you are likely to find quite firm restrictions and there are often periods when only fathers are allowed to visit.

One of the reasons for staying in hospital for a few days after the delivery is to ensure that you have some time when you can concentrate wholly on yourself and your baby without the distractions of household problems. This is just as important with a subsequent baby as it is with the first. If you are swamped with visits from well-meaning family and friends it can sometimes be difficult to relax and enjoy the new rituals of feeding and changing. It can be very tiring to feel you have to be polite to a constant stream of visitors, and your partner should tactfully try to cut down the numbers on any one day.

It is equally important that you are able to have time alone with your partner and the baby, so that the father feels fully involved in this unique experience. The first dirty nappy, the first bath, the early feeds are all great milestones which both mother and father should be able to share.

The care of mother and normal baby in the days after birth is traditionally the responsibility of the midwives, and if you are at home this will certainly be the case. Within a hospital unit the doctors will have a considerable influence over patterns of care although in practical terms they will concentrate on the problems and leave the care of normal babies to the midwives.

Each ward will have a Sister and Staff Midwives and if there is a midwifery training school attached to the hospital there are also likely to be pupils. You may find that day-to-day care of the babies on the ward is performed by nursery nurses rather than by midwives. These are girls who will not have done a formal nursing training but will have specialized in the care of newborn babies and infants.

It is not long since it was standard practice for women to stay in hospital for ten days after delivery. Now it is usually only women who have had complications who stay this long and even after a Caesarean section many women go home after only a week.

Your length of stay will have been discussed with you antenatally and you will probably have opted either for a 48-hour or five-day stay. If you are particularly keen to be at home you may even have arranged with your GP and midwife to go home as soon as six hours after the delivery (see p. 19).

If you are well supported at home and everything has been straightforward, then it is lovely to be able to leave hospital, but for many women a few days on the postnatal ward is a blessing even if it is rather noisy at night and the daytime is a bit regimented.

While you are obviously not keen to upset plans, do remember that a decision to take a 48-hour discharge is not binding and if you feel uneasy about handling or feeding your baby you should ask to stay a little longer.

EXAMINATION OF THE NEWBORN

Your baby will receive several examinations while in hospital. The first of these is performed by the midwife in the labour ward, (see above) and is performed to rule out obvious malformations, such as wrong numbers of fingers and toes, club feet (talipes), and the like. Thereafter the midwife will check the baby daily looking for any signs of minor infections such as spots and sticky eyes, or common problems such as jaundice. They will pass on any problems they cannot solve to the paediatrician,

who will be one of a team of doctors working under a consultant. He or she will make a routine daily visit to the ward.

In addition to the daily midwife checks, your baby will be thoroughly examined by a doctor. If you are staying for more than 48 hours there will probably be two such examinations, the first at about 24 hours and the second within 24 hours of your discharge. One of the examinations, usually the second, will be by a paediatrician and the other either by a pediatrician or a junior obstetrician. If you are being discharged at 48 hours the baby will probably only be examined once and that by the paediatrician.

If you have been delivered by your own GP and midwife within the hospital obstetric unit your GP will probably, although not inevitably, take on the responsibility of the newborn examination himself. He will certainly do this if you have your baby at home.

The purpose of these medical examinations is three fold; firstly, to identify any congenital abnormalities that the midwives may have missed or which were not apparent in the labour ward; secondly, to ensure that the baby is feeding adequately and that the systems such as bowels are functioning normally; and thirdly to give you, the parents, an opportunity to discuss any anxieties of your own. From this it is clear that the examination is incomplete unless it is done in your presence.

THE PHYSICAL EXAMINATION

The paediatrician will probably ask you to undress the baby yourself and will examine the baby either on your bed or in his cot. He is likely to watch the baby's general level of activity and alertness briefly while also noticing the colour of the skin and any obvious abnormalities, before proceeding to the more thorough examination.

When you yourself are examined by a doctor, he will usually look systematically at the heart and lungs, then the abdomen, then the nervous system, and so on. Examining a baby is rather different, as co-operation cannot be guaranteed! Things like listening to the heart and feeling the pulse which need to be done while the baby is quiet and relaxed are done first, while manoeuvres such as checking for congenital dislocation of the hip, which might make the baby cry, are kept till the end.

After watching the baby, the paediatrician will probably run his hand over the head, feeling the soft spot (fontanelle) on the top, which is of variable size, and checking that there are no obvious abnormalities of the head, or swellings such as cephalhaematomata which relate to the delivery.

THE HEART, PULSES AND ABDOMEN

The heart is listened to both at the front and the back, as some cardiac murmurs (uneven heart beats) are more easily heard at the back between the shoulder blades. You will also notice the paediatrician feeling in your baby's groin; this is to check the pulses in the arteries to the legs, which are difficult to feel if there is a narrowing (coarctation) of the aorta, the main artery coming from the heart.

The doctor will gently feel your baby's abdomen while the baby is still relaxed to ensure that there are no masses or lumps felt; such positive findings are extremely unusual but may represent one of the very rare neonatal tumours, or a congenital abnormality of one of the abdominal organs.

MUSCLE TONE

At this stage the doctor may lift the baby up, checking that there are no obvious abnormalities of the spine, and feeling the 'tone' of the muscles. Tone is really a description of the tension in the muscles; some babies who have suffered from asphyxia or babies with Down's syndrome tend to be floppy, rather like a rag doll, while other asphyxiated babies are more than usually stiff. Normally babies offer some, but not excessive, resistance as the limbs are moved to and fro.

REFLEXES

The paediatrician may then demonstrate some of the primitive reflexes which are present in normal babies at birth, such as the grasp reflex, when the baby grips a finger or pencil passed across the palm of the hand; or the stepping reflex, when the baby makes a stepping up movement when held upright and the top of the foot touches a surface, such as the rim of the cot. Other reflexes include the 'Moro response', when the baby throws out his arms and legs when startled; the walking reflex, when the baby 'walks' along a flat surface if held upright with feet touching it; and the 'rooting' reflex, which is important for feeding (see p. 152).

SPECIFIC AREAS

After this the doctor will look at specific areas more carefully. He may need to hold your baby's eyes open gently and shine a light into them, looking particularly for the rare cataracts which are sometimes visible as white specks in the lens of the eye. The roof of the mouth is felt with a finger and also examined with a torch to check there is no cleft palate.

Your baby's genitalia will be examined, ensuring in a girl that the vagina and the urethral opening are normally positioned, and in a boy that the penis is normal and that the testes are present in the scrotum. If one of the testes is not descended, this will be checked again at six weeks and later if necessary. Most testes come down by three months. Occasionally your doctor may suggest hormone injections to stimulate the descent, but if the testis has not come down by twelve months, an operation will be performed to bring it into the scrotum. This operation would take place in the hospital (see p. 258 for advice about this).

LEGS AND FEET

Attention now passes to the lower limbs and the position of the feet will be checked. A newborn baby's feet are often held in an unusual position, with the soles either inwards or outwards. This probably relates to the position of the feet while in the uterus and frequently causes anxiety in new parents. In the great majority of babies the feet are very mobile and the paediatrician will demonstrate to you how easily they return to a normal position. Only a very few have true deformities requiring referral to an orthopaedic surgeon.

EXAMINATION OF THE HIPS

Finally the hips are examined, either separately or together. You will see the paediatrician holding the leg with the knee bent as far as it will go, with the doctor's thumb in front and fingers behind the hip. With the baby lying flat on his back, the doctor will turn the leg outwards so that it comes to lie almost flat on the bed. The doctor is testing to ensure that the top of the thigh bone (the head of the femur) is within the socket of the hip joint (the acetabulum). If the joint is not correctly in place he will be unable to turn the leg out. This disorder is known as congenital dislocation of the hip.

Having ensured that the hip is in place a second manoeuvre is performed to check that it is stable and remains in place when gentle pressure is applied. It is common for slight 'clicking' of the ligaments around the hip to be noted during the first week or so and the paediatrician may comment upon this. This is thought to arise because the ligaments are relaxed as a result of the hormones of pregnancy crossing the placenta. These clicks are

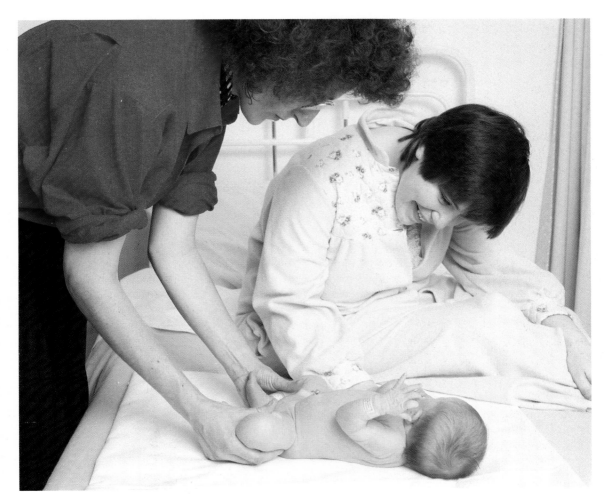

Testing for congenital hip dislocation is one of the most important elements of the medical check made on your newborn baby by the hospital paediatrician.

not serious. Genuine instability of the hip joint is much less common. If there is any concern about your baby's hips he will probably be referred fairly quickly to an orthopaedic surgeon. Congenital hip dislocation can be corrected over the first few months of life with the help of a special splint or plaster cast.

The examination of the hips is rather uncomfortable; not surprisingly, many babies object to this and may cry, so at this point in the examination you should be able to wrap him up and give him a comforting cuddle. Indeed, you yourself may find the hip manoeuvres rather distressing to watch. However it only takes a few seconds and helps to diagnose a problem which could lead to disability later in life if not treated.

POSTNATAL PROBLEMS

Occasionally babies who are well grown and who cause no anxiety immediately after delivery develop problems during their stay on the postnatal ward. The most common of these is jaundice, which does not usually appear until the latter part of the second day (see p. 121). Another frequent finding is that the baby makes repeated, quick, jittery movements of the limbs and startles a lot, which can be a sign that he has low blood sugar or calcium.

Similarly you or the midwives may notice a change in your baby's pattern of behaviour over the first few days in that he becomes sleepy or irritable and vomits, or goes off his feeds. Any of these signs may herald a problem such as an infection which, if not detected early, may become serious. In this case the midwives will quickly alert the paediatrician who will rapidly organize tests to try to find the cause of the problem. These will usually consist of blood tests together with the collection of a urine sample and frequently a lumbar puncture (removal of fluid from around the spinal cord) to exclude the very unlikely but important possibility of meningitis.

You may be fortunate enough to be in a hospital where these tests can be performed on the postnatal ward, so that you and the baby can stay together, but usually it will be necessary to take the baby to the Special Care Baby Unit. You may also find that if the staff are sufficiently concerned they will want to start treatment with antibiotics before all the results of the tests are available. In the newborn, it is not satisfactory to give antibiotics by mouth as they are not reliably taken up into the blood stream and so they have to be given into a vein. This too will probably mean that your baby has to be admitted to the Special Care Baby Unit (see p. 116).

Many of the common early problems such as jaundice or the frequently heard but usually insignificant heart murmurs in young babies are often not apparent until after the first 48 hours. With increasing numbers of women choosing to go home early the responsibility for identifying and managing these problems is being removed from the hospital staff and put on to your GP, midwife and later your health visitor.

TESTS ON BABIES

In addition to the examinations of your baby performed during the first few days of your baby's life, which are designed to detect anatomical abnormalities, other tests may be carried out during this time. These are designed to discover certain disorders not apparent on examination, or simply to monitor the extent of problems such as jaundice.

TESTS PERFORMED ON ALL BABIES

It is only justifiable to impose mass screening for a disorder if the diagnosis is not apparent upon routine physical examination and if there are advantages to be gained for the baby from early treatment. The only disorders for which all babies are screened in the United Kingdom are a very rare disease known as phenylketonuria, and the less uncommon condition of under-activity of the thyroid gland (hypothyroidism).

Babies with phenylketonuria are unable to use one of the amino acids present in milk; as a consequence the level of this amino acid in the blood rises and can cause damage to the brain. This problem is excluded by a test which will be performed on your baby by a midwife on the sixth day after starting milk feeds, probably when you are back at home. This test is commonly referred to as 'the Guthrie test'.

The baby's heel will be pricked and spots of blood collected on to absorbent paper. These papers are then sent to a reference laboratory where the blood is extracted from them and analysed. In the unlikely event of your baby's test being thought to be abnormal you will be contacted very quickly and a repeat sample of blood obtained for confirmation, before starting the baby on special milk.

Some blood collected at the same time is used for detection of under-activity of the thyroid gland. A few babies with thyroid problems will be detectable on physical examination but others with less severe impairment, which may none the less affect their later development, cannot be detected without a blood test and will benefit from early replacement with thyroid hormone.

SELECTIVE SCREENING TESTS

It is well known that some inherited disorders are more likely to occur in specific groups of people, and it is obviously helpful to detect them early in life. The most notable example of such a disorder is sickle cell anaemia which occurs predominantly amongst Afro-Caribbean people.

If you are black you will probably have had a special blood test during pregnancy (see p. 26) and if you are known to be a sickle cell carrier, your partner will have been checked too. This will enable the doctors to find out if your baby is at particular risk and a blood sample can be collected from the vessels in the umbilical cord after delivery. This blood is the baby's rather than yours, and it can be tested to determine whether or not your baby has sickle cell anaemia, and if so a course of treatment can be planned immediately.

There are inherited disorders of haemoglobin (the red pigment in the blood) other than sickle cell disease and if you live in a health district with a multiracial population you may find that all babies have blood collected from the umbilical cord in order to screen for these conditions.

The most common, serious inherited disorder amongst white children in this country is cystic fibrosis, (fibrocystic disease or mucoviscidosis). This chronic disorder results in chest infection, failure to digest food and reduced life expectancy. There are probably some advantages for diagnosing this condition early and it may be suspected after examination of the protein content of the baby's first bowel movement or by analysis of blood collected on to absorbent paper. Neither of these tests is totally reliable and they are not universally applied. If there is real anxiety about the possibility of cystic fibrosis a formal 'sweat test' is necessary at about six weeks of age.

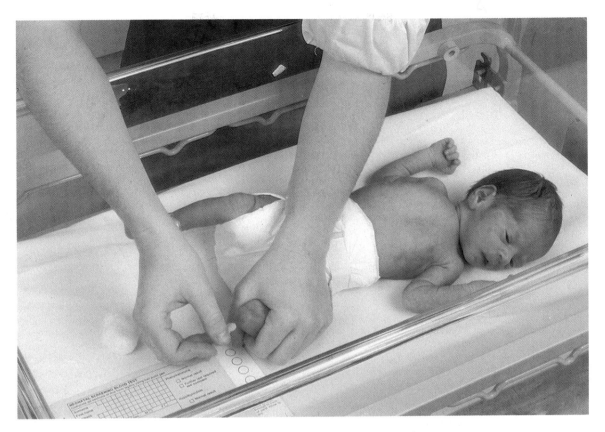

Your baby's blood will be collected by a heel prick on the sixth day, known as the 'Guthrie test', to be analysed for a rare metabolic disorder and for an under-active thyroid gland.

OTHER TESTS IN THE FIRST WEEK

The only reliable method by which to assess the severity of the very common problem of jaundice seen in the first week is to take a blood sample and to measure the amount of the yellow pigment, bilirubin, in it (see p. 121). Only a very small quantity of blood is required and it will usually be collected into a narrow capillary tube from a prick on the side of your baby's heel. The midwives will often perform such routine tests themselves and will only inform the doctor if there is a problem.

Similarly the midwives are ever vigilant for signs of infection and if your baby's umbilicus does not look completely clean, if his eyes are sticky or if there are any suspicious spots or red areas they will take swabs to look for bacteria, often before the doctors have examined the baby. If you are discharged early from hospital the community midwives who visit daily will take responsibility for organizing the routine screening procedures.

GOING HOME

Hopefully you will have been able to prepare home for the arrival of the baby during the late stages of your pregnancy. If your baby is delivered prematurely and you have been unable to make these preparations it may be a good idea to go home for one or two afternoons before the baby's discharge to make sure that everything is all ready so that you are able to relax with your partner during the first few days and concentrate on looking after the baby.

You will be bringing the baby home from the hospital in his own clothes so if possible you should put these out before you go into hospital so that your partner knows what is needed.

It is a good idea to give your baby a feed shortly before leaving the hospital and then if you are lucky you will have time to get things straight before you have to feed for the first time at home.

When you leave the postnatal ward your baby will be carried by one of the midwives and will be given to you at the hospital entrance, as they have responsibility for his safety until you leave the hospital premises. In the car the baby should be carried either in a carry cot strapped in the back seat or in your arms, sitting in the back seat.

THE SPECIAL CARE BABY UNIT

The technology of the modern Special Care Baby
Unit and how it helps low birth-weight babies

Most maternity units now have a ward dedicated to the care of babies with problems. Wards which offer full support for extremely tiny premature babies are increasingly referred to as 'Neonatal Intensive Care Units' (NICU), while the previously widespread title of 'Special Care Baby Unit' (SCBU), tends to be applied to units which are only able to support extremely ill infants for short lengths of time.

In Britain, the majority of health regions support at least one referral unit offering neonatal intensive care. The level of care offered in other regional maternity units will depend to a considerable extent upon local levels of paediatric medical and nursing staff. If your obstetrician has reason to believe that an extremely premature birth or a serious medical problem in the baby is likely, (see p. 61), you may be advised to transfer to the maternity unit with the NICU during your pregnancy. This may well necessitate a stay in the antenatal ward. Alternatively, if this is not possible or if unexpected problems arise after the birth, a team comprising a doctor and a nurse trained in neonatal intensive care (a 'flying squad'), will come with their equipment in a special ambulance to take the baby to the referral unit.

Having a baby taken into special care can be extremely worrying for parents. In many ways it is easier to understand if your baby is born very prematurely – and many NICUs regularly care for tiny babies born at 24 or 25 weeks' gestation. Having a basic idea of the likely reasons can help to allay fears, but more importantly you should talk to the consultant paediatrician in charge of the unit who will explain exactly why your baby needs special care and what the treatments are likely to be.

WHICH BABIES GO TO SCBU/NICU?

Admission to a special care baby unit depends largely on how much care is possible on the postnatal ward in terms of monitoring and attending to minor neonatal problems. The proportion of babies being admitted to SCBUs in recent years has tended to fall as blanket rules have been abandoned, such as the admission of all babies delivered by a Caesarean section or all infants of

diabetic mothers and babies in the 2-2.5kgs (4½-5lb) birth weight bracket. However, the pressure on these units remains very high and there has been a move in a few larger maternity units to establish 'transitional care' areas within postnatal wards. Babies requiring traditional 'special care' procedures, such as phototherapy treatment for jaundice (see p. 121), or tube feeding (see p. 127), can be looked after in transitional care, usually in close proximity to their mothers, thus avoiding unnecessary separation. This also enables the SCBU/NICU to concentrate increasingly on the most vulnerable babies.

The reasons for admission of babies to areas providing these different levels of care are summarized in the table overleaf, but it is important to emphasize that great local variations will be found.

PREMATURITY AND LOW BIRTH WEIGHT

The most common reasons for admission to SCBU/NICU are prematurity and low birth weight. These conditions often, but not always, co-exist. Some babies born at the expected time will have grown poorly in the uterus and be of low birth weight ('small for dates'); the baby of a woman with poorly controlled diabetes may be premature but large. Slightly premature babies and those of low birth weight can usually stay with their mothers on the postnatal ward, but if the gestational age is below 35 full weeks or the birth weight is below 2kgs (4½ lb), they will probably be taken into special care. The distinction between a small baby who is premature but well grown and a baby of the same weight who is mature and 'growth retarded' is important in terms of expected postnatal problems.

PROBLEMS OF PREMATURITY

A baby who is born before the expected time suffers from immaturity of several systems, which leads to a variety of medical and management problems.

The sophisticated technology of the Special Care Baby Unit continuously monitors the progress of the tiny babies in its care.

INEVITABLY ADMITTED TO SCBU/NICU	ADMITTED TO SCBU/TRANSITIONAL CARE
Birth weight less than 1.5kgs (3 lbs)	Birth weight 1.5-2kgs (3-4½ lbs)
Gestation less than 34 weeks	Gestation 34-35 weeks
Severe respiratory problems	Moderate respiratory problems
Severe birth asphyxia	
Severe infections	Minor infections
Convulsions	Low blood sugar
Severe jaundice requiring exchange transfusion	Moderate jaundice requiring phototherapy
Narcotic withdrawal	

TEMPERATURE CONTROL

All babies are at risk of becoming cold. This risk is increased in the premature baby because of the comparatively large surface area in relation to body weight. If babies are to grow properly they need to be able to put most of the energy from their food to that purpose and not to have to expend it on generating heat in order to preserve body temperature. Consequently one of the most important elements in their care is to minimize heat loss. Most premature babies are nursed inside incubators whose temperatures are adjusted according to the size and age of the baby and according to whether or not the baby is wearing clothes. As soon as it is practicable babies are dressed in ordinary baby clothes and usually wear a hat or bonnet. This not only brings pleasure to parents and staff but usefully helps reduce heat loss (see p. 130).

THE LUNGS

In the extremely premature baby, below 26 weeks' gestation, the airways within the lungs are very primitive, and actually create a barrier to the effective transfer of oxygen and carbon dioxide, essential if the baby is to survive outside the uterus. As the baby becomes more mature the airways become more fully developed in structure but often remain functionally immature. This means that they do not produce sufficient amounts of the substance surfactant, which enables the lungs to expand adequately for breathing. This produces the problem known as hyaline membrane disease or respiratory distress syndrome, which is the most serious respiratory problem in the premature baby. While this illness becomes less common with increasing gestational age, it can still occur in a baby born up to 36 weeks' gestation. Babies with this problem have to have help with their breathing in order to survive (see p. 126).

THE CENTRAL NERVOUS SYSTEM

Many aspects of the brain and nervous system are immature in the premature baby. The most important effects of this are upon control of breathing and the ability to suck.

Many premature babies experience frequent pauses in their breathing (apnoeic attacks), and may require help with breathing as a result, even if they do not have hyaline membrane disease.

While many very pre-term babies demonstrate sucking movements, very few babies below 35 weeks' gestation can feed effectively and many babies up to 37 weeks' gestation will not manage all their feeds themselves. This means the baby will have to be 'tube fed' – the administration of milk feeds via a tube passed either through the mouth or nostril into the stomach (see p. 127).

THE IMMUNE SYSTEM

The immune system, which comprises the white blood cells and the lymphoid tissue in the body, helps us to combat infection. During the last part of pregnancy some antibodies are transferred from the mother across the placenta (see p. 41), which help to protect the baby against a wide range of infections, including several months' protection against many of the common viral illnesses which the mother may have suffered, such as chicken pox. Nonetheless, even the well grown, full term infant is not as good as an adult at mounting an attack against infection and this problem is accentuated in the premature baby who has a very poor immunological response and who has not had the full benefit of placental antibody transfer.

As a result the premature baby is particularly susceptible to infection from a wide variety of organisms and may rapidly become extremely ill. Adult patients are usually persuaded that they do not need antibiotics unless there is definite proof of bacterial infection. However, a newborn baby, especially when premature, is so vulnerable that doctors leave nothing to chance and if infection is suspected, antibiotic treatment is often started immediately. Meanwhile the baby will be screened for infection by sending samples of blood, urine and cerebrospinal fluid, together with swabs from the baby's throat, umbilicus and rectum, to the laboratory for detailed analysis at the first suggestion that anything might be wrong.

THE SMALL-FOR-DATES BABY

The full term baby who is mature but small because of poor growth before birth has particular problems related to inadequate nutrition – the baby has literally been starved in the uterus. This may be due to a number of causes, such as poor placental function, or heavy smoking during pregnancy, (see p. 73), but the most notable results are poor temperature control and blood sugar maintenance.

TEMPERATURE CONTROL

During the last part of pregnancy the well grown baby accumulates 'brown fat' within the body, fat which, when put to use, generates significant amounts of heat. This tissue is lacking in small-for-dates babies, a deficiency which contributes to their tendency to become cold in comparison with normal babies. Even at full term a severely growth retarded baby might need to be nursed in an incubator as a result. Babies with lesser degrees of growth retardation will be nursed either on the SCBU or on the postnatal ward in cots with extra blankets. They require frequent temperature checks.

BLOOD SUGAR

Full term normally grown babies who are totally breastfed obtain comparatively little nutrition from the breast in the first few days and maintain their blood sugar by using up food stores laid down during pregnancy (see p. 49). The small-for-dates baby has failed to accumulate enough nutritional reserves and is liable to develop low blood sugar (hypoglycaemia) which if not attended to, can lead to convulsions that might damage the baby's brain cells. To prevent it, small-for-dates babies are

usually fed more than their well-grown counterparts and are given feeds more frequently. The blood sugar is usually checked regularly to ensure that the feeding regime is adequate. A tiny prick is made in the heel, similar to the Guthrie test (see p. 114) and a single drop of blood squeezed out for testing.

SPECIAL CARE OF THE FULL TERM BABY

Your baby may be taken to the SCBU for many other reasons even though he or she may be more mature. This can be bewildering if you have just given birth at the expected time, especially if you are still a bit groggy from drugs or very tired after a long labour. Your baby may need extra help on the resuscitator in the labour ward, and may be taken to the SCBU, the postnatal ward nursery or transitional care area for observation. It is difficult not to worry even though you should be trying to rest. Ask the staff on duty to make sure the paediatrician in charge comes to explain the problem as soon as possible; if your partner is with you he can make the necessary inquiries or find out for you later if you are still worried about anything.

RESPIRATORY PROBLEMS

The common respiratory problems in the premature baby, respiratory distress syndrome and apnoea, have already been described. However, there are many other causes of breathing problems which occur in more mature babies. Occasionally babies develop breathing problems because of a structural abnormality. Such defects are comparatively rare but early diagnosis is important as they may require surgery. These abnormalities can usually be ruled out by obtaining a chest X-ray.

Some babies develop an illness in the first few hours of life which is known as transient tachypnoea of the newborn. It is characterized by rapid breathing which may persist for several days. It is especially common in babies born after elective Caesarean section and is thought to be due to slow clearance from the lungs of the fluid which fills them when in the uterus. It is a less serious condition than hyaline membrane disease.

MECONIUM ASPIRATION

Meconium is the substance inside the bowel while the baby is in the uterus (see p. 109). If the baby is asphyxiated (deprived of oxygen) during labour, meconium may be passed before delivery as a sign of fetal distress, and there is a risk that the baby might inhale some at the time of delivery. If fresh meconium has been noticed by the midwife in the amniotic fluid during labour she will probably have called for a paediatrician to be present at the delivery, who will try to clear any meconium from the airways. However it is sometimes impossible to prevent some of this material being taken into the lungs, and if this happens the airways become plugged so that parts of the lungs fail to expand. Minor degrees of meconium aspiration do not usually create major problems but larger aspirations are serious as they impede breathing and may result in the death of the baby.

PNEUMONIA

A baby may suffer from pneumonia soon after birth, especially if the membranes have ruptured several hours prior to delivery, enabling bacteria to invade the amniotic fluid and cause an infection (see p. 78). It is also possible for the baby to develop pneumonia during the early neonatal period either as a primary disease or as a complication of the other lung problems which have already been mentioned.

A preterm baby aged four weeks and born nine weeks early (left), compared with a 'small for dates' baby aged two weeks, weighing only 1200g at full term (centre), and a normal newborn baby of only two days, weighing 3730g (8lb 4oz).

BIRTH ASPHYXIA

Birth asphyxia arises when the baby is short of oxygen around the time of delivery and is frequently predicted by the signs of fetal distress. The baby is liable to be born very limp with a slow heart rate and may not begin breathing without help. All labour ward staff are trained to resuscitate such babies – indeed it is one of their most important roles. The aim of neotatal resuscitation is to oxygenate the baby so that he or she becomes a normal pink colour with a normal heart rate, and to achieve this without letting the baby become cold.

Many babies who do not cry immediately at birth only require a little stimulation to start them breathing, such as a suction catheter being passed into the upper airway, after which they rapidly 'pink up' (see p. 102). However, babies who are severely asphyxiated will need more active intervention in the form of cardiac massage, and ventilation with oxygen either through a mask held over the face or through a tube passed into the trachea (wind pipe). This is obviously a situation which causes great anxiety to parents because of the possibility of brain damage. If the heart rate rises rapidly and the baby takes over his or her own breathing in the first fifteen to twenty minutes then the outlook is usually good, but if the baby fails to breathe on his own during this time even if he has become pink, then a

Babies with jaundice are treated with ultra-violet light, which changes the yellow pigment in their skin into a form which is more easily dispersed. Although severe cases may need to be taken to the special care baby unit, nowadays light therapy is often available either in a transitional care nursery or beside the mother's own bed on the postnatal ward.

more senior paediatrician is likely to be called to advise on the cause of the asphyxia and its likely result. He or she may want to discuss whether to continue resuscitation (see p. 100).

Babies who have been severely asphyxiated but successfully resuscitated are likely to be nursed on the SCBU. While asphyxiated the blood pressure is often low, which, combined with oxygen deprivation, may lead to a temporary failure of oxygen supply to crucial organs. This could result in swelling of the brain so that the baby may become semi-conscious, have difficulty in breathing properly or suffer from convulsions. It is also common to see a failure of urine production during the first few days. These problems require meticulous monitoring and treatment if adverse long term damage is to be kept to a minimum.

JAUNDICE

Jaundice is yellow discoloration of the skin and is extremely common during the first week of life. The characteristic yellow colour, which in mild form makes a fair-skinned baby look as if he has a sun tan, is due to the presence of a pigment known as bilirubin which is formed from the breakdown of haemoglobin within red blood cells. In adults, bilirubin is carried to the liver where it is converted into a form which dissolves in water, and is passed through the bile duct into the intestine to be excreted in the stool. Even at full term, the livers of newborn babies are immature and do not convert the bilirubin into a soluble form very efficiently. Since newborn babies also have an increased rate of red cell breakdown, a minor degree of jaundice occurs frequently in normal full term babies, but usually disperses without special treatment.

In the normal baby jaundice does not appear until at least the second day. It peaks at a modest level at about the fourth day and has disappeared by the eighth day. If the baby is well and the jaundice conforms to this pattern then no investigations or treatment are needed. In premature babies, it is common for jaundice to persist into the third week but in the absence of other worrying features this is usually regarded as normal.

Jaundice which deviates from these well recognized patterns needs investigation, because the level of bilirubin itself may be dangerous and the underlying cause may be significantly different from the description above. Before its conversion in the liver, bilirubin exists in a form which can cross into the brain and be deposited there. This does not occur to any significant extent in healthy full term babies, but if the bilirubin level becomes high in an ill baby then the amount being deposited in the brain is likely to be increased. This deposition in the brain is known as 'kernicterus' and may lead to a sudden and severe neurological illness. Previously this was most commonly seen in association with severe rhesus disease (see p. 22). If the baby survived, it often led to a severe form of cerebral palsy with associated mental retardation and deafness. However, severe rhesus disease is now mercifully rare, as is this particular form of cerebral palsy.

Some very low birth weight babies do develop deafness, although it is unclear whether this is attributable to jaundice. Even so, it is customary to treat jaundice once it has risen above certain levels or when its rate of rise suggests that it will reach high levels.

If your baby develops jaundice on the first day, your blood group and your baby's will be checked to exclude a blood group incompatibility. Injections of anti-D immunoglobulin to rhesus negative women before or after delivery have led to a dramatic reduction in the incidence of this problem but occasional cases do occur. Nowadays, incompatibility of the ABO blood groups is a more common problem – unlike rhesus disease it may arise in first pregnancies, and cannot be prevented by immunization.

If the bilirubin level rises very much then the baby will be examined closely for signs of infection and a urine sample will probably be collected to see if there is an infection of the urinary tract and to rule out certain very rare metabolic diseases. If jaundice has not disappeared by the eighth day the baby will be examined again and a blood test done to look for rare causes of prolonged jaundice such as structural abnormalities of the bile duct or hypothyroidism (an under-active thyroid gland).

TREATING JAUNDICE

Jaundice is usually treated by phototherapy (light treatment). The baby is nursed naked under a special ultra-violet light which changes the chemical structure of the yellow pigment in the skin so that it can be excreted. As a precaution the baby's eyes are covered with a pad during this procedure so that there is no possibility of them being damaged. Babies under phototherapy usually pass rather runny, greenish stools and they may need extra water to drink. In many hospitals phototherapy for full term babies can be given on the postnatal ward or in the transitional care area so that mother and baby do not need to be separated, important for both reassurance and convenience. Jaundiced babies are often very sleepy but need frequent feeding (perhaps even every two hours) which may be difficult and time-consuming. If your baby does need phototherapy, at least if it is taking place close by, you will not have to keep going to the special care baby unit to feed.

A severely jaundiced baby may require an exchange transfusion, which means that literally all the baby's blood has to be replaced with new blood. This is usually only necessary if the baby has rhesus disease, although it is occasionally required for other forms of blood group imcompatibility. The blood is usually exchanged through a catheter in the umbilical vein (through the navel), although other blood vessels may be used. This is a slow procedure which can take up to two hours, and may need to be carried out again.

PROBLEMS WITH FEEDING

Failure to suck may simply be a sign of prematurity, but some of the drugs commonly used for pain relief during labour have a sedative effect upon the fetus and may cause early suppression of sucking in a full term baby. If a baby who has been feeding well goes off his feeds, the paediatrician is likely to consider infection. A baby who is not feeding well may require admission to SCBU if tube feeds cannot be given on the postnatal ward.

A little vomiting during the first few days is common and provided the baby is otherwise well is unlikely to cause much concern. If however the vomit is green (bile stained), if it is associated with distention of the abdomen or the baby is otherwise unwell it is possible that there is an obstruction in the intestine and the baby will require admission to SCBU for investigations, including X-rays of the abdomen. Obstruction usually arises as a result of a structural abnormality of the bowel such as a narrow segment, a twisted bowel or a hernia in the groin, the latter being especially common in preterm babies. If the X-ray suggests that there is a blockage the baby will probably need to have an operation to clear it, which in many areas may involve transferring the baby to a specialist unit. Neonatal surgery is highly skilled, requiring the services of a specialist paediatric surgeon and of an anaesthetist experienced in treating the newborn.

The great majority of normal babies open their bowels for the first time ('pass meconium') in the first 24 hours (see p. 109). This may be delayed in preterm or ill babies. If there is no obvious cause for delay then the paediatrician will want to find out if there is an obstruction in the lower intestine such as an abnormal anus or a congenital abnormality of the large bowel which again may require surgery.

INTENSIVE CARE OF THE NEW BORN

Certain categories of ill babies are defined as requiring 'intensive' as opposed to 'special' care and they will be cared for in 'cots' (usually incubators) in the special care baby unit specially designated for this purpose. These have a higher level of equipment and staffing. Included in this group will be babies with severe lung disease requiring mechanical ventilatory support or who, although breathing on their own, are requiring constant attention, and babies requiring special procedures such as exchange transfusion. The majority of these babies will be pre-term, though not exclusively.

When a baby comes into intensive care, he or she will be looked after in an area of the ward where the lights are full on round the clock and the air temperature is between 25°-28°C (77°-82°F). The baby will probably have monitoring electrodes stuck on his or her chest and abdomen within minutes of arriving on the ward, and is likely to have tubes passed into the stomach through the nose or mouth. The baby will probably have a drip into an artery and another into a vein. These various leads and tubes will go into a variety of monitoring machines with 'beeping' alarms and flashing lights, and visual display units showing circulatory and respiratory wave forms. Large portable X-ray machines and ultrasound scanners will be moved in and out of the intensive care area during the often frenetic first hours while the support systems are established and the baby stabilized.

This activity is a thrill to the medical and nursing staff, many of whom will have a particular interest in the technology and it is too easy for them to forget that for the parents whose pregnancy has just abruptly and prematurely ended it is a catastrophic nightmare. Once the initial flurry of activity is over and the baby is stabilized in the incubator, the staff are careful to introduce you to the ward and its routines, and will explain the various pieces of apparatus. It is important to understand that the equipment is not actually doing anything to the baby, but rather it is collecting and displaying information so that the staff can assess the baby's clinical conditions without constant handling.

MONITORING BABIES IN INTENSIVE CARE

The baby's temperature will be monitored continuously by a probe on the baby's skin and/or a probe inserted a short distance into the anus. The recorded temperature may be shown continuously on a digital display. Heart rate and respiration are usually recorded from three small electrodes stuck on the baby's chest. Most monitors display the electrocardiograph (usually abbreviated to ECG) and the respiratory wave form on a visual display unit and usually give a numerical value for the heart and respiratory rates.

The oxygen and carbon dioxide in the baby's arterial blood are monitored carefully to ensure that the baby is being adequately but not over treated. (The level of oxygen and carbon dioxide indicate how well the lungs and heart are operating.) Blood for this purpose can be obtained intermittently by inserting a needle into an artery, usually at the wrist or behind the ankle. This is painful for the baby and causes disturbance, so in the first few days when the baby is at greatest risk most people choose to insert a line permanently into an artery (catheterization) so that samples of blood can be taken without handling the baby. The most common place to insert such a line in the first few days is into an artery at the umbilicus, where the line can then be threaded through so that it lies in the aorta, the main artery coming from the heart. After a few days the umbilical arteries close and become impossible to enter and if a line then needs to be inserted it is usually put into the artery at the wrist.

In recent years it has become possible to monitor the blood gases through the skin using 'transcutaneous' electrodes. These warm the skin beneath the electrode so that the tiny blood capillaries expand. The oxygen and carbon dioxide in the blood pass through the skin and can be measured at the surface. Transcutaneous electrodes may be unreliable in babies who are very sick but they have reduced the number of babies who need to have arterial lines inserted and have shortened the time for which those lines need to be left in.

Blood pressure gives a very important guide as to the baby's general condition and helps the medical staff monitor the effects of various treatments. Blood pressure can be monitored directly if there is an arterial line and the blood pressure trace may be displayed with the heart rate and respiration on the video screen. If there is no line it is possible to monitor the blood pressure with a small cuff around the upper arm which can be attached to an automatic inflation device, similar to that used for adults during surgical operations, which measures the blood pressure at preset intervals.

1 Oxygen monitor (monitoring oxygen concentration that baby breathes).

2 Thermometers, measuring air temperature in incubator.

3 Mouthpiece, connecting baby to ventilator.

4 Monitor display, showing heart rate and respiratory trace, can also show blood pressure waveform, temperature and transcutaneous oxygen and carbon dioxide in digital form.

5 Bag and mask, for hand ventilation.

6 Bag of intravenous fluid, with dextrose, sodium and potassium.

7 Porthole, for access to baby.

8 Syringe pump, for intravenous fluids, can also be used for giving continuous feeds.

9 Volumeter pump, for intravenous fluids.

10 Tilting tray, which can be pulled out for access to baby.

11 Skin temperature probe.

12 Conversion to fahrenheit.

13 Skin probe attachment.

14 Display of baby's skin temperature or air temperature.

15 Digital display control button.

16 Control to set air or baby's skin temperature.

17 Control and alarm buttons.

18 Humidifier, for moistening gases in ventilator.

19 Ventilator.

20 Display of pressure wave from ventilator.

APNOEA AND BRADYCARDIA

Apnoeic attacks are periods when the baby fails to breathe. They are particularly common in very premature babies but may occur in any baby as a sign that there is something wrong. Apnoeic attacks may be very brief, with the baby starting to breathe again on his own, or they may be prolonged, requiring intervention by the staff. The baby is resuscitated in the same way as a baby who does not establish breathing immediately at delivery, either by stimulation or by ventilating through a face mask or a tube in the airway (intubation).

Apnoeic attacks are important to prevent as they can be associated with a fall in the blood oxygen content and with circulatory disturbances which may occasionally lead to a long term handicap. If the attacks become frequent the medical staff will try to prevent them either by administering drugs which stimulate the baby's respiration, or by supporting the baby's ventilation either with 'continuous positive airway pressure' (CPAP), or 'intermittent positive pressure ventilation' (IPPV). Either of these techniques may involve the insertion of a tube (known as an endotracheal tube) either through a nostril or through the mouth, which is firmly held in position, probably attached to a hat on the baby's head.

Continuous positive airway pressure is a technique which involves the continuous application of low pressure to the airway. This may be applied either through an endotracheal tube, through a soft prong inserted in a nostril or via a face mask. It has the effect of helping to hold the baby's lungs open and of stimulating the baby's respiration and is very useful in the treatment of hyaline membrane disease and apnoeic attacks.

For intermittent positive pressure ventilation, a ventilator is actually inflating the baby's lungs. If the baby is very sick total ventilation can be used, inflating the baby's lungs many times a minute. As the baby improves the ventilator rate is turned down so that the baby is mostly responsible for his own breathing, receiving just occasional help.

Bradycardia is slowing of the heart rate, and is often seen in association with apnoeic attacks. Pre-term babies quite often suffer brief bradycardic attacks. The causes and implications are similar to those of apnoeic attacks and they will probably be investigated and treated in the same way.

PNEUMOTHORAX

Pneumothorax arises when a lung 'bursts' and a leak of air from the lung leads to an accumulation of air in the space between the lung and the chest wall.

If the leak is only small this may not affect breathing significantly, but if there is an increase in the accumulation of air, the lung is unable to expand adequately and will collapse. In the most serious cases ('tension pneumothoraces'), structures of the mid-line, such as the heart, are pushed over towards the other side and the lung on the opposite side is unable to expand properly. Large pneumothoraces can very quickly lead to cardio-respiratory failure, with the baby becoming blue (cyanozed) from poor circulation. The treatment in this situation is urgent.

Pneumothorax occasionally arises around the time of delivery in otherwise completely well babies. It is, however, more common in babies with lung disease especially when ventilation is required. The treatment is life saving and involves draining the air which has collected between the lung and the chest wall by putting in a tube (a chest drain) through the chest wall. This tube connects to a valve system so that if any further air collects it is drained to the atmosphere, but it is impossible for air to go back the other way.

CEREBRAL HAEMORRHAGE

Some of the blood vessels in the brains of babies born before 32 weeks' gestation seem to be rather primitive in comparison with those in more mature babies. In older babies and adults the blood flow through the brain is controlled in such a way that the brain tissue is protected against the effects of sudden surges and reductions of blood flow. The physiological processes affecting this control are less well developed in the premature baby so there may be sudden changes of blood flow through the primitive vessels, causing them to burst. The result is a cerebral (brain) haemorrhage. The parts of the brain where such bleeding is most likely to start are those around the cerebral ventricles, the fluid filled chambers in the centre of the brain. This is known as periventricular haemorrhage. If the bleeding continues, the haemorrhage may burst into the ventricles themselves (intraventricular haemorrhage) or into the surrounding cerebral tissue.

Such bleeding may occasionally occur in otherwise well premature babies but it is more likely to happen in those who have other problems, particularly lung disease with complications such as pneumothorax.

Haemorrhages are usually diagnosed by an ultrasound scan of the brain. Ultrasound scanning has become very much a part of the ordinary routine of neonatal care. The equipment is very similar to that used during pregnancy to look at the baby in the uterus, and the technique is both painless and safe. The images are obtained by placing the scanner over the anterior fontanelle, the soft part on the top of the baby's head.

A small haemorrhage is usually of no great consequence but more extensive bleeding is a serious event. In the short term the bleeding can lead to a drop in the baby's blood pressure and further deterioration of his general condition. Over the next days and weeks, particularly if blood has escaped into the cerebral ventricle, the fluid filled ventricles may progressively increase in size (hydrocephalus). This happens because the presence of blood within the ventricles interferes with the normal circulation of the cerebro-spinal fluid (CSF). As the size of the cerebral ventricles increases the pressure within may rise, preventing normal development of the surrounding brain tissue. Often this process corrects itself, but if not, the fluid has to be removed to relieve the pressure. This can usually be done by performing a lumbar puncture, which involves inserting a needle into the back and draining the fluid from around the spinal cord. (The fluid in and around the brain is continuous with that around the cord.) While this may sound a difficult procedure, it is easy and safe in a new-born baby and is commonly done while looking for infection.

The more extensive the haemorrhage and the more ventricles have been distended, the greater is the chance that the baby may develop some later neurological handicap, such as a problem with walking. This is a situation which causes concern both to parents and staff. It is extremely difficult at this early stage, when the brain is still growing, to predict what the long term prospects might be for a baby who has suffered cerebral haemorrhage and doctors are usually rather guarded in their advice to parents at this stage. If this happens to your baby, he or she will be monitored closely at the hospital clinic, where the picture will only become clear over the first few years. You will be offered all possible help if necessary (see p. 280).

PATENT DUCTUS ARTERIOSUS (PDA)

The ductus arteriosus is a blood vessel passing between the pulmonary arteries, which come from the right side of the heart, and the aorta, on the left. Before birth the fetus obtains oxygen via the placenta rather than the lungs so it is not essential for all the blood to pass through the lungs. The ductus arteriosus is important before delivery as it enables most of the blood coming from the right side of the heart to by-pass the lungs and to flow into the aorta and hence to the placenta.

The ductus usually closes within minutes of birth as the blood flow to the lungs increases and the baby becomes pink. It is however some time before the ductus becomes permanently closed; if the baby has respiratory disease and has a low blood oxygen level the ductus may re-open, a condition known as patent ductus arteriosus (PDA).

The doctor can diagnose this condition by hearing a typical heart murmur. The presence of PDA can lead to heart failure and may delay improvement in the baby's respiratory condition. If this is judged to be the case the medical staff may attempt to close the ductus by the use of drugs; if this fails, they might operate on the baby, to tie the ductus and then separate it.

FEEDING THE PRETERM BABY

Although extremely pre-term babies often make sucking movements, your baby is unlikely to take a whole feed by mouth much before 33 weeks' gestation, and unlikely to be taking all his feeds that way until after 35 to 36 weeks. In fact some babies do not do so until 38 to 40 weeks. Delay in establishing total oral feeding can often be the sole reason for keeping a healthy pre-term baby in hospital, and is often frustrating for parents.

TUBE FEEDING

The most common way to feed a small pre-term baby is to put the milk down a narrow tube, which is passed through a nostril into the stomach. This feeding tube will probably be secured to the face with some sticky tape and left in place between feeds. When inserting the tube, the nurse checks that it is in the right position by attaching a syringe to it and pulling back a drop of fluid. A sample of the fluid is then dropped on to a piece of litmus paper which turns red if the sample is acid, which shows that it comes from the stomach.

The milk feed is drawn into a syringe connected to the tube and held above the baby so that it flows slowly down by gravity. The amount of milk depends on the weight of the baby and his age – most units start with about 60ml per kilo (1oz per lb) body weight on the first day, 90ml per kilo (1½oz per lb) on the second, rising to about 150ml per kilo (2½oz per lb) over the first five days.

You may be able to hold the syringe and give the feed yourself. Depending on your baby's general condition, this can be done within the incubator or the baby may be cradled in your arms.

FEEDING BREAST MILK

If you eventually want to breastfeed your baby, you will be encouraged to express milk regularly from birth (see p. 154), and your own milk will be put down the tube. Any milk you produce in excess of the baby's needs can be stored in the deep freeze.

Maintaining milk production while the baby is too small to go to the breast can be difficult. Regular expression is the key, but even so you may find you cannot produce adequate milk and the baby might need topping up with formula. Remember that, even if your milk dries up before the baby is able to feed orally, the breast milk he has received will have been given to him at the time he most needed it.

PROGRESSING TO ORAL FEEDS

As the baby grows older and stronger and begins to suck more vigorously, the number of feeds which he is offered orally will be increased. If he tires during a feed it can always be completed by putting the rest of the milk down the tube. The manner in which the sucking feeds are increased will to some extent depend on whether you want to breast or bottle

feed. If you are keen to breastfeed then the staff may be reluctant to offer bottles at all. This is obviously a problem if you go home before the baby, and around this time you may find yourself being encouraged to come back into hospital for a while. If this is not possible you should try to increase your day time visiting so that the baby can be offered the breast during the day and be tube fed at night. Certainly before you take the baby home the staff will be keen to ensure that you can breastfeed successfully right round the clock.

If you intend to bottle feed, the organization is more straightforward and the baby will probably progress steadily through being offered a bottle on alternate feeds to total bottle feeding. If you are at home, the staff will try to arrange the feeding so that bottles can be offered at visiting times and you can feed your baby yourself. This is obviously much easier to arrange if you can let the staff know when you are going to visit. It can be very upsetting to

Even though your preterm baby may still be being tube fed, and his heart rate, temperature and respiration monitored, if he is otherwise well you may be able to take him out of the incubator to hold.

arrive on the ward to discover that the nurses have already had to give your baby his one feed of the afternoon.

Healthy babies of 32 or 33 weeks' gestation often appear eager to suck, and parents may be distressed that the staff do not push the feeding along faster. The reason for sometimes holding back a bit is that very few babies can achieve total sucking feeds before 35 weeks. Trying to increase the number of feeds before this will not bring foward the time when total feeding is achieved or the date of the baby's discharge from hospital, and occasionally results in the baby tiring and the number of tube feeds having to be increased again.

FEEDING IN INTENSIVE CARE

If your pre-term baby needs intensive care he may not absorb milk passed down a feeding tube. In this situation fluids will probably be given as a dilute solution of dextrose through a drip straight into a vein. However, such solutions do not provide a significant number of calories, so if after a few days there is still no likelihood of establishing milk feeds, your paediatrician may choose to drip-feed the baby with solutions of fat, amino acids and carbohydrate together with minerals and vitamins – a process known as 'total parenteral nutrition' (TPN). The nutrition is often administered via a 'long line', a very fine tube which is inserted under special sterile conditions into a vein in an arm or leg and then passed into one of the great veins in the trunk or even into one of the chambers of the heart. This way weight loss is minimized and the baby can begin to grow.

The proportion of very low birth weight babies fed intravenously varies between different units. Some paediatricians prefer to withhold milk until the baby is entirely stable and no longer requires intensive care, while others will begin to feed with milk while the baby is still requiring respiratory support from a ventilator.

TYPES OF MILK

When milk is to be introduced there is some dispute as to what type it should be. Many paediatricians favour using the mother's own breast milk, expressed and given straight to the baby. It is believed that the fine tuning of the content of such pre-term milk is ideal nutrition for the pre-term baby, that it is easily digested and that it contains immunological factors which are not available in any of the formula feeds. On the other hand, babies fed even with their own mother's milk do not regain their birth weight as quickly as babies fed on the formulae specially prepared for pre-term babies which are now available and which have a higher calorie content. As has already been mentioned, pre-term babies do not have the nutritional reserves which tide a full-term baby over the few days before his mother's milk comes in, and a pre-term baby may lose a dangerous amount of weight without these extra calories. However, pre-term babies fed on breast milk can have their growth rate increased by adding small amounts of carbohydrate and/or fat to the milk.

The long term significance of early rates of weight gain is very difficult to assess, which accounts for the variation in feeding regimes from place to place. The feeding regime should be fully explained to you and your feelings taken into account, especially if you have been keen to breastfeed. If you are not sure, ask the staff and make sure you understand their reasons. A mother can feel frustrated and powerless to help her tiny pre-term baby, so expressing milk is a way of positively contributing to her baby's care. If you want to express milk but your paediatrician thinks a special pre-term formula is more suitable for a while, you can always continue to express milk and freeze it. On the other hand, many mothers find continuous milk expressing tedious and tiring, especially if a baby is very premature and may be in special care for three or four months. There are other ways you can care for your baby to compensate for not being able to feed him yourself (see below) and if you can see the benefits of formula feeding in rapid weight gain it is easier to accept.

CARING FOR THE PRETERM BABY

The days of excluding parents from neonatal wards have gone and it is most unusual for a SCBU or NICU ward not to allow free visiting by the parents. Usually you will be asked to remove outdoor clothing and to wash your hands before entering the ward. Units vary as to whether or not they ask people to wear gowns all the time, but you are likely to be asked to put on some form of apron before handling the baby. Even when your baby is at his most ill you will usually be encouraged to touch him, since research has shown the benefit of this sort of contact in promoting growth, and at the earliest opportunity you will be able to hold him, maybe even while the baby still has many attachments in terms of tubes and electrodes. The degree of parental involvement is however at the discretion of the medical and nursing staff and occasionally if they are worried about the baby or if another baby in the same room is critical and requires urgent attention, parents may be asked to wait outside. There will probably be a sitting room within the unit for this purpose, where families can relax and spend time with their other children and prepare hot drinks for themselves.

Most purpose-built neonatal wards have the clinical area divided up so that there is a room, (often known as the 'Hot Room') which will be reserved for babies requiring intensive care, with a series of other rooms for babies requiring different levels of care, probably including some single cubicles for babies who are known to be infected with problem organisms which may be resistant to common antibiotics.

STAFF ON THE SCBU/NICU

The problem for parents in identifying staff within the ward is often complicated by the wearing of operating theatre clothes because of the heat. Some units have a helpful photograph at the entrance to the ward identifying the permanent members of the medical, nursing and support staff, and the staff often wear identifying badges as well. The nursing staff on the ward are likely to be a mixture of nurses and midwives who have done special courses training them in the care of ill newborn babies, and of nursery nurses, who have done a special course training them in the ordinary care of babies.

On the medical side there is likely to be a Consultant Paediatrician with overall responsibility for the running of the ward with a team of paediatric Senior Registrars, Registrars and Senior House Officers whose duties may be divided between the neonatal ward and general paediatric wards.

There will be other frequent visitors to the ward. Amongst these there may be a neonatal nurse or a health visitor who liaises between the hospital and the health visitors in the community. She will try to get to know parents while they are still on the ward and can be an invaluable support at the time of the baby's discharge.

Having a baby on such a ward for many weeks and often at a significant distance from the family home can impose terrible emotional and financial strains. There will be a social worker available who may be able to help with some of these problems. Ask the ward sister how to contact the social worker if you need financial or other support.

There will be other people working on the ward, such as a clerk and cleaners with whom parents often strike up relationships because they may not seem as busy or remote as the medical staff. In addition there are representatives of the support services, such as pharmacists and physiotherapists skilled in working with babies, who will have a commitment to the ward and will become familiar faces to parents whose babies have a long stay.

INVOLVING THE PARENTS

The nurses will be glad to teach you to take over much of the day-to-day care of your baby when you are able to visit the ward, even if he is still in the incubator. He will probably wear a nappy and be clothed in a stretchsuit or nightie – small babies usually wear hats as well to reduce heat loss through the head. First size baby clothes are far too big for pre-term babies and look ridiculous. Some people use doll's clothes for their babies and there are now specialist suppliers of tiny baby clothes specially designed for preterm babies.

The skin on a preterm baby's elbows and knees is very thin and sometimes active babies can rub it until it is quite sore. For this reason babies in some units are nursed on a sheepskin mat rather than on a sheet, which is liable to chafe the skin however soft it is.

You should always wash your hands before handling the baby; you can then open the portholes of the incubator to look after him. You will soon become quite adept at changing and dressing your baby in this confined space. Your baby will seem very small and fragile at first but in fact you will soon discover he is quite resilient.

At the equivalent of about 35 weeks' gestation, a healthy pre-term will be transferred from an incubator into an ordinary cot. From this point onwards his care is very little different from that of a full term newborn baby, except that he will usually be kept in a warmer room.

In the early days the baby is unlikely to have a bath as this is a great disturbance and may make him cold. Instead, he will be cleaned with cotton wool balls dipped in warm tap water. At about 35 weeks, however, he may receive an occasional bath. This is a great thrill for parents and staff, and is always seen as a significant landmark towards going home.

OTHER VISITORS

There is considerable variation as to who, apart from the parents, is allowed to visit the baby. Some units have observation corridors through which the babies can be seen, which eases the problem. Most departments are becoming more flexible in their visiting guidelines and whereas brothers and sisters used universally to be excluded, it is now very common for them to be allowed to come to see the baby and often to touch him. The extension of visiting to grandparents and other friends and family is often limited simply because the presence of large numbers of people makes the ordinary work of the unit very difficult.

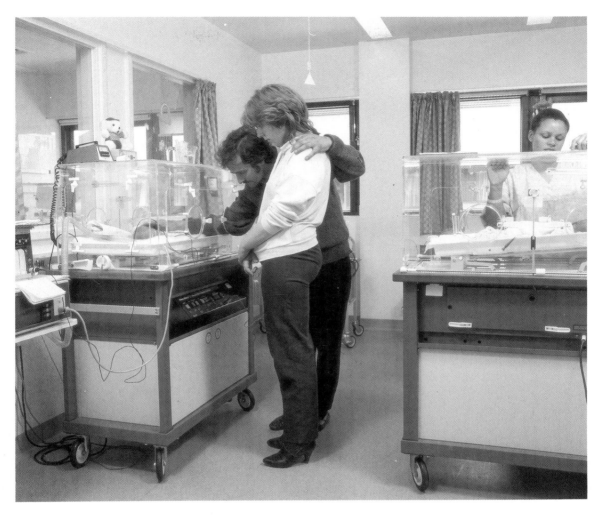

The special care baby unit often seems frightening to parents because of the amount of sophisticated technology used in the care of tiny and vulnerable babies. However most units now allow parents and sometimes other members of the family to visit as much as they like and encourage parents to help in the care of their babies as much as possible.

GOING HOME

One of the questions you will most want to ask about your pre-term baby after the birth is how long will it be before he is able to go home. The answer you are likely to be given is that he will be discharged at around the time you expected him to be born, so that if your baby was born at, say, 33 weeks, he will probably have been in hospital for about seven weeks. This sort of example is true in most cases, although if he has no complications at

all he will probably be home a little earlier. Twins usually go home together, but if you have more babies you might want to stagger their discharge.

You will almost certainly have gone home yourself long before your pre-term baby is ready to be discharged, so it may be helpful to come back into the hospital to room in with the baby for a few days before going home together. Most units have so-called 'mother and baby' rooms for this purpose on or close to the special care ward. This is particularly helpful if you live some distance away and have been unable to visit very regularly.

It used to be the case that strict criteria of age and weight were applied before pre-term babies were allowed home. Now things are much more relaxed. Most units prefer babies to be about 2kg (4½lb) before discharge. Sometimes babies who are mature and feeding well go home sooner. Most units do not apply rules in terms of gestational age but simply want to be sure the baby is feeding satisfactorily.

CHAPTER TEN

BACK TO NORMAL

Restoring your health and fitness during the six
weeks after your baby's birth

For the first few hours after your baby is born, you may find it difficult to grasp the fact that you are now a mother – you may be elated, dropping with fatigue, eager to talk to your partner, family and friends, or just want to be left alone with your baby. However you feel, your body is immediately working to return itself to the normal non-pregnant state.

For women, the postnatal period, known as the puerperium, is a time of adjustment after pregnancy, labour and delivery, during which there is a gradual return to normality in bodily functions. It can conveniently be divided into the immediate puerperium – the first 24 hours after delivery; the early puerperium – the first ten days during which supervision is usually undertaken by a midwife; and the late puerperium, which lasts until six weeks after delivery, at the end of which the postnatal examination is usually performed. The effects of pregnancy can, of course, continue after this time, but the involution of the genital tract – the uterus, cervix and vagina – will have been completed by this time.

THE POSTNATAL WARD

If you had your baby in hospital, your stay could be anything between a few hours for a 'domino' delivery, to seven or ten days for a Caesarean section. The average stay for a first baby is five to six days, depending on your own and your baby's progress. When you go home you will be looked after by your own doctor and a community midwife who will visit you every day until at least the tenth day after delivery. If you had your baby at home, the community midwife will visit every day, probably at least twice a day to start with.

Use your time in the ward to rest and to get to know your baby in the knowledge that there is help at hand whenever you need it. Most units nowadays prefer you to keep your baby with you at all times, and visiting is usually open for fathers apart from a rest period in the afternoon. The number of other visitors and visiting times are very much at the discretion of the individual unit – too many visitors can be extremely tiring.

As well as the midwives who are on hand at all times, you will be examined by an obstetrician every day, a paediatrician will check your baby's progress (see p. 102) and an obstetric physiotherapist will advise you about postnatal exercises and pain relieving techniques (see p. 139).

PHYSICAL CHANGES

While still in the labour ward, like most women, you may put your hands on your abdomen and be surprised and delighted by its softness and 'flatness'. However, this delight is often short-lived – in fact when you examine it properly your body will look saggy and stretched, and you will still look five or six months pregnant. However, this is a temporary state which changes rapidly as the uterus contracts and you begin to regain the strength of the abdominal muscles.

THE UTERUS

By the end of your pregnancy the uterus will have increased in size till it weighs about 1kg (2.2lb). Immediately after delivery the uterus will begin to decrease in size (involute) rapidly. This reduction is brought about by contraction of the muscle fibres, and by reduction in the number of muscle cells, but because of the stretching action of pregnancy the uterus never quite reduces to the size it was before your first pregnancy. On the first day after the birth, the uterus can be felt at about the level of your navel; after about the tenth or twelfth day of delivery it is no longer possible to feel its position in your abdomen.

THE LOCHIA

The vaginal loss that follows delivery is known as the lochia. For the first three to four days this is red and may contain some tiny clots. Subsequently it becomes brown, then yellow, before disappearing altogether. The duration of the lochia is very variable – the brownish loss can last for five to six weeks or can cease after two to three weeks.

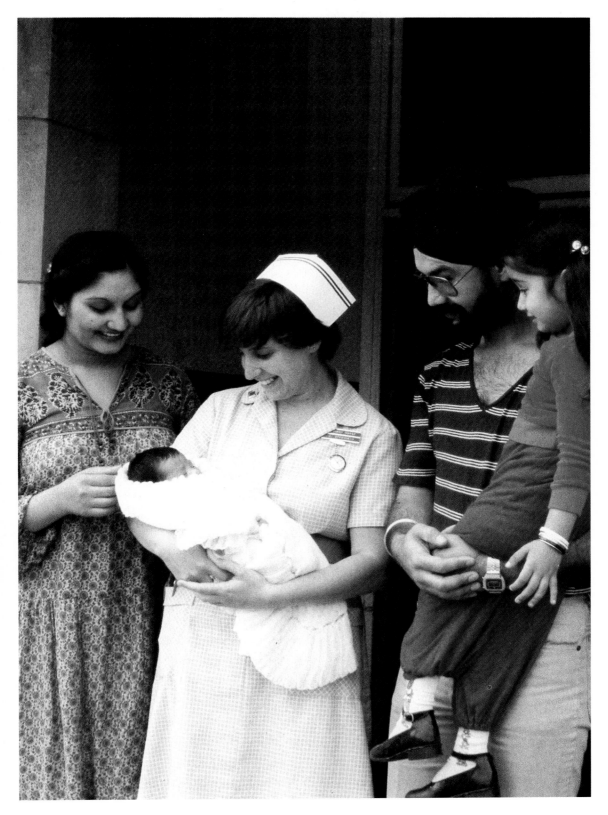

If you are breastfeeding, you may notice that the lochial discharge becomes heavier during a feed. This is because oxytocin, the hormone which causes the 'let down' reflex (see p. 150), also causes the uterus to contract.

Heavy bleeding with clots and abdominal pain is not normal, particularly if it happens after the lochia has turned brown, and should be reported to your doctor or midwife at once. It may mean that a small piece of placenta or membrane has been retained in the uterus and this may necessitate a small operation to empty the womb – an 'evacuation of retained products of conception' (ERPC).

THE BREASTS

Lactation begins about 48 to 72 hours after delivery, with engorgement of the breasts as the milk comes in (see p. 154). Before this time the breasts produce a yellowish substance called colostrum. Milk production is controlled by the hormone prolactin, and the release of the milk, stimulated by suckling, is regulated by oxytocin, as mentioned above. Both these hormones are produced by the pituitary gland in the brain. The mechanisms of milk production and breastfeeding, and the discomforts which may accompany the associated physical changes, are covered in detail in Chapter 11.

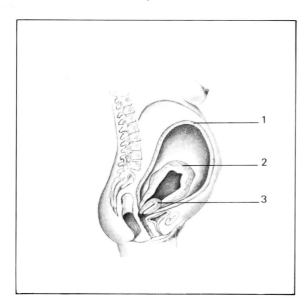

The uterus involutes (shrinks back) to its pre-pregnancy, normal size during the six weeks of the puerperium. 1 The uterus just before delivery. 2 Immediately after delivery; the uterus has shrunk down to about the level of the navel. 3 The uterus six weeks after delivery.

SUPPRESSION OF LACTATION

Some mothers may not wish to breastfeed, or may be unable to for medical reasons – either to do with themselves or their babies. Once the suckling stimulus has been removed then milk production will cease, but the breasts will still go through a period of being painful and engorged. Wearing a good supporting bra and the use of mild painkillers are usually the only treatments required for the few days that this process takes, and this natural suppression of lactation is generally preferred.

It is possible to assist the process with medication, and nowadays the usual treatment would be with the drug bromocryptine, which inhibits the production of prolactin, the hormone associated with milk production. It has to be taken for about fourteen days and tailed off slowly, otherwise lactation can start up again immediately the drug is withdrawn. It can also cause nausea, particularly on an empty stomach. If nausea becomes a problem for you, ask the advice of your doctor or midwife.

GENERAL PHYSICAL CHANGES

Following delivery the average woman loses about 4kg (9lb) in weight just as a result of the excretion of accumulated fluid – so you will notice a great increase in urine output. The circulation returns to normal, but the blood clotting mechanism is exaggerated, which accounts for the increased likelihood of thrombosis (a clot being trapped in a vein) at this time (see p. 72). Hormonal changes are abrupt – oestrogen and progesterone levels fall to non-pregnant amounts within a week.

ABDOMINAL AND PELVIC FLOOR MUSCLES

The abdominal muscles will have been greatly stretched during pregnancy – the waist measurement of the average woman increases from about 68cm (28in) to as much as 125cm (50in)! At first the muscles and their connective tissues stretch easily – but after a while the 1cm (½in) strip of tissue which holds together the two straight abdominal muscles (the recti abdominis) begins to split and the two sides of the abdominal 'corset' separate, leaving a gap which may be as much as 10-12cm (4-5in) wide. This is known as diastasis. The muscles will never again join, but muscle tone can be regained, particularly with the help of exercise (see p. 140).

The pelvic floor muscles will also have been stretched during your delivery and you will probably notice a distinct weakness in your perineal area. It is important to begin exercising these muscles as soon as possible after the birth (see p. 140) –

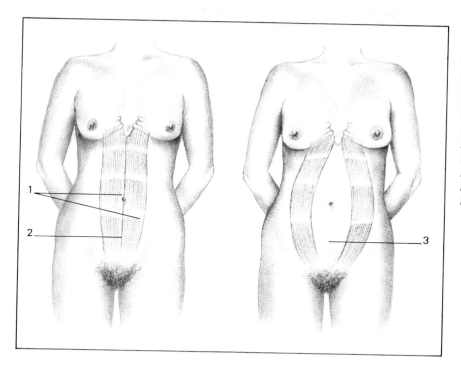

Far left: *The recti abdominis (straight abdominal muscles) before pregnancy (1).* **Left:** *The recti immediately after delivery showing how they have been stretched apart at the linea alba (2). The resulting gap (3) is known as the diastasis recti.*

because they are invisible, the pelvic floor muscles are often forgotten and are not exercised as vigorously as the abdominal muscles.

COMMON PROBLEMS OF THE PUERPERIUM

Even the most straightforward normal delivery can leave a woman feeling drained and tired, and few escape all the rather annoying physical problems associated with the postnatal period. If you have had to have stitches, or your labour was long and your baby quite big, you will probably have some discomfort to contend with after the birth. However, there are ways these problems can be alleviated – one of the most important being adequate rest!

PERINEAL DISCOMFORT

You may experience discomfort in the perineum (the pelvic floor area) even if you have no stitches, because of bruising, swelling and tiny lacerations caused by the passage of the baby. Usually the more stitches that were required the more the discomfort, but there are various ways of relieving it. The most obvious is of course analgesia – your doctor or midwife can give you pain-relieving drugs which will not harm your baby if you are breastfeeding.

Although you may be nervous because of the pain, try to begin your pelvic floor exercising – four tightenings held for a count of four at least every half hour (see p. 32) – as soon as possible. It will help

disperse the bruising and swelling and help to speed the healing process.

A short relaxing soak in a comfortably warm salt bath (a couple of handfuls of salt is sufficient) is very soothing, and cleansing the perineal area in a bidet, if available, is also extremely helpful. Ice packs applied to the area are also soothing, and you may be able to obtain an anti-inflammatory foam which you spray on to your sanitary towel. Ask your midwife about this. Most hospitals can supply an inflatable rubber ring to sit on so that you are not putting direct pressure on the painful area, but it is also a good idea to try and lie flat as much as possible, even for feeding (see p. 153).

If you are very badly affected, the obstetric physiotherapist can give you ultrasound treatment or pulsed shortwave, both of which have a very good effect on bruising and swelling. Infrared heat is another soothing technique which can be used if stitches become infected or are slow to heal. Stitches are usually of material which dissolves in ten to twelve days and so do not have to be removed. They may float away in the bath.

HAEMORRHOIDS AND CONSTIPATION

The action of progesterone on smooth muscle gives many women a predisposition to haemorrhoids (piles) during pregnancy, but they are also a particular nuisance after delivery. They often protrude through the anus as a result of the expulsive efforts of the second stage of labour and become engorged and painful. Your doctor may prescribe an ointment for local treatment plus pain-killers, and ice packs pressed against the affected area are also helpful. Try also to avoid constipation.

During the early puerperium you will probably be experiencing a change in your diet with hospital food, and may also need to take iron pills which tend to make the constipation worse. Try to eat high-fibre food, and a gentle laxative may be prescribed, although it may affect your baby if you are breastfeeding.

Perineal discomfort or haemorrhoids (or both) may inhibit you from trying to open your bowels at first, and some women worry that they may tear their stitches. Try supporting your perineal area with a spare sanitary towel or soft pad of toilet paper as you sit on the toilet – your stitches won't come apart and the support will give you confidence by making the first bowel movement much more comfortable.

'AFTER PAINS'

'After pains' are the cramping pains caused by contractions of the uterus after delivery. They are usually worse after second and subsequent pregnancies and are often most severe during breast-feeding, due to the release of oxytocin (see above). They can be relieved by mild analgesics and usually disappear within a few days of the birth.

BLADDER PROBLEMS

It is not uncommon to have difficulty in passing urine in the first day or two after delivery, particularly if you have had a long labour and a complicated delivery requiring forceps or a Caesarean section, possibly with epidural anaesthesia. This problem is caused by bruising to the bladder and urethra, and it usually resolves itself once you are up and about. Soaking in a warm bath often helps. Very rarely a urinary catheter may be necessary to drain the bladder for a short time.

Sometimes women have difficulty in controlling their urine flow and will notice leakage of urine on coughing and laughing – so-called stress incontinence. This is usually due to weakness of the pelvic floor muscles and can be considerably helped by pelvic floor exercises and other stimulative treatments that can be provided by the physiotherapist.

ANAEMIA

If you lost blood during your delivery, had a Caesarean section or were known to be anaemic before the birth, your haemoglobin levels will be tested on the postnatal ward and you may be given iron tablets. Occasionally a very anaemic mother may require a blood transfusion.

Anaemia is quite difficult to diagnose without a blood test, although severely anaemic women look pale and often complain of fatigue, which improves dramatically when the anaemia is treated. Most women are given a blood test routinely on about the fourth day after the birth from which any unsuspected anaemia can be detected. If you are found to be anaemic it is important to continue to take your iron tablets at least until your postnatal check-up, when your blood will be tested again. This is specially important if you are breastfeeding. If iron tablets make you feel sick, or you are constipated, talk to your doctor or midwife.

BACK PAIN

Backache can be troublesome and is often related to bad posture, exacerbated by ligaments loosened by the hormonal changes of pregnancy. Postnatal back pain is not restricted to any one part of the back and can range from upper back and neck pain, to lumbar or sacro-iliac pain, with very many women complaining of pain between their shoulder blades in the early days as well. If you have had an epidural anaesthetic, you may occasionally experience a little discomfort in your back over the site of its insertion – this is caused by slight bruising around the area and will disappear gradually in the same way that any bruising does.

Even women who did not have sacro-iliac pain antenatally may suffer it following the birth of their babies. It can be triggered by the movement of your legs into and out of the lithotomy position (the position required for forceps delivery or stitching). Try to make sure your legs are lifted into and out of the stirrups simultaneously.

If you experience sacro-iliac pain, your physiotherapist may be able to supply a simple elastic support for your back or an old 'roll-on' is helpful. The positions shown for the relief of sacro-iliac pain on page 49 may be necessary. If the pain fails to respond to these measures, assessment and treatment by a manipulative physiotherapist can be arranged.

The stabbing ache between your shoulder blades which comes on after a few days is almost always due to a bad feeding position such as sitting on the edge of your bed or chair and leaning forward over the baby. It's always worth an extra 30 seconds of crying to make sure you are properly supported (see p. 152). Remember that it is going to take four to five months for your ligaments to return to normal and they are easily strained until then.

Low back pain can also be due to mis-use of your back. Bending over a low cot or changing mat can cause intense pain in the lumbar region which can be aggravated by physical fatigue. Try to avoid this sort of bending, and always go down on to your haunches rather than bending at the waist to pick up something from floor level.

FATIGUE AND MOOD CHANGES

You may feel exhausted after having your baby, so try to get as much rest as you can during the day. Enlist as much help as you can from your partner, friends and relatives (see p. 164).

Mood swings are very common after having a baby, and you may find yourself feeling miserable and crying for no obvious reason. This is particularly likely around the third post partum day and is probably much influenced by the profound hormonal changes which are taking place around this time. It quickly resolves itself and needs no special treatment, except of course sympathy and understanding, especially from your partner and visitors.

Rarely, a very much more prolonged period of depression will occur after childbirth, with physical as well as mental symptoms, such as a disturbance of sleep pattern and loss of appetite as well as lack of interest in your baby and things around you. This is a serious problem and needs advice and treat-ment from your doctor. Indeed you may not realize yourself that it is happening – your partner however may be more vigilant and notice the signs of listlessness, fatigue and general inability to cope which may not be relieved by a reasonable period of rest. If a father does notice this in his partner, he should talk to the doctor or health visitor about it.

THE FATHER AND THE NEW FAMILY UNIT

One of the benefits of a home birth is that after the midwife and doctor have gone home, mother, father and baby can be together. It can be hard for the newly delivered father to have to leave his family in the hospital and go home to an empty house. The past few hours have been a time of stress for him too and he may well feel in need of support.

Pregnancy is a time for emotional as well as physical growth and maturation for both parents. But it would be an odd father who didn't at some stage worry about the impending changes in his life and in the relationship between his partner and himself. Here he is, his family unit suddenly increased by as much as 50 per cent (the first baby makes the most impact) and his whole way of life is about to change for ever. Any man who thinks things will return to exactly the way they were before his partner was pregnant is deluding himself and is going to be disappointed.

A new father finds the task of getting to know and cherish his newborn baby is just as thrilling and emotional as it is for the mother who actually gave birth.

The mature and understanding father will be prepared for tiredness, turmoil and disorganization – he can be a great source of strength and support during what can be a trying and exhausting time for both partners. He may have to show his caring and love in different ways for a while and accept that his partner's sexual desire is at a very low ebb.

AFTER A CAESAREAN SECTION

The most important thing to remember if the baby was delivered by Caesarean section is that you have had a major abdominal operation which will restrict your mobility and require the administration of post-operative analgesia (pain relief). You will need help with feeding and changing your baby every time for at least the first 48 hours, and it may be worth asking if your partner, mother or a friend can stay with you in the hospital to help you during that time.

The physiotherapist will show you the most comfortable way to get in and out of bed and how to support your wound if you need to sneeze, cough, laugh or move. She will show you the early breathing, foot and leg exercises which are routine following any form of abdominal surgery. Having a Caesarean section doesn't mean that you can't breastfeed, although this may be slightly more difficult. If you support the baby on a pillow so that he is not resting directly on your wound, or feed him lying down (see p. 153), you will find that breast-feeding can proceed quite successfully.

Common problems after Caesarean section are difficulty in passing urine and abdominal 'wind', which tends to be worst on the second or third day after delivery. Deep breathing while pulling your abdominal muscles in firmly and gentle pelvic rocking (see p. 32) are both helpful.

You are likely to be in hospital for seven to ten days after a Caesarean section. Many women are grateful that modern birth technology has given them a healthy undamaged baby, but others may feel very disappointed after a Caesarean, especially if they had been hoping for a normal delivery until the last minute. It is helpful to talk to your obstetrician before you are discharged and go over again the reasons for your Caesarean operation to clarify whether this is something that might need to be repeated in a subsequent pregnancy.

COMPLICATIONS OF THE PUERPERIUM

After delivery, most women experience little more than the minor disorders that have already been mentioned above. However there are a few more serious complications which can occur in a few cases.

HAEMORRHAGE

During the immediate puerperium there is a danger of haemorrhage from the site of the placenta within the uterus (see p. 91). After the first 24 hours, the likelihood of severe haemorrhage lessens but may still occur if a small piece of placental tissue or membrane is retained. This is called a secondary post partum haemorrhage; if it happens after you have been discharged from hospital you will have to be readmitted at once and usually have an ERPC (evacuation of retained products of conception).

INFECTION

The genital and urinary tracts are particularly susceptible to infection after childbirth. Urinary infections are likely if you have a long labour or repeated bladder catheterizations. The genital tract is vulnerable because the cervix is open, the tissues are bruised and the lochia neutralizes the normal acidity of the vagina. Other common sites for infection are the breasts, the sites of perineal lacerations or episiotomy and a Caesarean section wound.

If your temperature rises at all, it will be taken seriously by the medical staff as a sign of infection and will be fully investigated. Once the source of the infection has been found you will be given suitable antibiotics to clear it up.

THROMBOSIS

Blood clotting mechanisms are enhanced after delivery, causing a predisposition to thrombosis (blocked circulation caused by a clot in a vein). If this occurs, it is usually in the deep veins of the lower leg, causing pain and stiffness in the calf muscle. Thrombosis in the pelvic veins is also possible, although this usually does not have any symptoms. It usually occurs about ten days after delivery.

Thrombosis is a rare but very serious complication of the puerperium as blood clots can travel to the lungs to cause a pulmonary embolus. Risk factors for thrombosis include a past history of thrombosis, obesity, smoking, age over 35 years, operative delivery especially by Caesarean section, a prolonged labour and dehydration. Superficial varicose veins do *not* predispose to this condition however.

The risk of thrombosis can be reduced by early mobilization, so the midwives will be keen to see you up and out of bed within hours of the delivery. Leg exercises also help (see p. 31), and certain mothers may be given anticoagulant treatment.

PSYCHIATRIC PROBLEMS

Postnatal depression has already been mentioned, but it is worth bearing in mind that it can have an insidious onset and only become manifest weeks or even months after delivery. There is also a very rare complication of the puerperium known as puerperal psychosis, which is characterized by hallucinations, restlessness, insomnia and sometimes expressions of harmful intent towards the baby. This condition needs expert psychiatric help and usually involves in-patient treatment.

BEFORE YOU LEAVE HOSPITAL

While you are in hospital (or are under the care of the community midwife) you will have daily checks of temperature, blood pressure, involution of the uterus and inspection of your stitches. The baby's general health and progress will also be monitored (see p. 111).

RHESUS NEGATIVE MOTHERS

If your blood group is Rhesus negative (see p. 22) then the blood group of your baby will also have been checked by taking a blood sample from the umbilical cord at delivery. If the baby is Rhesus positive then you will be given an injection of Anti-D immunoglobulin within 72 hours of the delivery to prevent you forming antibodies against rhesus positive cells which could cause severe anaemia and jaundice in your next baby.

RUBELLA IMMUNIZATION

If you were not immune to rubella when routinely tested at the start of this pregnancy (see p. 22) then you will be offered immunization by injection. You should avoid pregnancy for three months after this has been given.

THE POSTNATAL EXAMINATION

When you leave hospital or are discharged from the care of your community midwife you will be given an appointment six weeks after delivery for a postnatal check-up. It is frequently seen as the 'signing-off' consultation, whether it is with your own doctor or the hospital obstetrician. Although this check is primarily concerned with the physical aspects, most good doctors will be equally interested in you as a person; remember that the postnatal check is to establish *your* state of health, not to find out how your baby is progressing, which is done separately at the child health clinic or hospital paediatric clinic (see p. 190).

It is important to keep this appointment – in the flurry of looking after a newborn baby it is easy to ignore your own state of health, but ultimately both yours and your baby's well-being may depend on it. Use the check-up to air any worries you have about yourself – write them down beforehand like you did at antenatal visits in case you forget when the time comes.

THE PHYSICAL EXAMINATION

The postnatal check is very like your early antenatal visits. Blood pressure, weight and urine are all checked and you may have a blood test as well if you were anaemic immediately after the birth. Your breasts will be examined, whether you are breast-feeding or not, and the doctor will check your abdomen to see that the muscles are returning to normal.

You will be given an internal examination to check the uterus, cervix and vagina, ensuring that any stitches or laceration have healed and that the vaginal walls are neither too tight nor too lax. The doctor will also take a cervical smear for testing if this was not done antenatally. If you have resumed intercourse let the doctor know if you have experienced any discomfort and he or she will advise you on the best course of action.

The doctor will also want to know when the lochia ceased and if you have had any subsequent bleeding or discharge. He or she will also want to know if menstruation has begun and will probably discuss contraception with you or refer you to the family planning clinic.

The doctor will also want to know how you are feeling about your baby, whether you are eating properly and getting enough rest, and how the rest of the family have reacted to the new baby. If any problems, physical or emotional, remain, make sure that a further appointment is made to assess your progress. There is no need to put up with backache, perineal discomfort, pain during intercourse, stress incontinence or a feeling of constant fatigue or depression. Your doctor is there to help you return to physical and emotional comfort and strength, so don't feel that you are bothering him with your anxieties.

POSTNATAL EXERCISES

Most women will find that quite a lot of regular exercising will be necessary to firm and strengthen weak stretched muscles – and during the first few postnatal weeks this may be the very last thing you feel like doing or have time for. However, one of the causes of fatigue following your baby's birth is the fact that your abdominal and pelvic floor muscles aren't able to carry out their normal role of supporting your internal organs properly. Nor are they able to give proper support to your spine, which, together with the softened state of its ligaments, makes it much more vulnerable to injury.

Apart from the immediate aims of reducing fatigue and the risk of back damage, the long term aims of postnatal exercises are also important. Every woman wants to regain her figure or even improve on the shape she had before pregnancy – the tape measure and her old clothes are cruel critics of the state her body is in. If she looks good, the chances are she'll feel good too. So much for the exterior figure; but there is an interior 'figure' as well – the shape and strength of the pelvic floor muscles, the vagina and all the connective tissue and ligaments which go to make up this incredibly important part of the female body. Even when clothes fit and visible muscles are firm and strong again, because the pelvic floor area is out of sight it is often out of mind, too, and a woman can be storing up long term trouble for herself in terms of stress incontinence, prolapse and sexual dissatisfaction if the pelvic floor remains lax.

EARLY DAYS

Unless you have been following a rigorous exercise programme during the whole of pregnancy your motto for postnatal exercising must be 'slowly but surely'. A sudden return the aerobic workout of a year ago is ill advised and foolhardy.

For the first few days concentrate on foot exercises and pelvic tilting (see page 32), which you should now do lying on your back with both knees bent, standing up, or sitting on a chair. (Omit pelvic tilting on all fours until your vaginal loss is no longer red or brown.) Pelvic floor tightening and relaxing (see page 32) can be started while you are still in the labour ward. Some women will have reasonably normal sensation in this area, while others may find it difficult to control these muscles at all during the first few days!

'Little and often' is the best way of dealing with the early postnatal exercises. Pelvic floor and abdominal muscle work can easily be carried out whilst you're feeding, day or night. Progress the strengthening effect of these gentle exercises by holding your tummy muscles in while you count slowly – first up to six – then eight, ten, and finally twelve. Vary your pelvic floor work too; sometimes draw the muscles inwards and upwards, then relax at once; other times, contract the muscles – count up to four and then release slowly.

Postnatal exercises
1 Curl ups
Lie on your back with your knees bent up high. Draw your abdominal muscles in, lift your head and shoulders from the floor and curl up as high as you can, reaching your hands towards your feet. Try not to jerk upwards, and don't tuck your toes under something heavy or hold on to your legs. Hold the position for a moment, without holding your breath, then lie back slowly.
Increase the strength of this exercise by staying curled up for longer each time – up to 30 seconds.

2 Curl downs

Sit on the floor with your knees bent up high, your ribs lifted, abdomen pulled in and your arms stretched out in front of you. Gradually round your back and curl down slowly; stop when you reach half way – hold the position a moment then return to your starting position without holding your breath. Increase the time you hold the position gradually to 30 seconds.

3 Side bends

Lie on the floor with your knees bent up high. Draw your abdomen in firmly and stretch your right hand towards your right foot, bending sideways – then return to the middle. Repeat to the left. At first, bend to one side and then rest in the starting position; as you get stronger move from side to side like a clock's pendulum, but make sure your abdominal muscles are held in firmly all the time.

4 Twisters

Once again, lie on the floor with bent knees and abdomen well drawn in. This time stretch your right hand towards your left foot, twisting your body from the waist – then return to the floor. Repeat to the other side.

POSTURE

The way you sit and stand after birth can reduce the size of your waist by as much as 10-12cm (4-5 in)! Slump in your chair or walk about with rounded back, drooping breasts and sagging abdomen and it will take you much longer to regain your normal shape. Sit well in to the back of your chair, with a cushion behind your waist and bosom lifted, and you'll be five centimetres 'thinner'; stand and walk 'tall' – breasts and ribs lifted, bottom tilted under – and centimetres drop off your waist measurement! Your body has forgotten its normal upright posture after months of adapting to an increasing abdominal bulge, so make use of mirrors and shop windows constantly to check on your posture. It is important, too, to choose a stroller or pram with handles that are not too low for you (see p. 176).

STRONGER EXERCISES

Hopefully an obstetric physiotherapist will have seen you in hospital, assessed the strength of your muscles, shown you the gap between your abdominal muscles (see page 135), and will have helped you cope with problems such as perineal and back pain. She will have suggested exercises to be done regularly at home which will strengthen your abdominal and pelvic floor muscles and close the gaping space in front. The width of the gap between the recti abdominis varies from woman to woman – a lot depends on her height and pelvic shape, and the size and number of babies is important too.

To check your own abdomen, lie on your back with your knees bent up high. Put two or three fingers in the midline just below your umbilicus and press them into your abdomen. Then draw your abdominal muscles in firmly, curl your head and shoulders up from the floor and reach for your feet with your other hand. You will feel your two recti come together as you lift up and then move out sideways again as you lower back. Some women may have a wide gap – as much as ten centimetres (four inches) or more to start with. Others will find that the space is only a couple of fingers wide.

Eventually, the two recti muscles should lie side by side, about 1cm (½in) apart, and should feel firm and strong when they work.

WHEN TO EXERCISE

The amount of spare time for exercises will be strictly limited at first – there are many other demands on your time – so restrict yourself to the four illustrated on pages 140 and 141, and do them as often as possible. However, don't neglect your pelvic floor exercises which can be done at any time.

Try to find three or four short periods during every day to lie down and do these exercises. Start by doing each one eight times and gradually increase up to 20. Once again, 'Little and often' is better than fifteen minutes late at night once a week when you're feeling guilty because you haven't thought of exercising for days!

These exercises are designed gradually to improve your muscle control and strength so that when your baby is a few months old, you will be fit for whichever form of normal exercising you prefer. It can be dangerous to go to an intensive exercise class to get fit – only start when you are fit and your muscles are strong again. Make sure you tell your exercise teacher or coach that you have recently had a baby when you do take up any new form of exercise. Some local health centres offer postnatal exercise classes given by a physiotherapist, so it might be worth checking this.

RESUMING SEXUAL INTERCOURSE

There is no reason to wait until after your six-week postnatal check before resuming sexual intercourse, unless your doctor advises it because of a particular problem. Resumption of intercourse is very much a personal decision and most men these days understand that, physically and mentally, their partners may not feel like full coitus for quite a long time. Apprehension, the soreness from stitches or bruising and vaginal dryness may make the first attempt rather uncomfortable.

When sex becomes attractive again (after a considerable time for many women), it's worth bearing one or two points in mind to make things more relaxed. Use a smear of KY jelly or another lubricant just inside the vagina and vulva and forwards to the clitoris. Post partum dryness can sometimes be a transitory problem, but if you are breastfeeding your oestrogen levels are low which may make the vagina slightly inflamed and tender.

A nervous woman will feel more confident if she is on top so that she can control the amount of penetration that feels comfortable. Both partners may be unable to relax for fear of waking the baby – if this is the case it will not do any harm to move the cot into another room for a while.

Ovulation does not normally resume until two or three months after delivery in mothers who are not breastfeeding, but can occur as early as six weeks, so contraception does need to be considered. In breastfeeding mothers the return of ovulation is delayed and menstrual periods may not return for many months. However it is important to remember that it is possible to conceive while breastfeeding.

CONTRACEPTION

Contraception may be the last thing on your mind when you have just had a baby, but if you want to space your family then it makes sense to consider various options at this time.

The midwife or doctor advising you on family planning will often start by discussing the method you used before becoming pregnant. In some circumstances it may be possible merely to return to this exactly as before, but in others certain modifications are needed because of changes brought about by the pregnancy.

THE PILL

If you are breastfeeding then the combined oestrogen-progestogen pill is not usually recommended as it can reduce the amount of milk produced – the progesterone-only pill, sometimes known as the 'mini pill' is suggested instead as it has no effect on lactation. It is usually started around the twenty-first day after delivery and must be taken daily. It is not quite as effective as the combined pill and a change is generally recommended to alternative contraception once breastfeeding is discontinued. For non-breastfeeding mothers either pill is suitable.

THE INTRAUTERINE DEVICE (COIL)

If this is your chosen method of contraception then it can be fitted at your six-week postnatal check. Insertion before this time is not recommended because the uterus has not regained its normal size. The fitting of an intrauterine device is much easier once you have had a baby as the cervix has been stretched. This makes it a method worth considering even if, in the past, you may have rejected it.

THE CAP OR DIAPHRAGM

Even if you have used this method in the past you will need to be fitted for a new diaphragm once you have had a baby. This is best done at the six-week postnatal visit, as by this time the genital tract should have returned to normal. The stretching of the vagina during delivery, however, will probably mean that you will need a slightly larger sized diaphragm than before.

THE SHEATH

This popular method of contraception is often a sensible choice for the early post partum months. No preliminary fitting or insertion is required and it may be a relief to transfer the responsibility for contraception to your partner for a while. This method is most effective if used in combination with vaginal spermicidal cream or pessaries.

INJECTABLE CONTRACEPTIVES

It is possible to prevent pregnancy by the injection of a long-acting hormone, progestogen (Depo Provera). This is commonly used in developing countries and its effects last for about three months. However it sometimes produces rather irregular vaginal bleeding and the return of fertility can sometimes take up to a year, so its use is recommended only in special circumstances.

STERILIZATION

You may consider that after this pregnancy you do not want any more children and are looking for a permanent form of contraception. If you are thinking of sterilization then you should discuss this with your obstetrician and your GP before the birth.

Nowadays it is very unusual for a sterilization operation to be performed straight after you have delivered. This is because the procedure is associated with more risk and produces an unsightly scar. If a sterilization has been agreed, it is much more likely that you will be asked to return to the hospital when the baby is about six to eight weeks old and have the operation performed via a laparoscope – a telescopic instrument which is inserted just below the umbilicus (navel). This procedure can be performed as a day case or with just an overnight stay and you can usually bring the baby with you.

It may be that your partner has decided he will be sterilized, in which case he will undergo the operation of vasectomy and will need to discuss this with his doctor and the local hospital. Vasectomy operations are not immediately effective and so you will have to consider alternative methods of contraception until the stored sperm supplies have been ejaculated.

Although the operations of both male and female sterilization are meant to be permanent and reversibility cannot be guaranteed, they are associated with a small failure rate.

THE RHYTHM, TEMPERATURE AND MUCUS METHODS

These rather unreliable methods of contraception are based on the avoidance of intercourse around the time of ovulation. Because regular ovulation may take some time to re-establish itself after delivery these methods are inappropriate for use in the postnatal period.

FEEDING THE BABY

The essentials of feeding for the young baby,
whether you choose breast or bottle

Apart from the birth itself, feeding is probably the aspect of babycare that most preoccupies new parents. Feeding is fundamental to the well-being of a new baby and is a positive symbol of the love and care that parents can give to their child. Whether your baby is fed by breast or by bottle, if feeding is going well you can see the benefit to your baby by the way that he is thriving, and the pleasure he obviously derives from it.

You will probably be asked at the antenatal booking clinic how you intend to feed your baby. Many women will have made the decision already; others may not like the idea of breastfeeding or may be undecided. The midwife will probably discuss the pros and cons of breast and bottle feeding with you during your pregnancy, and there is usually a session on feeding in preparation classes run by hospitals, clinics and others. If you haven't made up your mind early in your pregnancy, you still have plenty of time to think about it before the birth. The following guidelines may help you.

BREAST OR BOTTLE

Every woman is naturally equipped to feed her baby, yet as recently as twenty years ago, as many as 75 per cent of all babies in the West were bottle fed. This statistic is now changing, as the advantages of breastfeeding are being re-established, and women are becoming able to make informed decisions for themselves. The two most powerful reasons for favouring breastfeeding are the nutritional suitability of breast milk for the human baby, and the great psychological pleasure which successful breastfeeding brings to mother and child. But there are other factors which also need to be considered, such as allergy, medication, convenience and expense.

NUTRITIONAL FACTORS

Human milk is by definition precisely formulated for the nurturing of human babies, and, provided that breastfeeding is successfully established, is always completely satisfying. There is no doubt that un-treated cow's milk as delivered from the dairy is an unsuitable feed for human infants on several counts – not surprisingly, since it is perfectly formulated for calves!

It has a higher protein and lower carbohydrate content than does human breast milk, and although the contribution of fat to its overall calorie content is similar to that of breast milk, there is a higher proportion of saturated to polyunsaturated fat. Just how significant some of these differences are is still unclear, but there is no doubt that the high protein content makes it quite unsuitable.

Another great area of difference is in the mineral content. In contrast to other mammals, human milk has a particularly low sodium (salt) content. The young baby's kidneys have difficulty in dealing with too much sodium and in trying to get rid of it, the baby loses water as well, subsequently becoming dehydrated. This can be dangerous. Human milk has a fairly low iron content but iron is particularly well absorbed from it. Untreated cow's milk has an even lower iron content and far from being well absorbed, it provokes bleeding from the intestine. As a result a baby fed with doorstep milk is likely to become anaemic.

All the basic infant formulae are based on cow's milk, although they may have vegetable fats or products from other animals added. The formula manufacturers have paid meticulous attention to modifying cow's milk so that it more closely resembles human milk. The protein content has been reduced to the minimum levels recommended by the World Health Organization, although these still exceed the protein content of breast milk. The nature of the protein has been changed so that it is more easily digested. The carbohydrate content is increased, the ratio of polyunsaturated to saturated fats is adjusted and the sodium reduced. Iron is less well absorbed from formula feeds than from breast milk, so most have iron added, as well as other minerals and vitamins, usually having a higher level than human milk.

When looking at the crude values of protein, fat and carbohydrate in infant formula, it appears that there is little significant difference between formula

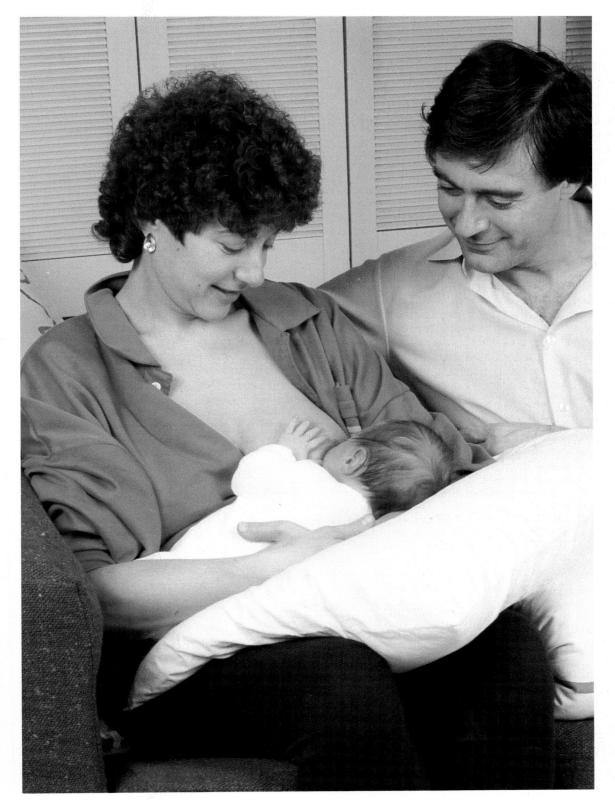

milk and breast milk. However, there are inevitably many more subtle differences that remain, simply because formulae are not based on human milk.

PSYCHOLOGICAL FACTORS

In recent years particular emphasis has been placed on the evidence that a stronger mother/child relationship is forged between mothers and breastfed babies, particularly when the baby is fed soon after delivery. This does not of course mean that the bottle fed baby is at a psychological disadvantage; in very many individual instances, this is clearly not the case. There is no doubt however that the great majority of women who breastfeed do enjoy the experience and feel especially close to their babies as a result. Once breastfeeding is established it can be the most simple, relaxing and pleasurable activity for both parties. Indeed, some women continue to breastfeed well beyond twelve months just because of the pleasure it brings, for in the West at least, by this age there is no nutritional advantage in continuing to breastfeed.

However, it would be wrong to ignore the fact that some women do not enjoy breastfeeding and that they suffer it out of a sense of duty which can easily turn to a feeling of guilt when they stop. It is difficult to see how this benefits the developing relationship; if you feel like this, bottle feeding would probably be a better option, since you can still hold your baby close and cuddle him while feeding from a bottle, and the baby enjoys feeding from the bottle because that is what he is used to.

A small proportion of women who have a genuine desire to breastfeed find that they are not natural breastfeeders: they appear to have a poor supply, or they find the sensation of feeding unpleasant. Women like this often eventually change to the bottle with a significant feeling of sadness.

FATHERS AND BREASTFEEDING

Fathers, too, often have ambivalent feelings about breastfeeding. Rationally, they will agree that 'breast is best' when presented with the facts, but first time fathers especially, who have been used to thinking of their partners' breasts in terms of sex, may have difficulty in making the psychological shift to seeing them as much more functional objects. Some men also resent the closeness of breastfeeding, as their partners seem to be utterly absorbed in the baby to the exclusion of the father. Yet others miss the chance to be able to contribute to their baby's care in a positive way.

A surprising number of women worry about starting to breastfeed, or give it up, because of their partners' reaction. If this seems to be the situation when you are thinking about breastfeeding, or once you start, it is best to try to talk it through. Your health visitor or doctor may be able to help if you feel that your relationship as a couple is suffering. Bottle feeding does sometimes solve this type of problem without doing any harm to the baby and being able to share the feeding can be a positive advantage (see below).

PROTECTION FROM INFECTION

It is worth bearing in mind that even breastfeeding for a few days can give your baby the benefit of antibodies in the milk that will protect him from dangerous infection. On the world scale, the overriding reason for advocating breastfeeding is the avoidance of gastroenteritis. The breastfed baby has the advantage of receiving milk which is itself clean and contains specific factors which increase the baby's resistance to infections of this sort. These immunological factors are particularly abundant in the colostrum produced by the breast in the first few days after delivery; infant formulae obviously cannot contain these immunological factors, are themselves easily contaminated by bacteria and could be fed to babies in bottles which have not been properly cleaned.

In developed countries, however, which have good water supplies and sterilizing equipment readily available (see p. 158), it is easier to be sure that bottle feeds are not contaminated. While it is still true to say that infantile gastro-enteritis is more common in bottle than breastfed babies, babies in the West do not usually succumb to the problems of chronic infection.

ALLERGY

Within some families, there is a significant incidence of allergic problems, such as asthma, eczema and hay fever. Such families are known as 'atopic' (see p. 270). Mothers in this situation are often advised to breastfeed their babies, for while it does not offer total protection against the development of atopy, it might 'limit its severity. The evidence in this area is rather conflicting; some research seems to suggest that breastfeeding might actually predispose a baby to atopy. Certainly you shouldn't feel guilty if you are in this situation and you elect to bottle feed.

If young babies are fed ordinary cow's milk, a significant proportion are found to be allergic to the protein in it. A sign of this is if the baby passes blood-stained stools; less commonly, the baby may develop swelling round the mouth and throat which

Breastfeeding is very convenient as you can feed your baby more or less anywhere, helped by discreet use of a bulky jumper, coat or shawl. Even a trip to the local playground with older children need not be curtailed when your baby is hungry.

may lead to difficulty in breathing. These reactions were relatively common with early infant formulae, but as these have been improved, reactions like this have become very rare. Babies who are found to be sensitive to cow's milk protein should either be breastfed or given an alternative formula. Some doctors advise the use of a soya milk but this is not always the answer, as a significant proportion of babies who are sensitive to cow's milk are also sensitive to soya. In this case there are special milks available on prescription.

Babies often grow out of cow's milk sensitivity and in later childhood cow's milk products can be reintroduced. Your doctor will advise you about this. If one child of a couple has had this problem there is an increased chance that subsequent children will also be affected, and breastfeeding should be seriously considered.

MATERNAL MEDICATION

You may assume that any medicines that you are taking will appear in the breast milk. Often however the concentration of the drug in the milk is very low and will not cause any problems for the baby. If you

do have to take medicines you should discuss with the medical staff whether breastfeeding is advisable: the answer will usually be 'yes'. Once you have left hospital, if you have to go to the doctor for any reason while breastfeeding and he is likely to prescribe drugs, let him know that you are breastfeeding. There are often several alternatives which he could prescribe for a given condition, and he will choose one that is safe to take while breastfeeding.

CONVENIENCE

One of the great attractions of breastfeeding is its convenience. It needs no special preparation, and there is always enough available for your baby's needs. By contrast, bottle feeding needs organization and forethought; bottles have to be sterilized every day, feeds have to be made up in advance, or you have to make a hungry baby wait while the feed cools down.

If you breastfeed, you can feed your baby almost anywhere and at any time. But while many women will happily breastfeed in public places and at social gatherings, it should be remembered that there are others who are more inhibited and who prefer privacy. For these women breastfeeding can be slightly more restricting. In addition, although it is probably becoming less common, it is also the case that many people still feel uncomfortable in the presence of breastfeeding women, and while this may seem preposterous, it should be respected.

Buildings such as airports and railway stations usually incorporate a room for feeding and changing babies, but the appearance of such facilities in the more traditional restaurants, cafés and shops frequented by nursing mothers is lamentably slow, even when the establishment specifically caters for babies and children. This is something worth campaigning for.

Even if you are breastfeeding, when you go out with your baby you do need a certain amount of paraphernalia with you in terms of changing equipment and clean clothes. However, the problem is greater if you are bottle feeding. You need enough bottles to cover the time you are going to be out and you need to be particularly careful about hygiene. In addition you may feel that you need to be able to warm the milk before giving it to your baby, although this is not strictly necessary (see p. 161).

Bottle feeding is convenient however in that it can be done by another person apart from the mother. In terms of cementing the family unit, it is a great help for the father to be able to give some of the feeds, and if you are going back to work within a few weeks of the birth or simply want to go out somewhere without the baby, his feeds can easily be arranged. Some women do organize their lives so that they are able to leave expressed milk to be bottle fed to their babies while they are out, but this requires very considerable motivation (see p. 154).

EXPENSE

It is interesting how rarely people bring the question of expense into the decision as to how to feed their babies. In fact the outlay on bottles and sterilizing equipment, together with the continuing cost of infant formula, is quite considerable, while breast-feeding is of course free.

OTHER FACTORS

The stools of a breastfed baby are usually soft and inoffensive, whereas some bottle fed babies' stools are occasionally rather smelly. It is also true that the stools of a breastfed baby are more acidic and that they tend to have fewer nappy rashes.

Although they probably rarely influence the decision on how to feed, some other important points are worth mentioning. Breastfeeding helps the uterus to contract efficiently in the days after delivery (see p. 132) and, as it uses up fat specifically laid down during pregnancy to promote the production of breast milk, breastfeeding speeds up the regaining of your figure.

THE CHOICE

The majority of women make the choice about feeding their babies not because of the finer points of protein concentration or stool acidity but as the result of attitudes which will have developed from those within their own families and environment. Many women who are currently of child bearing age will themselves have been bottle fed during the fifties and sixties when breastfeeding was at a low ebb, and they will never have contemplated feeding their own babies. Conversely, it will never have occurred to other women that they will do anything other than breastfeed. The choice must be your own but it is inevitable that in the present climate you will be encouraged to breastfeed. What is essential is that this encouragement does not turn into pressure, and that it is backed by helpful support during the first two or three weeks after the birth while breastfeeding is being established. It is worth remembering that modern infant formulae provide an excellent food and the choice of feeding method should not become a battle ground.

BREASTFEEDING

Breastfeeding is a natural part of the physiology of child bearing; women do not have to do anything to make their breasts produce milk once the baby is born. Babies are also born with the ability to suck (see p. 104). However bringing these two in-built processes together especially for the first time often needs some guidance. Understanding how breast-feeding works through some knowledge of simple anatomy and physiology is an important start.

THE STRUCTURE OF THE BREASTS

The breasts lie over the muscle on the front of the chest; before pregnancy they are largely composed of fatty tissue, formed into a roughly circular shape except where they extend up towards the armpits. Each breast is divided up into about eighteen segments. Within the fatty tissue of each segment is a series of tiny sacs, each of which has a lining of cells which are potentially milk-producing, surrounded by muscle cells which can squeeze the milk from the sacs. All the sacs within a segment drain into a milk duct which extends towards the nipple, so that there are about eighteen openings at the nipple. Just behind the nipple each of the milk

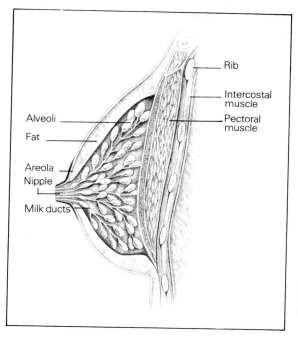

The structure of the breast. During pregnancy, the number of milk-producing sacs increases. The breast is divided into eighteen segments, with milk draining from each to a separate duct.

ducts has a slightly widened part where a limited amount of milk may collect.

The pigmented area around the nipple is known as the areola, upon which may be seen small raised areas, known as Montgomery's tubercles. These are thought to secrete lubricants which help to protect the skin of the nipple and keep it supple.

During pregnancy the breasts increase in size and the nipples tend to elongate under the influence of hormones, in particular the oestrogens produced by the ovary and placenta which promote an enormous increase in the number of milk-producing sacs within each segment of the breast. During the last two or three months of pregnancy the sacs begin to produce colostrum, the 'pre-milk' which is produced until the baby is a few days old.

Once the baby has been born, the levels of oestrogen fall dramatically and enable the main milk-producing hormone, prolactin, to make its presence felt so that the cells lining the sacs within the breast begin to manufacture milk. This happens even if the delivery is very premature.

HOW BREASTFEEDING WORKS

The more often the baby goes to the breast the more rapidly the prolactin levels rise and milk production is established. It is thought to be exceedingly rare

When the baby suckles on the areola (1), nerves send messages (2) to the pituitary gland in the brain (3) which secretes the hormone oxytocin. This causes the muscle cells of the alveoli to contract (4), squeezing milk down into the ducts and out through the nipple.

for the breasts to fail to produce milk at all, but where some difficulties can arise is in the transportation of the milk from the sacs where it is made, down the ducts to the area behind the nipple from which the baby can suck it. This movement of milk is known as the 'let down' or 'draught' reflex, and can be felt as a tingling or prickling sensation.

The nipple area is richly supplied with nerve endings which are stimulated when the baby sucks upon the areola. Messages are carried along the nerves to the pituitary gland at the base of the brain which secretes a hormone called oxytocin (the same hormone which causes the uterus to contract during and after labour). There is a sharp increase in the concentration of this hormone in the blood stream and this causes the muscle cells around the milk producing sacs to contract and squeeze the milk down the ducts. (It also induces uterine contractions at the same time, which is why you may experience 'after pains' during breastfeeding in the early days after delivery – see p. 136).

The 'let down' reflex has well-defined neurological and hormonal components; however it does appear that it can easily be affected by the mother's mood. Many women do not actually need the baby to suckle directly on the breast to stimulate the reflex, but have merely to hear the baby cry or even to think about it for 'let down' to occur. A mother who is perhaps held up in traffic when hurrying home to feed her baby may find that her breasts are leaking quite involuntarily. Other women who are anxious about some aspect of feeding may find that the reflex is inhibited so that not enough milk comes down to satisfy the baby, despite his suckling and the presence of plenty of milk within the breast.

When a baby feeds he takes the whole nipple into his mouth until his gums are round the areola. Then he rhythmically squeezes it between the tongue and the roof of the mouth until he has obtained all the milk from behind the areola. He will then pause while more milk comes down the ducts, after which there will be another burst of sucking. Once feeding is established, the baby will get most of the milk in the first five or six minutes, although in practice most women feed their babies for about ten minutes on each side. Babies derive a great deal of pleasure just from suckling and being close, so this does nothing but good. After the feed the breasts will usually be full again within two or three hours.

CAN ANY WOMAN BREASTFEED?

It is probably true that any healthy woman can breastfeed, but it is clear that not everyone who sets out to do it is successful. In maternity units where there is particular energy put into the encouragement of breastfeeding and women are fully supported during the postnatal period, most women learn to breastfeed their babies successfully – but without this sort of support, breastfeeding rates fall away with regrettable speed. Breastfeeding comes easily and naturally to many women, but for others it can be a struggle to get it established.

In rural parts of underdeveloped countries where a baby's survival is dependent upon successful breastfeeding, virtually all women breastfeed with no problems. In the West, some women do genuinely seem to fail to feed. It seems unlikely that this is due to a simple organic failure; rather, it is probably due to doubts and anxieties within these particular women about their ability to produce adequate amounts of milk. These often have their roots in jibes about flat chests or flat nipples at school, and widespread talk of 'under-production' of milk, often by mothers and grandmothers who can insidiously undermine the efforts of midwives and others, and the confidence of the breastfeeding mother.

Small breasts are said to be more prevalent among twentieth century emancipated women, but there is no evidence that women with small breasts are poor milk producers. If anything the reverse is true. Similarly, a flat nipple should not be a problem as the feeding baby does not latch on to the nipple but fixes on to the areola. A true inverted nipple (see p. 157) can cause difficulties but it is a fairly rare condition that is much over-diagnosed, causing unnecessary worry.

BREAST CARE DURING PREGNANCY

Care of the breasts during pregnancy with a view to breastfeeding is one of the areas where you are likely to be given conflicting advice. Some people will advocate rolling the nipples regularly between the thumb and forefinger to help draw them out, and if you have rather flat nipples you may be encouraged to wear rubber shells inside your bra which are thought somehow to help this process. There is no scientific evidence that any of these activities help successful breastfeeding; pregnancy itself will prepare the nipples for feeding and it is quite possible that undue attention to the shape of the nipples may sow the seeds of anxiety, leading to later problems.

Another controversial question is whether colostrum should be actively expressed during the last week of pregnancy. Some people feel that this makes the milk flow more easily later on and that it ensures that the duct openings at the nipple are clear at the time of delivery. Again there is no evidence that this activity is of any benefit. It may worry you during your first pregnancy that you can't

To establish breastfeeding successfully, make sure the baby has the whole nipple in his mouth and that his gums are firmly gripping the areola, the dark area that surrounds the nipple. This ensures that the 'let down' reflex is stimulated and helps to avoid sore or cracked nipples.

see the duct openings but you should rest assured that the openings are certainly there and that they will allow the milk through. There is no doubt that at the end of pregnancy the breasts will be full of milk-producing tissues and that as soon as delivery has occurred milk manufacture will accelerate at a great pace irrespective of whether you expressed colostrum antenatally or not.

It is sometimes thought that in order to prevent cracked nipples, moves should be made to toughen up the skin around the areola, especially if your skin is fair. Drying the breasts with a rough towel is a common suggestion and even more drastic abrasives have been encountered! Topless sunbathing is also advocated for this purpose, and for healing a cracked nipple. While there is probably something to be said for the latter in that fresh air probably aids healing, for the former it won't make any difference either way, while care should be taken as a sunburnt breast could be a disaster!

None of these measures is necessary – indeed they may have the opposite effect in that excessive dryness may make the skin more liable to cracking. Pregnancy prepares the breasts for breastfeeding and the cause of cracked nipples is not fair skin but the baby not being properly at the breast.

DIET

Most of the calories you require for breastfeeding will have been laid down during pregnancy. As has already been described, breastfeeding is of course the last part of the normal reproductive cycle and is the most physiological method of getting your figure back to its original dimensions.

You do not need to 'eat for two' while breastfeeding, any more than you did during pregnancy. However, it is obviously sensible to eat a normal, well-balanced diet and in particular to eat protein and iron-rich foods. If your doctor finds that you are anaemic after the birth (see p. 136) you may need to take iron tablets for a while as well. In terms of quantity you should just eat what you feel you need. Similarly you should only drink when you feel thirsty; indeed, excessive drinking sometimes seems to reduce milk production. Neither is it a good idea to drink large amounts of cow's milk as some of the protein might cross into the breast milk and can very occasionally lead to problems of cow's milk allergy.

ESTABLISHING FEEDING

It has been observed that female monkeys isolated in zoo cages do not feed instinctively and they have to be taught how to put their young to the breast. The same is true of women. In contrast to lower mammals such as the domestic cat, who feed by instinct, it appears that the higher order primates learn by watching and that women raised in small families who might never have seen other women breastfeed quite simply do not know what to do. This is fine provided that you are surrounded by skilled friends, relations or midwives to offer support. However, for women on postnatal wards often short of midwives, whose families are scat-

This is the most popular position for breastfeeding, with the baby's head cradled on your arm and his body across your chest. To put the baby to the breast, rest his head in the crook of your arm and turn his whole body towards you. At first it helps to guide the nipple into his mouth with your free hand. Support your arm and his body with a pillow or cushion to bring him up to the level of your breast.

tered and whose own mothers bottle fed, it is tragic how many who set out to breastfeed abandon their efforts in the first few weeks, demoralized by having to struggle behind curtains on the ward with painful nipples, and confused by conflicting advice.

It really need not be like this. With a little patience and good will, breastfeeding can be established with the minimum of fuss in most cases and it will not be long before you will be wondering why you ever thought it could be difficult in the first place. The most important thing is to make sure the baby is latched on to the breast properly, with his gums round the areola as described. This is best achieved if you are holding him properly and you are comfortable yourself.

HOLDING THE BABY

To start with, while everything is still new, it is often helpful to wrap your baby up in a shawl so that his hands and arms aren't in the way. Later on, when breastfeeding is well established your baby will have his hands free and may hold the breast and play with it, while feeding.

Sit propped up in bed or in a good supporting chair with arms. The best position is to cradle your baby across the front so that he is almost horizontal, but his face is turned up and in so he can look at you. If you are right-handed you will probably feel most comfortable if the baby is lying along your left arm while feeding from the right breast, and vice versa. It is important however that you do find a comfortable way of holding the baby on both breasts otherwise one of the breasts might not be regularly emptied of milk. To enable you to hold the baby comfortably close to the breast without having to lean forward, lay a pillow across your knee to raise him higher. Put a pillow behind the small of your back as well to avoid back ache.

PUTTING THE BABY TO THE BREAST

It cannot be emphasized too strongly that the key to successful breastfeeding is putting the baby correctly to the breast. If the baby is not on properly the nipple is liable to become painful or even to crack. You will then dread the baby sucking on it, which will interfere with the 'let down' reflex, the baby will become frustrated and everyone will be in tears.

One of the first challenges for many mothers is to get the baby to open his mouth. However this is really simple since the baby will be ready to suck on anything if you take advantage of his 'rooting reflex'. If you tickle the side of the baby's mouth with the nipple or a finger he will turn in that direction and 'root' for the nipple by obligingly opening his mouth to receive it. He needs a little help at this stage; cradle his head in one hand, turning his whole face towards the breast while you hold the areola with the other to ensure that not just the end of the nipple but the whole of it plus part of the areola are in his mouth (see the illustration on p. 151). For the first few feeds it is a good idea to hold the baby's head and the breast in position; this is where an experienced helper and strategically placed pillows can provide invaluable assistance.

It is comfortable to breastfeed lying down in bed, with your baby lying alongside you. This position is useful for night feeds (don't worry if you both fall asleep in this position afterwards). It is particularly helpful to feed in this position after a Caesarean section or if you had stitches after the birth, since it avoids putting any weight on the painful area.

You can avoid aching shoulders by breastfeeding with your baby tucked under your arm like a Rugby football, his head resting on a pillow by your side. If you have had a Caesarean section, this is another useful position to avoid pressure on the wound during breastfeeding.

WHICH BREAST FIRST?

It is usually recommended that you offer both breasts to the baby every time, alternating the breast you offer first at each feed. In this way it seems likely that each breast is emptied at least at alternate feeds which will help milk production on each side to settle down to fit the demand.

LENGTH AND TIMING OF FEEDS

It used to be thought that if the baby stayed on the breast for too long in the first few days that the nipples were liable to crack, so strict guidelines for the number of minutes on each side were laid down. It is now felt that provided the baby is on the breast properly, the breast will not become painful and so the amount of time you have the baby on each breast is entirely up to you and your baby. Once milk production (lactation) is established, the milk flow is greatest in the first few minutes of the feed and if the baby feeds from the first side for eight to ten minutes, that side should be emptied. You may find that your baby often remains at the breast for much longer than he needs to for strictly nutritional purposes. He simply enjoys it, he is warm and comfortable and takes pleasure from the proximity of your body.

It was only relatively recently that strict feeding regimes were abandoned. There is now much evidence that if a baby is fed on demand, that is, put to the breast (or indeed, given the bottle) as often and for as long as mother and baby want, there are fewer problems with engorgement (see below) and that a feeding routine will be established more quickly.

When demand feeding was first advocated, it was argued that it was difficult to achieve on postnatal wards because it made it impossible for the midwives to organize their time. In practice this has not been borne out, partly because in most hospitals the baby's cot remains by the mother's bed at all times, and partly because the adoption of demand feeding has drastically reduced the number of breast-related problems on the ward.

The length of time between feeds will gradually extend as the baby grows. However, whether he wakes up hungry after two, three or five hours depends on individual factors, and you cannot force a baby into a rigid routine – he will cry when he is hungry and if you leave him longer than about ten minutes he will become distressed. A distressed baby is more difficult to feed successfully.

During the first week of life he will want to feed very frequently which helps to build up the milk supply, but by the end of two weeks he may have settled down to a rough schedule of six to seven feeds in 24 hours. This will gradually decrease so that by three months many babies have dropped one late night feed and most do not require feeding during the small hours of the night from about six months.

WHEN THE MILK COMES IN

At the time of delivery the breasts are large but soft, containing small amounts of colostrum. Under the influence of the hormone prolactin and increased blood supply, there is a speeding up of milk production during the first few days so that, around the third day if you have had your first baby, and a little earlier with subsequent babies, the breasts rapidly fill with milk, becoming stiff and engorged.

This can be uncomfortable as the breasts may feel very hard, lumpy, hot and tender. At this time it can be very difficult to get the baby on the breast because the nipple and areola become distended with milk. It is helpful to express a little of the milk by hand before putting the baby to the breast. This relieves the tension a little and allows the nipple to be manipulated into the baby's mouth.

Although it may be difficult, the best treatment for engorgement is frequent feeding. The discomfort in the breasts may be relieved by holding hot flannels on them or by lying in a warm bath. Ice packs are also helpful between feeds and discomfort is eased if you wear a supportive bra at all times. If your breasts are very uncomfortable your midwife or doctor may suggest a mild pain-killer. Mercifully

this stage does not last long; if you continue to feed regularly, within 24 hours the breasts will be softening again and it will be easier to feed once more.

WINDING

Breastfed babies usually have less problem with wind than bottle fed babies, although occasionally there is so much milk in the ducts at the start of a feed that it may cause the baby to splutter and choke, thereby swallowing some air. If you think your baby has wind, the simplest way to 'burp' him is to set him on your knee with his back straight and his head supported under the chin with one hand, while you gently pat or rub his back with the other. Alternatively you can hold him against your shoulder. If no wind comes and he is comfortable, it is not worth pursuing it.

EXPRESSING MILK

At the time the milk is coming in it is often helpful to express a little milk at the beginning of the feed prior to putting the baby on the breast (see above). You will probably find that the supply of milk settles very quickly to fit your baby's needs over the first ten days or so, but some women do seem to overproduce for a little longer than this and they find it helpful to use a pump to remove excess milk. Simple hand pumps are adequate for this purpose.

If your baby is ill and unable to feed but you anticipate being able to resume feeding when he is better, it is important that you express both breasts regularly, five or six times a day. If you don't do this your milk supply might begin to diminish. For total expression it is preferable to use an electric pump. These are expensive but they can often be hired from hospitals or voluntary organizations like the National Childbirth Trust or the La Leche League.

CARE OF THE BREASTS AFTER DELIVERY

It is not necessary to wash the breasts with soap and water after every feed; if you do this you are likely to wash away the natural lubricating secretions which help to protect the nipple. Just wash your breasts normally in the bath or shower every day.

There are various sprays available which are said to protect the nipples from cracking and are mildly antiseptic. Some also have a light local anaesthetic effect which may deaden the pain of a cracked nipple. However they are of no real benefit; in fact they tend to sting initially if your nipples are sore and they mask the natural smell of your breasts which is one of the ways in which your baby's instinct to suck is aroused.

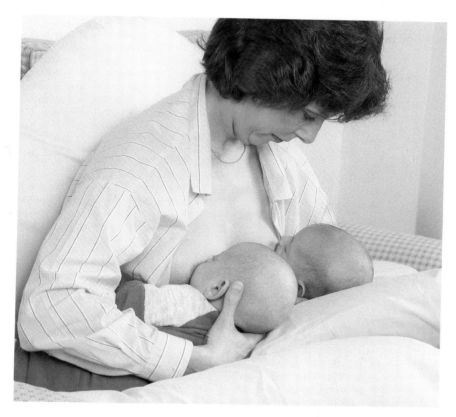

Breastfeeding twins is best achieved by tucking a baby under each arm, with his head forward, in the 'football position' shown on page 153, and supported by as many pillows as possible.

BREASTFEEDING AFTER A CAESAREAN

If your baby has been delivered by Caesarean section you are likely to be uncomfortable for the first few days and you might not be able to cope with holding the baby horizontally as he may press on the wound (see p. 138). However there is no reason why you should not breastfeed successfully. You will need extra help from the midwives or from a friend but there are various tricks which might be helpful. Sometimes it is enough to put a pillow on your lap to support the baby as already described. Some mothers manage to feed comfortably lying on their side with the young baby lying beside them, as illustrated on page 153. Many mothers find this restful, whether they have had a Caesarean section or not, and it is particularly useful at night. Another popular choice is to feed sitting up, well supported, with the baby lying on a pillow at the side from which he is feeding. You then tuck him under your arm with his head beneath the breast (see p. 153).

BREASTFEEDING TWINS

Breastfeeding twins is a practical possibility if you can feed them at the same time. This is usually achieved rather in the same way that you might feed after a Caesarean section, with one baby at each side, their bodies tucked under your arms. You need to be well supported with pillows or cushions to achieve this and you will need lots of help while you are learning how to do it.

When breastfeeding is established some mothers of twins alternate between breast and bottle feeds, breastfeeding each twin in turn and letting the babies' father or another person give a bottle to the other baby. However many mothers of twins have successfully breastfed both babies for some months without recourse to complementary bottles. Enough milk is produced because the babies create their own demand. However, breastfeeding twins is tiring and you need to pay particular attention to the quality of your diet.

BREASTFEEDING A BABY WITH CLEFT PALATE

It is difficult for babies with cleft palate to breastfeed as they cannot suck with the nipple against the roof of the mouth and there is a tendency for milk to come back down the nose. It is sometimes possible to have a special plate made for the baby which makes breastfeeding easier. Alternatively some women in this situation express their milk and feed it to the baby on a spoon. This sounds extremely tedious, but in fact babies cope very well. A cleft lip without a cleft palate is not usually a significant problem with breastfeeding.

COMMON BREASTFEEDING PROBLEMS

There are some common problems associated with breastfeeding which may be off-putting if you don't know how to deal with them. The midwives on the postnatal ward are there to help you in the first few days, and your community midwife will continue to advise you when you get home. Your health visitor and doctor will both want to encourage you to continue breastfeeding and are available for advice as well. An experienced friend or relation who has successfully breastfed can be just as good, if not better, since she will understand your doubts and fears and may seem more sympathetic than a professional health worker. Alternatively some organizations like the National Childbirth Trust have volunteers who act as postnatal support and breast-feeding counsellors who will call on you if you need help with breastfeeding at home.

IS THERE ENOUGH MILK?

One of the things that most worries some women who are breastfeeding for the first time is that they cannot see the amount of milk that the baby is getting. During the first few days before the milk comes in the baby will only receive small amounts of colostrum, so during this time he uses some of the stores of carbohydrate that were laid down in his body during the last part of pregnancy. It is natural for him not to receive all his nutritional needs by mouth during this time; a normal full term baby should not need extra feeds. If he does not seem to be satisfied just put him back on the breast.

There is a great temptation during the early days of breastfeeding to offer the baby a bottle feed 'just in case he isn't getting enough milk' and 'would like a bit more'. It is very likely that he will drink it but it does not mean he really needs it and it will not help your supply of milk to settle down to match his needs. It can lead to confusion and the ultimate abandonment of breastfeeding.

The best way to prevent this situation is quite simply not to have any formula milk or bottles in the house. While you are in the hospital the midwives may offer to give your baby a bottle to let you rest, or if your nipples are sore. Try to resist this, for it is in these early days, when your baby may be coming to the breast as many as ten or twelve times during 24 hours, that milk production is established; supplementary bottles will simply fill your baby up so that he doesn't want to come to the breast.

CRACKED NIPPLES

Cracked nipples almost always arise because the baby has not had the areola properly in his mouth but has been chewing on the nipple itself. A cracked nipple is very painful and is a great disincentive to breastfeeding, so prevention is extremely important. Various sprays and lanolin based creams are available to help this problem, but they are of limited use.

You should be able to feed with a cracked nipple provided that the baby is properly latched on so that he is not actually gripping on the crack. The moment that the baby latches on is usually the worst, so it is worth trying to breathe through it as you may have done during labour, as the pain is transitory. Once the milk is flowing feeding is not painful. Be careful when removing the nipple from your baby's mouth – always insert your finger to release his grip as described earlier.

If it is really too painful to feed than it is worth trying to use a nipple shield for a few feeds. Your baby might not like this as it is sometimes quite difficult for a baby to suck efficiently on it. If all else fails, the solution is to express milk and to feed it to the baby on a spoon or in a bottle until the crack has healed. Mercifully, cracked nipples heal very quickly and are usually better within 24 hours.

BLOCKED DUCTS

Occasionally you will find that a segment or sometimes a larger section of the breast becomes locally firm and tender. The most likely reason for this is that the ducts leading from those segments have become blocked, so that when the 'let down' reflex occurs the milk collects in the ducts which become swollen and tender. As with many feeding problems this situation probably arises because the baby is not properly on the breast, so special attention should be paid to this.

The pain can sometimes be relieved by applying a warm flannel to the breast and gently massaging in a downwards direction. It is most unusual for the blockage to persist for long. It is a good idea to put the baby to the affected breast first when he is hungry and sucks most vigorously as this encourages faster milk flow and helps clear the blockage.

MASTITIS

If a part of the breast becomes red and tender and you find that you have developed a temperature it is probable that you have an infection in the breast and you should contact your doctor as soon as possible, who will prescribe a suitable antibiotic.

This sort of infection is known as mastitis. It is particularly likely to occur if you have a cracked nipple which can act as an entry portal for bacteria or if you have a blocked duct in which the milk has stagnated. If the part of the breast which is infected is in the upper, outer quarter you may be aware that the tenderness is extending up towards your armpit, where you may feel inflamed glands.

Mastitis is not a reason to stop breastfeeding; in fact it is most important that feeding continues regularly so that the breast is emptied. The antibiotics prescribed will not affect the milk or harm your baby.

Rarely, mastitis develops into a full-blown breast abscess. In this situation, a part of the breast becomes very red, swollen and tender and it might be possible to express pus from the nipple. This might require admission to hospital for drainage of the abscess and antibiotic treatment. Again it is important that the breast is emptied of milk regularly but in this instance the milk from the infected breast has to be expressed and discarded until the infection has subsided, while the baby is just fed from the non-infected side.

INVERTED NIPPLES

If you have a true inverted nipple it is worth trying to encourage it to come out during pregnancy by rolling it between finger and thumb and wearing a nipple shell under your bra. The midwife at the antenatal clinic can advise you about this. If your nipples are still inverted after delivery (and this is very rare) you may still be able to feed, but if there are problems you could wear a nipple shield.

LEAKING

The extent to which different women leak milk from the breast varies. You may find that during feeding milk drips from the opposite side. At one time there was interest in collecting this milk for hospital milk banks, but in fact it is of low nutritional value. If you do drip in this manner you will need to wear a breast pad during feeds.

Leaking tends to be more of a problem in the first few weeks of lactation before the supply settles down to fit the baby's demands. You will quickly learn whether or not you do have a tendency to leak milk when the breasts are full or if you hear your baby crying, and if you know this is likely to happen it is worth always putting a pad inside your bra and keeping a few spares with you as they can quite quickly become saturated. Cup-shaped breast pads are more efficient than rectangular ones and fit more neatly inside your bra.

THE BABY THAT FIGHTS THE BREAST

Occasionally the first few days of breastfeeding are made particularly difficult because the baby appears to resist going on to the breast and becomes stiff and angry, sometimes arching his back and crying even though he is hungry. This is a curious phenomenon. One theory is that it may be due to the baby's nose having been restricted during feeding at some point so that his breathing was obstructed. The unpleasantness of this sensation may condition him to resist feeding. Whether this is true or not it really can be a most frustrating experience for mother and baby.

If your baby seems to be behaving in this way you need to make sure that his nose is free so that he can breathe and you need to seek some moral support as it can be a distressing time. Remember that it is not your fault, and your baby is not doing it because there is anything wrong with your milk. If your baby fights in this way it is a good idea to lift him off the breast and carry him about for a minute or two over your shoulder or cradled in your arms until he is calm again. If he has already shown an obvious preference for one side or the other, put him to the preferred side first for a while until the problem passes. Don't despair, this behaviour is always temporary.

GOING OUT

Once you are home, going out with your baby while you are breastfeeding is not difficult, since in theory the baby can be fed anywhere. While your baby is still small it is usually easiest to take the baby with you if you are going to somebody's house. Make sure you wear something in which it is easy to feed – either front fastening or easy to lift from the waist. It can be very uncomfortable having to strip in order to produce a breast in a strange, possibly cold house!

Breastfeeding can be a hindrance while the baby is still feeding frequently if you want to go somewhere such as a theatre or cinema where you cannot take the baby, especially if it involves going out for longer than the period between two feeds. In the early weeks this time period may be difficult to predict anyway. In this situation it is important that you have some breast pads with you as you may well begin to leak at about the time the baby's feed is due.

Some women who are extremely well organized are able to express milk which can be left behind to be given to the baby from a bottle. If your feeding is going so well that this is no problem then it is probably the best thing to do, provided that the baby will take a bottle – and some breastfed babies are reluctant to do this once breastfeeding is established. Breast milk freezes well, and if you use bottles with disposable bags (see p. 146) one of these can be defrosted and placed in the holder with the minimum of fuss. On the other hand, if your baby will take a bottle it really is not going to do any harm to give the occasional bottle of formula milk, and this is the preferred course of action for many women. If breastfeeding is well established, it is a myth that once the baby is offered a bottle he will no longer like the breast.

CHANGING FROM BREAST TO BOTTLE

If you want to wean your baby from the breast before six months you will need to use bottles. Usually this produces no problems, but some babies do take a little time to get used to them, so don't leave the change-over until the last minute if you have a deadline such as going back to work. You may need to experiment a bit with teats before you find something he likes (see opposite).

If you breastfeed up to or beyond the age of about six months you may be able to wean your baby straight on to a cup with a spout and avoid ever having to use bottles. It is a surprise to many parents how well babies cope with these cups. It is probably best to continue on a formula milk until the age of about nine months, but if you do change to whole cow's milk, you must still pay great attention to hygiene. The cup needs washing and sterilizing as you would a bottle, paying special attention to cleaning the little holes in the spout.

It will be much more comfortable for you to affect the change-over to bottles gradually, stopping one or more breastfeeds every two or three days; this will help you not to become too engorged. If you have already started to introduce solid food into your baby's diet (see p. 200), it makes sense to start by dropping the breastfeed that accompanies the meal your baby is most enthusiastic about, such as breakfast or lunch. Some mothers manage to maintain the bedtime 'comfort feed' for some weeks even when all other breastfeeds have been dropped.

If for some reason you do have to stop feeding suddenly you will probably need to express a little milk occasionally. Try not to do this more often than you need and within three or four days you will be through the worst.

BOTTLE FEEDING

Bottle feeding requires far more practical forethought than breastfeeding, whether you are intending to bottle feed from the start or are changing from breast to bottle before your baby is six months old. You will need to decide on the type of formula you are going to use, which bottles and teats and how many, and make sure you have sterilizing equipment and know how to use it.

CHOOSING BOTTLES AND TEATS

While you are in hospital you will probably be provided with milk prepacked in small glass bottles. Once home, you have the choice between two main types of bottles. The traditional rigid bottle (now usually made of plastic) is still used by the majority of people with no problems. However, with these bottles the air pressure inside inevitably falls as the baby sucks, so that the teat has to be released from time to time so that air can enter the bottle. Increasingly, however, women are using disposable, polythene bags which are mounted on a plastic holder with a large rubber teat over the top. This type of 'bottle' has two advantages. First, the inside of the polythene bag is already sterile so only the teats and tops have to be sterilized at home, and secondly, the bag collapses as the baby sucks so that there is no vacuum to release and the baby holds the teat in his mouth continuously as he would on the breast.

You have to buy the right teat for the type of bottle that you choose. Rubber teats are larger and firmer than the human nipple and areola and it is generally easy for the baby to feed from them, but you may have to experiment to find the right hole size. For most newborn babies the size is right that allows a steady stream of drips when the bottle is held upside down. If the flow of milk is too slow the baby may become frustrated and angry during the feed, while a hole that is too large will produce a flow of milk so fast that the baby will splutter and choke.

STERILIZING EQUIPMENT

Bacteria can easily grow in formula milk so it is essential that they are sterilized before use and cleaned thoroughly afterwards, before being sterilized again. Great care must be taken to prevent stale milk from accumulating in the bottle, especially in the grooves around the neck.

Bottles should be rinsed out directly after every feed, washed and scrubbed in soapy water with a special bottle brush and then rinsed thoroughly in running water before being sterilized. Some people suggest rubbing the teats with salt to remove the last vestiges of milk, but this is probably not necessary provided the teat is rinsed with the bottle immediately after use.

All the parts of the bottle – teats, caps and covers

Sterilizing equipment
Before sterilizing, always wash bottles, teats and other equipment thoroughly in hot water and rinse under the tap. Use a bottle brush for bottles.

Fill the sterilizing unit or other container with the required amount of cold water and add sterilizing tablets or solution according to the manufacturer's instructions.

Place all bottles, teats, covers, spoons and dummies (if used) in the sterilizer, making sure that all are completely immersed and that no air bubbles are trapped in the bottles.

Leave the bottles and other equipment in the sterilizer, covered, for the length of time recommended by the manufacturer of your sterilizing preparation. Change the solution every 24 hours.

solution which kills bacteria. This is prepared by diluting a strong liquid or by dissolving tablets in tap water. Chemists, specialist baby departments and large supermarkets usually stock a variety of agents for this purpose so you will be able to choose one most suited to your needs. It is important to read the directions carefully so that you get the strength of the solution right, and also have the bottles and other equipment completely immersed in the solution with no air bubbles for at least the prescribed length of time – for some brands this is now as little as half an hour. The solution should be changed every day.

When the bottles and teats are needed they should be removed from the sterilizing solution very carefully, holding the outside edges only. The bottles should be filled with milk and sealed directly without being rinsed.

Any other objects or utensils such as dummies and feeding spoons should be sterilized in the same way. The solution corrodes metal so is only suitable for plastic utensils, and the sterilizer should also be plastic. You can buy special sterilizing kits although these are not strictly necessary. What is important is that the container is large enough to hold at least four bottles at a time completely immersed and that it has a well-fitting cover. Other equipment such as a measuring jug and bottle brush should be kept very clean and only used for your baby's feeds.

MAKING UP FEEDS

If you choose to bottle feed from the time of the baby's birth your midwife should teach you how to make up feeds. If you change from breast to bottle after going home and are uneasy about making up bottles contact your health visitor for guidance. A feed made up incorrectly can be dangerous.

In Britain, formula milk is sold almost exclusively in powder form although liquid concentrates are available. Formula is available in most chemist shops and large food stores or you may buy it at your child health clinic. Some people may be able to obtain supplies cheaply; check with your health visitor about this if you have a low income.

You should always be careful to follow the manufacturer's instructions when making up a feed. If you are at all confused ask for guidance from your health visitor. Each formula packet or tin is provided with its own scoop – only use the scoop provided for that particular brand.

As long as you have a refrigerator in which to store the bottles, it is sensible to make up the whole day's supply of bottles at one time. It is particularly useful to have bottles ready for night-time feeds so that you can feed the baby with the minimum of

as well – need sterilizing. The most basic way to do this is to boil them in a pan of water for at least five minutes, then to pour off the water and leave the bottles in the pan with an airtight cover or until needed, preferably in the refrigerator. Very few people now use this method as a routine, but it is always good to remind yourself that you can achieve adequate sterilization quickly and without sophisticated chemicals or equipment, should you need to.

Most bottles are now sterilized by leaving them for a prescribed length of time in a chemical fuss. Some people suggest making up the day's supply in a large measuring jug and transferring it to the bottles, but you have to add a large number of scoops and it is very easy to lose count.

Boil the kettle and, while you allow the water to cool slightly, wash your hands thoroughly. Then remove the bottles from the sterilizer, shake off any excess sterilizing solution and stand the bottles on a firm, flat surface. While the boiled water is still hot, pour the required amount into the bottles. Most bottles are now calibrated with millilitre and fluid ounce measurements so there is no need to use a measuring jug. Then drop the required number of scoops of dry formula into the bottles. Each scoop should be full to the top but not pressed down – level it off with the edge of a knife to be sure. Cover the bottles then shake them vigorously to dissolve the powder. Allow them to cool and place them in the refrigerator if you don't need to feed immediately. If your baby doesn't finish the bottle at any one feed don't keep it for later, but throw it away and start afresh next time. You also should discard the milk in unused bottles at the end of 24 hours.

Only put in the number of scoops advised for the amount of water you are using – never be tempted to add an extra scoop because you think your baby may sleep better or because you think he isn't gaining weight fast enough. Seeing that your baby is growing well provides deep satisfaction, and some people have been led to believe that if a little more powder is to be added then the baby will become bigger and stronger. This is not the case; on the contrary, if the milk concentration is too high it is dangerous because of its high sodium content.

There has been some recent attention focused on the practice of using bottled mineral water instead of tap water for making up formula. This is not recommended. The powder contains all the minerals your baby requires and there are potential risks in increasing them by using mineral-rich water.

It is not advisable to take a bottle-fed baby to a part of the world where the water is liable to be contaminated and where you do not have free access to a kettle. If you have to travel to an area like this and bottled water is the only source of safe water, seek medical advice as to what type to use.

HOW MUCH TO OFFER

Some guidance as to how much milk to offer will be given on your tin or packet of formula, and your health visitor can also help you here. To start with, during the course of the day your baby will take about 180ml per kilo body weight (about 3fl oz per pound) spread over several feeds during the day. He may take as little as 30ml (1fl oz) at any one feed to

It is helpful and satisfying for both parents when a father is able to help with night feeds – usually only possible if you are bottle feeding your baby. Make sure the bottle is always held at enough of an angle to ensure that the teat is full of milk. Never leave a baby alone with a propped bottle.

Making up a feed

To make up a feed, remove the bottle from the sterilizer and shake off excess liquid. Fill the bottle with the required amount of hot, boiled water.

Add the formula, a scoop at a time, levelling each scoop off with the back of a knife. Do not press the powder down and never put in more than the recommended number of scoops.

Put on the teat and cover. Shake the bottle vigorously to make sure the formula is completely dissolved. Allow to cool before feeding, and store in the refrigerator if not needed immediately.

start with, but by a week, a baby of average birth weight may be taking about 90ml (3 fl oz) per feed.

Don't try to force your baby to finish his bottle every time. If he fights the bottle while still obviously hungry, try winding him, make sure the teat is not blocked or change position to settle him down again. The same principles of demand feeding should apply to bottle fed babies as have already been described for breastfed babies (see page 153). Provided he is growing normally you should not be too concerned about variation of intake between different feeds. He will probably settle down to six feeds a day till about eight weeks of age, and by the age of three months he will probably be taking about 250ml (8 fl oz) per feed – the equivalent of a full bottle – with about five feeds during 24 hours.

GIVING THE BOTTLE

Right-handed people usually feel most comfortable holding the baby in their left arm with the bottle in the right hand. The bottle should be held at an angle so that the teat is always full of milk, otherwise the baby will tend to swallow air as well. If the milk is in a rigid bottle the baby will need to release the teat periodically so that air can bubble back into the bottle to replace the milk he has drunk. If this doesn't happen it will become progressively more difficult for him to suck and he may become frustrated. Babies learn quite quickly to pause and release the teat themselves, but in the early days you might find it helpful occasionally to remove the teat from his mouth. This isn't necessary, however, if you use bottles with disposable bags, since the bag collapses as the milk is sucked from it.

WINDING

There is a tendency for bottle fed babies to have more wind than those fed on the breast. If your baby does seem to be swallowing a lot of air you should check that the bottle is always held at the right angle and pay attention to the size of the hole in the teat.

It is customary to interrupt bottle feeds about half way through to bring up wind, but this is only worth doing if you find that your baby does usually burp at that time. If not, he may become frustrated that his feed is being interrupted. When the feed is finished he may need to be winded, so hold him like a breastfed baby, either sitting him on your knee with his head supported, or against your shoulder. A little milk often comes back with the wind so make sure you have a cloth handy. However, you can expect stained clothes occasionally!

Babies sometimes do seem to become very uncomfortable with wind and if you are having a lot of problems you should have a talk with your health visitor (see p. 187). Sometimes changing from a rigid to a collapsible bottle can help.

THE TEMPERATURE OF THE MILK

When the milk is first made it is very hot and must not be given to the baby until it is cooled down at least to blood temperature. The temperature of the milk can be gauged by letting some drops of milk fall on to the back of the hand. The milk should feel neither hot nor cold.

In hospital bottles are usually given to babies cold. At home most people warm the milk to blood heat by standing the bottles in a jug of hot water or a bottle warmer. Some people do this because it is believed that the baby is less likely to get colic. There is no real evidence to support this and if you find that your baby is happy with cold milk there really is no point in wasting time heating it. If you do feel you want to warm it you must be careful not to let it get too hot.

THE YOUNG BABY

Caring for your baby's physical and emotional needs in the first three months of life

Taking on the responsibility for a newborn baby is both exciting and unnerving. If the baby is your first, you will have all the usual apprehensions of anyone embarking on a new task, and even if he or she is not, there is always a certain amount of upheaval in introducing a new person into an existing family unit. Having a baby requires adjustment on all sides – mother, father and baby have to get to know each other – and if there are other children they also need to have it made clear that their needs and anxieties are taken into account too.

EARLY DAYS

If you had your baby in hospital, you will have had the security of knowing that there was always someone to call on if you were anxious about yourself or your baby. At the same time, you will probably be longing to come home to be in familiar surroundings and among your friends and family, so that you can begin to fit your new baby into your everyday life. Even so, you may feel lonely and frightened at first, particularly if you were on your own. In addition you may still be feeling physically uncomfortable as well as tired. The stress of coping with exhaustion from broken nights and constant emotional demands should not be underestimated. But mothers having their second babies will tell you how inexperienced they felt first time round, and how much more confident they felt about the second. They may tell you how they used to look in on their sleeping baby every few minutes just to check that he was still alive, and how worried they felt when he would not settle.

All babies have different personalities – differences may even be apparent in late pregnancy – and they all have different rhythms of eating and sleeping. Some babies cry more than others, some sleep more than others, some are more contented than others. Your friends' babies will behave differently from yours; if they happen to be easier babies, that is just good luck, not better management, whatever your friends may say.

The early weeks are likely to be chaotic. There may be no pattern at all to your baby's needs for food and sleep and it is impossible to stick to a rigid timetable. Feeding and lack of sleep become the over-riding features of this period, and both parents need to recognize this and try to organize life to accommodate it. However, your baby will soon begin to settle into some kind of rhythm, although this is unlikely to be tailor-made to suit you. If you manage to satisfy his needs during the course of the day, feeding him when he is hungry, changing him when he is wet or soiled, comforting and cuddling him when he is upset or bored, you are doing very well indeed. Finding time for anything else at this stage may be impossible.

After a few weeks your baby's rhythms may become a little more predictable, and you might be able to start planning your routine around his needs. If he wakes you several times at night, you may be able to set aside an hour during the afternoon when he usually sleeps to have a rest yourself. The essential thing is to be flexible; your baby's requirements at this early age have to take priority over yours because he is unable to alter them to suit you. As the weeks pass you should be able to manipulate his routine to fit in with yours. Once he feels secure in the knowledge that you will always be there when he needs you, you might for example be able to lengthen the time between feeds, and to cut out the night feed. With luck, his timetable will gradually approach the one which suits you best, although this does not always seem to happen.

During the first few months – especially if you are breastfeeding – you may find it very difficult to concentrate on any intellectual activity. This is not a permanent loss of function but a normal feature of early motherhood, caused by a combination of your natural concentration on your baby and lack of sleep. It always gets better within a few months, so do not let it worry you.

FATHERS AT HOME

Fathers are sometimes able to get paternity leave or take a holiday for a week or two after the baby is born. It means that both partners can share the early

Many fathers like to be at home in the early days after the birth so that they can be with their new family and take over the household chores to help their partners recover fully from the birth.

joys of your baby, and you can get to know your baby together. It also means that he will be able to take over the household chores to enable his partner to rest properly.

A father often feels elated when his partner comes home from the hospital with the baby, and needs to be aware that she might not be feeling the same way. She may be tired, weepy and irritable, or may be totally absorbed with the baby to the exclusion of everyone and everything else. In addition she may not be feeling the expected surge of maternal feelings and love for the newly arrived member of

the family, which can lead to feelings of guilt which spill over into her relationships with others. These feelings are normal – loving your child does not always happen instantly but develops gradually as you get to know him. In this situation it is not surprising that some fathers feel rejected. A man may feel that all his partner's affection and interest has been transferred to the baby, or may worry that his own feelings of love for the child are not fully shared by the baby's mother. After a while things do settle down and life begins to return to a familiar pattern. Until then a father needs to be especially tolerant and understanding. In turn, mothers need to understand that their partners also may feel overwhelmed by the changes in their lives.

With the understanding that perfect mothering and fathering do not come instantly and automatically, and that the first weeks are always difficult, you will be able to experience together all aspects of your new baby – the rewards, the enjoyment and the fun, as well as the anxieties, the tiredness and the sheer hard work.

During these early weeks when your life revolves totally around your baby's needs, any help you can get in running the home will make life easier for you and free you to concentrate on your baby. Friends, grandparents and other members of the family, or paid domestic help can all be valuable, depending on your circumstances.

With or without extra help, you should not feel bad about taking short cuts with cooking and housework. If you normally keep your home spotlessly clean and tidy, you may need to adjust to lower standards for a few weeks. Alternatively, if you can afford it, you may prefer to pay someone to keep your home as you like it. This is a worthwhile expense if you can budget for it, even if it is only for a couple of hours a week for the first few weeks. If you are a single parent, or have several other children and your partner cannot take time off, or if you have any other social problems at home, you may be able to get a Home Help through your local Social Services department. When your Health Visitor comes to see you for the first time (see p. 187), ask her advice about this and she will be able to help you arrange it.

You may, however, feel that buying a large, labour-saving item like a washing machine, tumble drier, freezer or microwave would be more useful in the long run, if you don't have them already. Sometimes grandparents offer to buy large items of equipment for the baby to help out, so if they can afford it, suggest they contribute one of these to make your life easier, rather than some expensive item of baby furniture. As you will see from the next section, your baby's needs are few to start off with and you can build up the equipment gradually, much of which can be obtained secondhand.

Your priorities are attending to your baby and looking after yourself. Try to get some rest during the day and try to eat regular healthy meals in between feeding and changing – this will more than fill your day. If you can avoid being overtired you are more likely to be able to enjoy your baby to the full.

EQUIPMENT FOR YOUR BABY

Choosing clothes and equipment for your new baby can be a difficult task; the choice is vast and bewildering. There has been an enormous develop-

ment in 'baby technology' in the past decade and the result has revolutionized the design of items such as prams, strollers and high chairs. It has also resulted in the invention of a large number of attractive but expensive items which are not really necessary. For instance, a special changing table helps to confine the changing equipment to one area, but a simple changing mat on a convenient table or chest costs a fraction of the price.

Start looking round the shops several weeks before the baby is due, as you will feel increasingly tired as your pregnancy nears its end. Think very carefully about what you are likely to need before you spend any money. Your choice will depend on the time of year the baby is born and on your way of life, as well as on your budget. Do you usually drive a car, or do you walk to the shops or take a bus? Do you live in a house with stairs or a flat with a lift? Will your baby be born in winter or summer? Talk to friends with babies about what they found useful. Staff in some of the larger department stores are usually experienced and helpful in guiding you round the market. Check all items for safety.

Equipment need not be expensive as many of the larger items can be bought secondhand. You can look at advertisements in the newspaper, or check in your local baby clinic where notices of items for sale are put up. Friends and relatives are often delighted to hand on a pram or carrycot which has been taking up space in the attic, but do check especially carefully for safety on older models. Friends and family may like to give clothes as gifts for the baby; if they ask you what you would like, don't be afraid to tell them exactly what you need – this avoids duplication and helps your budget. The tables included in this chapter are designed to help you choose what you need.

Buying children's clothes is much more fun now than it used to be. Colours and styles are fresh and bright, and there is a broad range from which to choose. Babies grow very rapidly, so don't buy too many first size clothes. Budget to allow for some second size as well so that you will have something available as soon as the baby needs it. Babies born in winter or summer will obviously have different immediate requirements. In cold weather several layers of clothes are warmer than one thick layer.

Choose fabrics which are easily washable – preferably machine-washable – and can be tumble-dried. If you do not have a washing machine or tumble drier you may need one or two extra garments, especially in the winter when everything takes longer to dry. Woollens are more difficult to

FIRST CLOTHES

Vests	3-4 cotton or fine wool. Envelope necks are easier to pull over the baby's head than round necks. Wrap over vests tend to be fiddly. Some vests are like 'body-suits' which fasten over the nappy with poppers; these are snug in winter.	**Pramsuit**	Usually made of quilted polyester. Similar in style to the sleepsuit, but warmer, a pramsuit will keep your baby warm in the buggy or baby carrier, or when he or she is sitting up in the pram. Smaller babies may feel warmer in a pram with blankets and a quilt than with a pramsuit.
Shawl	Useful as an extra wrap for night feeds, but if lacy, avoid wrapping the baby in it in bed in case fingers are trapped. A lightweight blanket does just as well.	**Stretchsuits**	6 at least. These are comfortable, warm and practical. Those with poppers all down the front and inside the legs make nappy changes easier. Beware of stretchsuits with small unshaped feet, they may constrict your baby's feet as they grow, and cause damage. Most have shaped feet. If these appear to be getting too tight, you can always cut them off and dress your baby in socks and bootees instead. Fold-back mittens on the sleeves are useful in cold weather or if your baby is inclined to scratch himself. Stretchsuits with short sleeves and no legs are useful in hot weather. It is a good idea to have at least one second size stretchsuit – better slightly too large than slightly too small.
Nightdresses	4. Useful as they make night-time nappy changes easier. Some have a drawstring through the hem to stop them riding up.		
Sleepsuits	1-2 for cold weather. Usually made of synthetic fleecy fabric. Some are like a sleeping bag with arms and a hood and have a zip opening which makes it easy to lift the baby in and out. Others have legs, less easy to put on but still snug. Useful for night feeds or for keeping warm in the pram.		
Cardigans or matinee jackets	2 wool or acrylic. These are not essential unless you find it difficult to keep your home warm. Those which button all down the front are warmer than those with one button at the yoke or neck. Be careful of the fastenings and avoid any styles with drawstring tie fastenings at the neck as these can be dangerous. Close-knit ones are better than loose lacy ones in which little fingers can get trapped.	**Hats, mittens, bootees**	Wool or acrylic. 1 hat and pair of mittens in winter. A cotton hat is essential in summer to protect your baby's head and face from the sun. The weather can be very cool even in summer and you may need a warm hat and mittens. Scratch mittens made of soft cotton are sometimes recommended; keeping the nails trimmed is an alternative. Bootees over a stretch suit keep a baby's feet extra warm. Beware of loose threads which may constrict fingers.

wash than cotton or synthetic fabrics. Avoid clothes which need ironing, as you will have difficulty finding time for this. Clothes should be easy to get on and off, bearing in mind that nappy changes and soiling will be frequent.

BATHS AND NAPPIES

A baby bath is not an essential item; babies can be bathed in a washing-up bowl, a large basin or an ordinary bath. However, it is practical, safe and the easiest place to bath your baby during the first few months. Use a mat in the bath if it doesn't have a non-slip surface.

There are several different designs of baby bath made out of rigid plastic. Some have plugs, which makes them easier to empty into a bucket. You may need a separate bath stand if you do not have a good surface on which to put the bath – check that this fits properly and is stable. Some baths are designed to fit over the big bath; these can be easily filled and emptied without having to be carried.

Baths made out of soft plastics are also available, which have their own stand. This type of bath is very useful if you are short of space, as it can be folded away, and it does not need to stand in the bathroom. It can be filled from a bucket and emptied back into the bucket through an outlet tube. Some designs have an attached changing mat which fits on top, and a shelf for toiletries.

The big decision is whether to buy terry towelling nappies or disposable nappies – or both. Terry nappies can be cheaper in the long run. They are more absorbent and softer than disposables, and they will fit babies of all shapes and sizes. Their main disadvantage is that they have to be washed and dried. If you do not have a washing machine this is a very laborious process, and even with a machine more work is involved than with disposables. Terries must be completely dried and properly aired, so you need plenty of space, or a tumble drier. Nappies come out softer from a drier than if they are air dried. For terry nappies you will also require extra equipment such as nappy buckets, sanitizing powder or liquid, washing powder, pins and elastic pants.

Disposable nappies are quicker to put on – they do not have to be folded. However they do take up a lot of room, they are bulky to buy and store and they create large volumes of rubbish. They do not always fit very well and they can leak or cause chafing. They are also expensive, and with approximately 2000 nappy changes to look forward to in the first year this may be a major disadvantage.

Most parents find that a combination of terries and disposables suits them best. The terries are fine for home use while the disposables are useful for outings, when convenience is the top priority.

CHANGING NAPPIES

Although changing nappies is usually regarded as one of the most unpleasant aspects of parentcraft, yet it provides a wonderful opportunity for you and your baby to be close. Once your baby is comfortable in a clean nappy you can both enjoy spending a little time together playing and talking, getting to know one another. Parents often find that they notice their baby's first smiles while changing his or her nappy.

The decision whether to use terry nappies or disposables is discussed above, but the basic procedure for changing a nappy is the same, whichever type you decide to use. Although disposables are quicker to put on, it takes the same amount of time to cleanse, and, if necessary, to dress your baby in clean clothes whichever type of nappy you use.

In general, a baby's nappy should be changed when it is very wet, and as soon as it is soiled, in order to avoid nappy rash. Of course, you do not need to wake your baby at night just for a nappy change, but it is worth checking the nappy if he wakes for any reason. Sleeping through the night in a wet nappy does not matter as long as the baby is not cold or uncomfortable.

You will probably need to change your baby's nappy at every feed and at other times to start with – as many as twelve times a day in the early weeks. Some babies open their bowels before a feed, others during or after a feed. There is little point in changing the nappy before a feed if your baby is likely to produce a stool by the end of it. Your baby may prefer to be dry and comfortable before a feed, or may be too hungry to wait despite having a full nappy. You will soon learn which pattern suits your baby best.

After a few weeks your baby will enjoy spending a period of time during the day kicking around on a towel or mat in a warm room without a nappy on. This is a particularly good idea if he or she has sensitive skin or a rash.

Most babies pass urine around the time of birth and about three to four times a day during the first few days. By ten days of age they will be passing urine about ten to twelve times per day. The colour of the urine depends on how much the baby drinks; the less fluid he drinks, the more concentrated and darker ('stronger') will be the urine. If the urine always appears dark and is passed less frequently, the baby probably needs more to drink.

The frequency and consistency of babies' stools varies greatly. The stools of breastfed babies are soft and yellow, with the consistency of scrambled egg. Sometimes they are green and very loose and contain mucus. Most breastfed babies pass several stools a day, though it is not unusual for several days or a week to go by without a stool being passed. This is because breast milk is designed to fit your baby's requirements and there is very little waste matter left over.

The stools of bottle fed babies tend to be harder than those of breastfed babies. These babies do not usually go for more than one day without a bowel movement (see p. 109). The stools are greyer in colour and their consistency is more like clay. They can sometimes also be green. Very hard stools may indicate that the baby is not being given enough water to drink.

Folding terry nappies
Kite method: 1 Lay the nappy in a diamond shape and fold corners inward 2 Fold points in neatly 3 Pin on each side, as shown.

Origami method: 1 Fold nappy in two with free edges uppermost 2 Pull left-hand corners across 3 Turn folded nappy over 4-5 Fold the two middle layers in and over twice. Pin as for the kite method.

HOW TO CHANGE A NAPPY

Assemble all the equipment you will need: changing mat, nappy, and nappy liner, pins and plastic pants (if required), clothes, if necessary, cotton wool and baby lotion or warm water, or baby wipes, barrier cream, nappy bucket filled with nappy sanitizing solution and waste bin. It is easier at home to set aside an area for changing so everything is close by.

If you are using a terry nappy, fold it and put a nappy liner in place before you remove your baby's clothes and soiled nappy. Then remove the wet or soiled nappy and any of the baby's clothes which may also be soiled or wet. Wipe the baby's bottom with cotton wool dampened in warm water or baby lotion. (If soiled, clean the baby's bottom with a tissue first.) If the baby has nappy rash it is a good idea to put a teaspoonful of very mild antiseptic solution in the water. If there is no soreness and especially if you are away from home, baby wipes are a convenient alternative. Girls must always be wiped from front to back to prevent germs from entering the vagina or bladder from the anus.

Dry the area thoroughly but gently, then lift the baby's legs and slide the nappy underneath. Apply a barrier cream if the baby's bottom is sore or chafed. Some parents prefer to use some form of barrier whether their baby has a rash or not – vaseline or

When pinning a towelling nappy, always make sure that you place your fingers behind the nappy, between the point of the pin and your baby's skin, so that there is no danger of pricking your baby even if he wriggles.

petroleum jelly are soft and spread evenly without clogging and so are more suitable for use at every nappy change. Zinc and castor oil cream or other medicated creams are thicker in consistency but are more effective in forming a waterproof barrier if your baby has a rash (see p. 193). Try to avoid using too thick a layer of cream as it can clog the one-way action of nappy liners. Which cream you use is

CLEANSING EQUIPMENT

Terry nappies	You will need at least two dozen. Buy the best you can afford as the cheaper ones wear thin very quickly. Terry nappies are traditionally square; you can also buy shaped nappies but they are more expensive and less efficient. You will need nappy pins with safety heads.	**Baby oil**	This is useful if your baby's skin is very dry. Baby lotion can also be used for this purpose. Talcum powder is not necessary after a bath. It can cause irritation, especially if applied to wet skin, and it must not be sprinkled too near the nose or throat as it can be inhaled.
Disposable nappies	All-in-one disposable nappies are plastic-backed and therefore do not need plastic pants. There are also disposable pads which fit inside plastic pants. These pads also provide useful extra protection at night for the older baby, worn inside terries or disposables. Disposables should *not* be put down the lavatory but placed in plastic bags, sealed and disposed of in the dustbin.	**Soap**	Pure soap or special bath-care liquid. This can also be used as shampoo for the first few months, but is not always necessary at first.
		Cotton wool	This is for cleaning your baby's face and bottom. After a few months you can use a small sponge or flannel for the face, keeping a second one for the rest of the body.
Nappy liners	Disposable one-way liners are worn inside terry nappies. They help to keep the baby's bottom dry and also protect the nappy from soiling. They can be flushed down the toilet. You can also use them inside disposable nappies.	**Bowls**	Any small container – for example a yoghurt pot – can be used to hold boiled, cooled water for your baby's face and eyes. 'Top-and-tail' bowls can be bought, with two separate compartments for water and cotton wool.
Plastic pants	The choice is between snap fastening, elasticated and tie fastening pants. The snap type are easy to put on and are most efficient, but tend to chafe. The tie fastening type are easily adaptable to different sizes and shapes.	**Baby lotion and baby wipes**	These are for cleaning the baby's bottom. Baby wipes are easy and convenient when you are out, but may sting if your baby has a nappy rash. Baby lotion or warm water on a piece of cotton wool is sufficient at home.
Nappy bucket and nappy sanitizing solution	One or two buckets with lids are needed for soaking terry nappies, one for wet, one for soiled nappies (see opposite). Also useful for soaking white clothes or bedlinen (the solution tends to bleach coloureds).	**Baby bath**	With stand if necessary.
		Towels	Cotton towels are best. Some have a hood at one corner to keep the baby's head warm. One or two smaller towels are useful in addition to pat the baby dry.
Gauze squares (muslins)	One dozen should be enough. These have many uses: for extra protection inside a terry nappy, as a bib, to put under your baby's head in the cot or over your shoulder to absorb dribble or regurgitated milk.	**Plastic changing mat**	A changing mat at home saves soiling towels or other surfaces when changing. A holdall which opens out to make a mat is useful. One variety has the mat attached to but separate from the bag.
Barrier cream	To form a protective barrier between your baby's skin and the wet nappy which prevents soreness, and protects your baby's bottom if it develops a rash (see p. 193).	**Storage**	You will need to store the toiletries near the nappy changing area, on shelves, in a box or basket or in a set of pockets hung on the wall. A box or basket is useful as you can carry it around; you may like to keep it near the crib at night.

SLEEPING

Once again, your choice of equipment will depend on your lifestyle. You will definitely need a cot for your baby to sleep in until about two years of age. For the first months, however, you may prefer your baby to sleep in a crib, a Moses basket or a carrycot. These are more easily made draught-proof and are more snug and secure for newborn babies, although a Moses basket may not be rigid and is therefore not safe for use in the back of a car.

Bedding

Cribs and cots are usually sold complete with a mattress, which must fit properly otherwise your baby could become wedged in a gap or trap his hands or feet at the side. Non-allergenic foam is the best filling. Some are partially covered with a waterproof plastic covering, leaving one end porous to avoid the danger of suffocation. A pillow is not necessary for the first year and can be dangerous for a small baby. Small sheets and blankets can be made from full size bedding, or can be bought. Fitted stretch bottom sheets usually made in towelling or flannelette, are more expensive but are easier to put on and more comfortable for your baby. Top sheets in flannelette are warm and cosy and need less ironing than standard cotton sheets.
A newborn baby will be swaddled in a shawl, light blanket or sheet for the first few weeks, and will need tucking in with a light blanket. The best blankets are made of cellular cotton, wool or acrylic; wool is warmer for winter, acrylic is cheaper and easier to wash. A satin or polyester edge prevents the blanket from irritating the baby's skin.

Cot

Once your baby grows out of the crib or carrycot he or she will sleep in a cot. This must conform to British safety standards. It must be well made with sides high enough to stop the baby climbing out. The bars must be close enough together to stop a little head getting stuck between them. If painted, the paint must be non-toxic. It is important to check this on a secondhand cot. Cots with a wooden base are very good; some have adjustable bases so that a small baby can sleep higher up and be more easily lifted out and put down. Drop sides also make it easier to put your baby in the cot, but check that the catch is not too easy to operate.

Crib

A wicker or wooden crib can be very attractive, though it is not an essential item. Cribs should be lined to make them draught-proof. Some have stands, others swing, which is useful for soothing a crying baby. These can be fixed so that they cannot swing when the baby is alone. Cribs are not really portable.

Carrycot

(see also p. 272)
If you often travel in the car, a carrycot is extremely useful. Many designs and sizes are available. One of the most useful comes with a transporter which can be neatly folded or converted to a buggy. This type is usually quite small, light and easy to carry. Your baby will grow out of the carrycot by about nine months of age, although the buggy should last for about two years. Carrycots are versatile; they serve as a bed for the baby at home, they can be put in the back of the car (see below), or they can be used as a pram.

Moses basket

A Moses basket is cheap and is light to carry around. However, it is not safe in the back of the car, and is not waterproof, unlike most carrycots.

Travel cot

If you often stay with friends or relatives you might consider buying a travelling cot. These are light and quite compact when folded. They have a firm base and strong fabric sides. Sometimes these are available for hire locally.

Baby alarms and intercom systems

If you are worried because you may not hear your baby crying, you might consider installing an intercom system. Some models do not require any wiring and can be plugged into a socket. An intercom should be sensitive enough to pick up soft crying or the sounds of a restless baby turning over. You can plug your receiver in wherever you are and feel reassured that you will hear your baby as soon as he wakes.

for routine circumcision of the newborn. Moreover, there is no relationship between the incidence of cervical cancer in women with uncircumcised partners, so this cannot be considered as a reason for circumcision of an infant. The medical reason for circumcision is usually a condition known as phimosis, which is severe scarring of the foreskin caused by forcible pulling back or repeated infection. Phimosis does not usually appear until well into childhood or later.

SLEEP

Babies vary in their sleep requirements just as adults do, depending on their personality. Newborn babies spend at least two-thirds of a 24-hour day asleep. At first they have little notion of night and day, and their pattern of sleep is quite random. Gradually they settle into a regular pattern of wakefulness and sleep. After a few weeks they become more aware that night differs from day and will sleep for longer periods at night, with more wakeful periods during the day. At about three months most babies will have three or four periods of sleep during 24 hours.

Some babies are active and wakeful, needing very little sleep. Hunger is not the only reason for being awake; the surroundings are fascinating and there is company and entertainment at hand – too much to see and hear to be asleep. Babies with a more placid personality sleep much more, and at four to five months of age may still be sleeping through much of the day time. Both patterns are normal; there is no set length of time a baby should spend sleeping each day. It is pointless to try and impose longer sleeping times on an active baby who does not need more sleep.

As your baby gets older you can try to adjust his or her pattern of sleep. For example, if he sleeps for long periods during the day but is wakeful at night, you could shorten his day time naps or space them so that he is more sleepy by nightfall. But do not worry about the total amount of time your baby sleeps, as long as he is contented.

A wakeful irritable baby who cries a lot may be uncomfortable or unwell. If you cannot find a reason for his irritability don't be afraid to seek the advice of your health visitor or doctor. Similarly, if his sleep pattern has changed, ask your doctor to check that all is well.

WHERE TO SLEEP

For the first month or two when he or she is still needing night feeds, you will probably prefer your baby to sleep in your bedroom. The room should be warm – about 21°C (70°F) for a tiny baby – and should be free of draughts. By two or three months of age the temperature can be lowered gradually to not less than 15°C (60°F). The room should not cool down too much at night, so the window will need to be kept closed in winter.

In a warm room, a baby wearing a stretchsuit or nightie should only require one or two light blankets or light duvet to keep him warm in a crib or carrycot. Babies who are too hot will probably wake and cry; those who are too cold may not. Overheating and overcooling can both be dangerous. Small babies are less well able to regulate their body temperature, and can become very cold very rapidly, being unable to shiver or move about to keep themselves warm. Check your baby's temperature by feeling his abdomen; it will feel cold if he is too cold, and warm and sticky if he is too hot. When you lift your baby out at night for a feed or nappy change, you may need to wrap him in a shawl or blanket to keep warm.

With the cot or crib near your bed, you can easily take your baby into your own bed for a feed, if you wish. Don't worry if you fall asleep during or after feeding; your baby will not suffocate and you will not roll over on top of him. A baby will naturally move his face out of the way if his breathing is obstructed. Parents filmed asleep at night with their baby between them have been shown to roll away from the baby each time the baby touches them. However, you may find that your baby gets too hot in your bed and is happier back in the cot after the feed. A note of warning: do not let your baby sleep in bed with you if you have taken alcohol or any kind of sedative drug, as your reflexes will be dulled. Babies wearing a splint (for example for a dislocated hip) should not sleep with you either because they are unable to roll over.

You may prefer your baby to sleep in a separate room from yours from the beginning. Babies snuffle quite a lot when they are asleep and parents can find this very disturbing. If there is no separate bedroom, there is no reason why he or she should not sleep in the living room or even on the landing, as long as it is warm and free of draughts and you can hear when the baby cries. You could let the baby sleep in your room until you go to bed, then move him to another room, though this obviously becomes more difficult as the baby gets older.

SLEEPING POSITIONS

For the first two or three weeks babies in Britain are usually swaddled, that is, wrapped up firmly in a sheet or blanket before being put into the cot on their side. They feel secure like this, being enclosed

A fretful baby can be worrying for parents, but there are ways you may soothe him. Try laying him across your knee and stroking his back gently (above), or putting him against your shoulder and walking about or gently rocking in a chair (below).

as if they were in the uterus.

After this time babies prefer to have their limbs free to move. They should no longer be put on their side as this position is unstable, but should lie on their back or stomach. The safest position is lying on the stomach with the head to one side. Any regurgitated milk will dribble out of the mouth, so there is less risk of choking. A pillow should not be used for the first year, as there is a risk of suffocation during the first few months.

If your baby wakes and is unable to roll over on to his back to look around, he may get bored and will cry until someone comes to the rescue. Toys or a small mirror where he can see them may help.

DISTURBED NIGHTS

After a few weeks, settling your baby to sleep may be easier if you establish a familiar routine. This may be different for daytime and night time sleeps. For example, your baby may feel sleepy in the evening after a bath and a cuddle, so you can establish this as a bedtime routine.

Babies who are overtired find it difficult to get off to sleep and may cry for a long time before they finally settle. Rocking your baby in your arms for a while often helps. However, your baby may fall asleep happily in your arms, only to wake and cry as soon as you put him down again. If this happens, you could try cuddling him in the cot without picking him up, laying him down gently when he is asleep. Sometimes your baby just needs to get his crying done before he can go to sleep.

Babies who wake frequently at night are exhausting for their parents, but this is inevitable during the first few weeks. If you are bottle feeding you can take it in turns with night feeds. If you are breastfeeding but exhausted, it won't hurt to let your partner give the baby a bottle at night once or twice, once breastfeeding is established (see p. 158). If one or both partners is working while night feeds are still a regular feature, it might be worth discussing sleeping in separate rooms occasionally. During the day it is important for you to have a rest in the afternoon when your baby is sleeping.

When your baby wakes in the night it is best to deal with his needs immediately – but as briefly as possible. Prolonged playing or cuddling sessions will encourage your baby to believe that waking you in the night carries a special reward. Once he learns that he will be fed or comforted as needed but is unlikely to get extra bonuses, he will begin to modify his behaviour.

When your baby is fast asleep, nothing is likely to disturb him. It is better not to aim for a silent household whenever your baby sleeps, or he will

TRAVELLING

The amount of driving, travelling by public transport or walking you do and the time of year your baby is born will affect your choice of equipment. Babies born in winter will be warmer in a carrycot or pram than in a stroller or buggy. For those born in summer the newer designs of stroller suitable for tiny babies are excellent.

Sling

A sling is a wonderful way of carrying your baby about, indoors or outdoors. In a sling he can snuggle up against your chest leaving your arms free. For very small babies a sling must provide good head and back support; some styles have a detachable headrest, others enclose the baby almost completely – these are usually very good. Check that those with a headrest do in fact provide adequate support. Choose a sling with wide, comfortable shoulder straps which are adjustable, and with an easy fastener at the back – don't be afraid to try on the different types in the shop.

Back pack

Once your baby has good head control he or she will enjoy going for walks in a back pack carrier. This is very light, has a tubular aluminium frame and can be used until two to three years old, depending on the weight of the child and the strength of the parent! Some have adjustable supports for the smaller baby, and others have a stand so that the baby can be propped up on the ground without having to be lifted out of the back pack.

Pram

If you intend to do a lot of walking with your baby, and you have a large area at home in which to park a pram and not too many steps to reach it, you will probably find a pram very useful. A pram is larger than a carrycot and will therefore last longer. Prams with a well-sprung chassis and large wheels are extremely comfortable for your baby, and less bumpy than the smaller-wheeled pushchairs. This type of pram is usually higher than the average carrycot and stroller so is more comfortable to push if you are tall. When old enough the baby can sit up and look around, and will be high above ground level where the view is more interesting and he is at your level. When he is tired you can simply lie him down to go to sleep. In the summer your baby can sleep out in the pram, as it is more stable than a carrycot on wheels. You will need a cat and insect net. Another advantage of a carriage-built pram is that it can hold a toddler seat, useful if you have two children quite close together. When choosing a pram, check that it is balanced and stable, has fittings for a safety harness and efficient brakes. Check that it is easy to manoeuvre, and whether a shopping tray can be fitted.

later wake at the slightest sound. He will not be disturbed by background noises, but will find them reassuring. Your routine of daytime noises and night-time silence will help him to adjust to a similar routine, especially if you do not seem to be interested in playing with him at night.

CRYING

A crying baby exerts a profound emotional effect on his parents. A placid baby who cries infrequently and is easily soothed, sleeping most of the time between feeds, makes his parents feel relaxed and gives them time to rest and catch up. A baby who cries for long periods during the day and night may induce enormous anxiety in his parents, especially the mother. She feels inadequate in dealing with his needs; nothing seems to settle him. She becomes more and more exhausted and irritable and her baby senses this and cries even more. A mother feels very much to blame when her baby cries frequently – other people's babies seem to be so much 'better behaved'. Society's expectations of the perfect mother and housewife, always organized,

Stroller and pushchairs	Ordinary non-adjustable strollers or pushchairs are unsuitable for newborn babies, who are unable to sit up. Several newer designs adjust to a reclining position so that a tiny baby can lie down flat. These can usually be adjusted so the baby can either face you or face forward. This type of buggy is small, and your baby will have grown out of it by six to nine months of age. As soon as he can sit up for a reasonable length of time he can use an ordinary buggy. Some of these do recline to some extent, and this is an advantage since babies prefer to sleep lying down. Strollers are much easier to take shopping as they are narrow enough to push through a supermarket checkout. Collapsible strollers are light, easy to fold and compact to store in the boot of the car or at home. If you are likely to go for long walks along roads and pavements, you might prefer to buy a traditional reclining pushchair with a high back and large sprung wheels. These are heavier and less compact but are very comfortable for your baby.
Stroller accessories	Buggies are unstable when heavy shopping is hung on the handles, but some models have a firm shopping tray underneath. A waterproof cover is worth having for rainy days, and you will need a hood and apron if it does not already have one. A hood will also protect the baby from strong sunshine, or you can buy a parasol which fits on the handle. A parasol is cooler than a hood in hot weather. In cold weather a warm quilted bag for the baby's legs is useful.
Carrycot	If you do not have a car safety seat suitable for a small baby (see below) you should only use a carrycot in a car, secured in the back seat with a carrycot restraint that conforms to British safety standards. The advantage is that you can drive to the shops then put the carrycot on its transporter to take inside the shops – all without waking your baby. Check the model you choose for stability and for efficiency of the brakes. Check also that it is easy to remove the carrycot from the frame and that it is easy to fold the frame. See that the separate parts are light enough for you to carry.
Car safety seat	Not all babies are content to sleep in a carrycot in the back of the car; at times they would much prefer to sit up and see what is going on around them. Several designs of car safety seat have recently come on the market which are suitable even for tiny babies. These are secured in the front passenger seat with an ordinary safety belt. They can be adjusted to a lying down position and can face backwards or forwards, so that you and your baby can look at each other. This type of seat will last until your baby is about six to nine months of age. Standard car safety seats are designed for babies from six to nine months of age until two to three years. These fit in the back of the car and are fixed by a special anchorage system which is usually bought separately.

fully rested and never flustered, smiling at her invariably calm and happy baby, are unlikely to be fulfilled, especially during the first few months.

The fact is that some babies simply do cry more than others. Studies have shown that some babies aged two weeks cry for about two hours a day; those aged six weeks may cry for almost three hours a day. By about three months crying time has fallen to about one hour a day. A few babies cry excessively throughout their first year, which can be very trying for their parents. Crying is most frequent in the late afternoon and evening (see 'Colic' on page 191).

WHY DO BABIES CRY?

Babies cry for a variety of different reasons. These include hunger, thirst, discomfort from a wet or soiled nappy, boredom or frustration, loneliness, fear, feeling too hot, or feeling unwell or in pain. Parents can usually distinguish different types of cry in their own baby. The hunger cry differs from the cry of temper or tiredness. It often begins as a weak but restless whimper, gradually developing into an insistent, angry wail. The cry of a distressed or uncomfortable baby is different again. Mothers hearing this cry know they have to see to their baby immediately; with the hunger cry they know they can afford to wait a few minutes. You will soon learn to recognize what the different cries mean.

If hunger is not the cause of your baby's crying, check whether he or she is uncomfortable in a wet nappy, or feeling too hot or too cold. If you fed him recently, he may be thirsty rather than hungry. Pick him up and talk to him and cuddle him for a few minutes; if he stops crying and looks happier, he may have been feeling bored or lonely, want to change position or simply feel the security of being close to you. Check for obvious causes of pain or distress such as an open nappy pin. Pain is very difficult to assess (see p. 255 and 256).

Sometimes you will be unable to discover any reason at all for your baby's crying, and will feel frustrated because you do not know how to soothe him. Indeed there may not be any specific reason, other than perhaps a need for him to release tension and energy before going to sleep. Babies will usually settle down before long if they are not unwell. If your baby cries persistently for a long time, don't be afraid to telephone your doctor for advice, especially if he refuses to feed or seems otherwise unwell (see p. 255).

HOW TO COPE WITH A CRYING BABY

Although you cannot avoid feeling distressed if your baby cries a lot, you must try to accept that it is not your fault. Your baby is struggling to adapt to his surroundings, and it will take you a while to learn all the reasons for his cries. Don't try to keep your anxiety to yourself; share it with your partner and perhaps with your own mother, a friend with small children, or the health visitor. This will help you to keep things in perspective. It helps too, if both parents can share the daily routine, and if grandparents or relatives are able to take over if the situation becomes fraught.

FEEDING TIMES

Feeding times will not be rigid during the first few weeks (see p. 153). Some babies require more frequent feeding than others, and you will find it very difficult to keep your crying baby waiting for an hour just because he had a feed only two hours before. Just as adults' appetites vary, so do babies', and the time they take to feel hungry again between feeds. Nor does giving a larger feed necessarily mean a longer sleep before the next one. Feeding and sleeping are independent activities to some extent, and your baby's rhythms depend more on his personality than how much milk he has taken.

There is evidence that the close proximity to a parent which babies derive from being carried in a sling actually increases their sense of security and makes them less clingy when older.

'SPOILING'

There is absolutely no danger of 'spoiling' a tiny baby by picking him up or feeding him when he cries. On the contrary, this is essential, in order that he develops a sense of security and a feeling that he is loved. Babies who feel insecure are likely to be much more demanding; they soon learn how to get their parents' attention, while a secure baby is much more willing to accept discipline later on. Most young babies respond very well to the security of being carried in a sling, which has the added advantage of leaving your hands free to do other things.

After the first two to three months you may become aware that your baby is crying not because he is hungry but because he knows he will be picked up or put on the breast. He will rapidly learn how to manipulate you in this way if you let him. However if he feels secure in the knowledge that you will respond to his needs but not necessarily to his every whim, you will have more peaceful nights.

ROCKING

Motion is often helpful in soothing a crying baby. Rocking your baby in your arms, over your shoulder or on your lap is traditional and effective. Babies who cry frequently may enjoy being carried around in a sling or sitting in a bouncing chair. Many babies are soothed by an outing in the pram or in the car.

PACIFIERS

Pacifiers (dummies) can be useful if your baby wants the comfort of sucking rather than a feed. With twins they are particularly useful when one twin has to wait while the other is fed.

Pacifiers are not harmful unless they are sweetened by dipping into honey, syrup or any other sugar-based substance, since this can damage the teeth even before they have appeared. They will not cause teeth deformity if they are discarded at a fairly early age. The disadvantage is that when a pacifier falls out of the baby's mouth, someone has to find it and put it back again, and a pacifier should be sterilized at least for the first three or four months. The practice of attaching a pacifier to string to make it easier for the baby to find is dangerous, as a mobile baby could be strangled.

The picture of a baby or a toddler with a dummy constantly in his mouth is not a very attractive sight, and may even be impeding the normal desire of a child to talk. Tempting though it may be to plug in a dummy every time your baby starts to cry, this may not satisfy all his needs for stimulation and company, and he may be inclined to seek more attention as a result. It is better to spend a little time trying to find out why your baby is crying than merely trying to stop the noise.

THUMBS AND FINGERS

Many babies enjoy sucking their own fingers and thumbs from birth and even before, if they happen to reach the mouth, and later, once they learn how to bring their hands to their mouths. This is normal and safe, and certainly more aesthetic than sucking a pacifier. The only disadvantage of a thumb is that it cannot be taken away (unlike a pacifier) when you think your child is too old to suck it. Intensive thumb-sucking in older children can cause dental malformations; pacifiers are thought to cause less pressure against the teeth. Neither thumbs nor pacifiers are likely to cause any problems at all in infancy.

LEAVING YOUR BABY TO CRY

Your small baby has been fed and changed, cuddled and comforted, and still will not stop crying. Should you leave him to cry? If you are feeling exhausted and angry, your baby will probably sense this, and you are unlikely to be able to soothe him. In these circumstances it is better to leave him for a short while, returning every five to ten minutes to check that he is coming to no harm. Small babies should not be left for longer than this at a time.

Better still, let your partner or a friend deal with the problem once in a while. An occasional evening out leaving your baby with a reliable babysitter may result in a calm baby as well as calm parents. (See page 196 for advice about this.) Leave the telephone number where you can be contacted with the sitter, as well as your doctor's telephone number, and brief the sitter carefully on what to do if problems arise or if the baby does not settle. If the crying persists, it may be because your baby is unwell and you should telephone your doctor for advice.

GROWTH AND DEVELOPMENT

From birth to two years, babies grow and develop very rapidly, especially during the first six months. It is exciting to watch your baby developing new skills almost every week, and growing into a toddler with a unique personality. Babyhood is short-lived, and all the joyful moments when new achievements are reached are easily forgotten. Photographs and a regularly kept diary will provide you with a fascinating record of these milestones. You will also be able to compare the progress of a sister or brother, and see how very differently each child grows and develops.

Regular assessment of growth and development is important because any delay can be detected early and a cause found, thus avoiding or minimizing any permanent problems and helping your child to reach his or her full potential. Growth and development influence and affect each other.

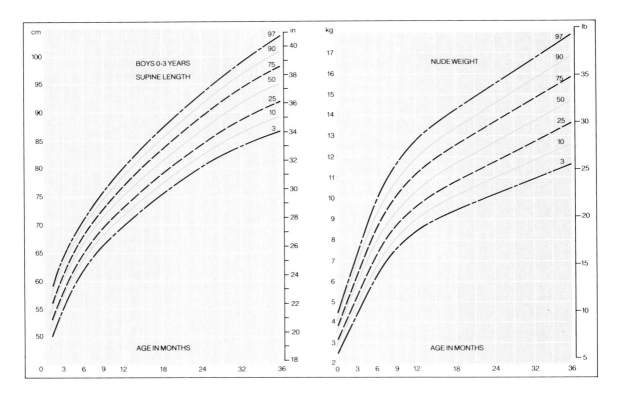

GROWTH

Growth is one of the most sensitive indicators of well-being in childhood, although your doctor or health visitor would never take it in isolation, always taking your child's physical and mental development into account as well. It is easier to measure than development, and is done by measuring weight, height and head size.

The size of a baby at birth depends mostly on the function of the placenta, through which the fetus is nourished. This in turn, depends on the health and environment of the mother during pregnancy. For example, pre-eclampsia (see p. 70) reduces the efficiency of the placenta, and babies born of mothers with this condition may be smaller at birth. Babies born of mothers who smoke also tend to be smaller (see p. 72). Babies whose mothers are diabetic are usually large (see p. 74). A mother who is small in build is likely to produce a smaller baby. This is simply because her small size limits her baby's growth in the uterus.

After birth growth is extremely rapid in the first two years. During this time the antenatal factors which help to determine birth weight gradually wear off, giving way to inherited growth patterns. Taller than average parents will usually have taller than average children, but this effect may not be seen until after the age of two.

GROWTH CHARTS

Your baby's growth will be plotted at the child health clinic (see p. 187) on special 'centile' charts, derived from the measurement of hundreds of babies. There are separate charts for girls and boys; for each sex there is a standard chart for weight, height (or length lying down for babies under two) and head size. There is a chart from birth to two years, one from about three to nine years and from about ten to nineteen years, since the rate of growth varies throughout childhood.

The charts show that there is a very large range of normal weights and heights at any given age. The 50th centile can be regarded as the average, since 50 out of every 100 children will have a weight or height less than that level, and 50 will have a weight or height greater than that level. A child whose weight is on the 3rd centile is still normal; 3 out of every 100 children will weigh less than him or her, whilst 97 will weigh more.

Children growing normally will grow along a line parallel to one of the centile lines; it is the rate of growth which is important, not any single measurement at a particular age. Several measurements need to be taken over a period of time before the rate of growth can be seen. A child who is growing rapidly will have a steep growth curve, crossing centiles upwards. A child who is growing slowly will

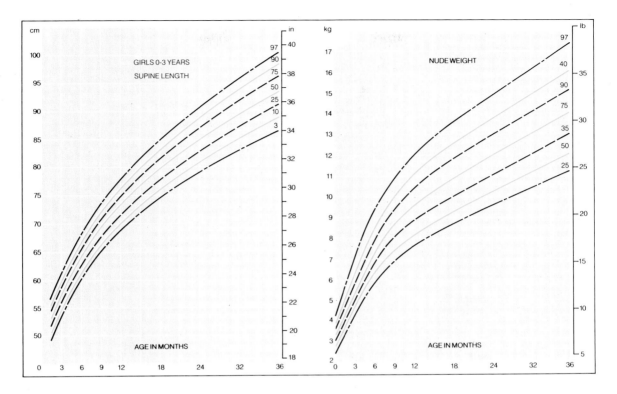

Examples of centile charts for growth, for boys (left) and for girls (right). The measurements of weight and length at birth and during the first three to five years are plotted on a chart similar to these. Each line represents a different centile. Although the range of normal is extremely wide, most babies and children will follow roughly the same centile during this period, although they may dip below or rise above it at different times, since growth rates vary. Any significant dip or imbalance between weight and length or height will be examined more closely by your health visitor or doctor.

have a flatter curve, crossing the centile curves downwards.

Centiles may also be crossed during the first few months of life, when a baby may be 'catching up' on slow growth in the uterus and adjusting to his inherited growth rate. This is quite normal, as long as weight, length and head size all increase at the same rapid rate.

Allowance has to be made for premature babies, whose actual birth weight should be plotted before the age of '0' on the chart. For example, the weight of the baby of four weeks old born four weeks early would be entered at age '0' on the chart. Parental size also has to be taken into account when interpreting charts. Children who appear to be abnormally large may be well within the normal range when the size of both parents is considered.

If a child's growth curve crosses centile lines (apart from during the first few months) he or she should be investigated by the doctor. Investigations should also be done if there is a big difference in the growth curves for weight, height and head size. For example, if a child's curve for head size is along the 97th centile, this is normal if the curves for weight and height follow a similar centile. However, if the weight and height curves follow a much lower centile, close observation may be needed, unless one or both parents clearly had a similar pattern of growth in infancy.

MEASUREMENT OF WEIGHT

Your baby's weight is a useful guide to his well-being, but should not be overrated as an indicator that all is well. Too frequent weighing is likely to cause anxiety, especially since a baby's weight varies considerably from day to day, and at different times of the day. A baby weighs more immediately after a feed, and less after he has opened his bowels or passed urine. Babies should always be weighed naked; wet nappies are quite heavy! Weighing scales are often inaccurate, too.

Newborn babies nearly always lose weight during the first week (see p. 108), but are usually back to birth weight by the tenth day. During the next six months they gain on average 142-170g (5-6oz) per week. An average-sized baby will be approximately double the birth weight in the first six months, and treble it by one year, though this may not be true of babies who are smaller or larger than average at birth.

Although you may find it reassuring to take your baby to be weighed every week, it is not really necessary to do it more often than once every three to four weeks. A contented energetic baby is a better indicator of good health and satisfactory progress than weight gain.

MEASUREMENT OF LENGTH

Under the age of two, babies prefer to lie curled up, which makes it more difficult to measure their length. In the clinic they are usually measured on a special table or mat with a headboard at one end. One person holds the baby's head straight, touching the headboard. A second person gently straightens out his legs so that they lie flat on the table, then brings up a moveable footboard against the heels. It is quite difficult to get an accurate measurement of length with a moving, crying baby – and almost impossible with only one person. Measurement of length is not always done routinely at the clinic, so don't be surprised if your baby is not measured in this way. Over the age of two children can be measured standing up. (This is usually done as part of the programme of pre-school developmental checks organized by your doctor or health visitor, and described on page 189.)

MEASUREMENT OF HEAD SIZE

This is simply done by measuring the circumference of the head at its widest point with a tape measure. The head grows at a very rapid rate during the first twelve to eighteen months, reflecting the growth of the brain. A baby's head is very large relative to the rest of the body, being about a quarter the size of the trunk at birth, becoming about one eighth in adulthood. The skull bones do not join together until the rapid phase of brain growth is over, and the 'soft spot' (anterior fontanelle) on the top of the baby's head does not usually disappear before about twelve months. The smaller posterior fontanelle closes by about three months.

INFLUENCES ON GROWTH

Weight loss is likely to accompany even minor illnesses such as colds or diarrhoea. More prolonged and serious illness or malnutrition will affect length as well as weight. Unless it is very prolonged (exactly how prolonged is not known), this slowing of growth will not be permanent, and will be followed by a period of rapid 'catch-up' growth when the child recovers. Slow growth in the absence of obvious illness may be due to a hormone deficiency or a failure to absorb food, for example due to an allergy to cow's milk (see p. 146).

Failure to gain weight may be simply due to insufficient food, and your health visitor will be able to advise you if this is the case, or if there may be other problems (see p. 00) which need investigation. However, overfeeding will lead to obesity and this is not healthy. Fat babies may grow into fat adults, and may also be more prone to infection. Again, your health visitor will be able to discuss your child's growth charts with you and advise you about feeding.

Disturbances in the rate of growth of the head are rare but it is important to detect them early, in order to arrange treatment to avoid brain damage.

DEVELOPMENT

Development is more difficult to assess than growth. There is no standard rate or age at which milestones are reached, and the range of ages over which babies and children achieve various skills is very wide indeed. It is common for your baby to be ahead in one area of development and behind in another. Even within the same family two children will probably have very different patterns of development. Keeping a simple baby book or diary for each child is an interesting source of comparison.

Development in one area depends on development in other areas; vision, hearing, language, movement, intellectual, emotional and social development are all interconnected. For example, if a child does not hear well, his or her language and communication will be affected, which in turn will affect social development. This is why healthy children are regularly assessed to see if there is any developmental delay. The earlier any such delay is detected, the earlier it can be treated.

As parents, you are in the best position to observe your children's development. You can tell if your child is not seeing or hearing properly much earlier than anyone else, and your comments and anxieties should always be taken seriously. When reviewing your baby's progress, your doctor or health visitor only sees the baby for short periods of time, and babies and children do not always present themselves at their best if they are tired, hungry or irritable, or simply frightened of strangers. The table of simple questions and observations given opposite will help you to assess your own baby's progress particularly in the areas of hearing and vision during the first year of life. They are meant for reassurance – if you are at all doubtful contact your own doctor or the health visitor or clinic doctor who will check your baby in more detail. Development checks can easily be arranged in addition to those done routinely at the child health clinic.

If your child seems to be walking or talking later than you expect, the chances are that he will be advanced in other ways. Children are constantly learning and developing new concepts, and sometimes their understanding is far ahead of, say, their manipulative skills or their ability to move around. Development usually follows a certain sequence – for example sitting, crawling, pulling to stand and then walking. However, some children find that they can get around quite well on their bottoms, instead of crawling. These 'bottom-shufflers' often start walking later than usual (see p. 208) simply because they have found a very efficient way of getting around without needing to stand up.

INFLUENCES ON DEVELOPMENT

Your baby's development depends not only on his or her inherited characteristics, but also on the opportunities he or she has to learn and practise new skills. A baby will not be able to sit up before his nervous system has reached a sufficient stage of maturity, no matter how hard you try to teach him and encourage him. Moreover, he or she will sit up sooner or later without any encouragement at all. However, a lack of stimulation is discouraging and slows down progress.

Instead of trying to influence your baby's development in a particular area, it is much better to provide a generally stimulating and loving environ-ment in which to encourage development. Don't try to push too hard to achieve a new skill. Learning should always be fun, and should give you and your baby great pleasure. Your delight in day-to-day achievements will be a further incentive to learn. Play is an essential part of learning – indeed, play *is* learning and vice versa.

Prematurity influences development only in that allowances have to be made for the age at which milestones are reached. Actually the development of premature babies tends to be speeded up, so that a baby born six weeks early, who might be expected to smile at the age of twelve weeks, may smile at around ten weeks.

Development may be delayed for a period of time by illness. Sometimes a child may even revert to an earlier stage of development after an illness or an emotional upset. For example, a child may start bedwetting again following the arrival of a new baby (see p. 240). This usually expresses a need for love and attention when the child is feeling insecure. Normal behaviour is resumed when a feeling of security returns.

The more time you can both spend with your small baby, playing with him, talking to him and loving him, the more independent he or she will become later. Within a strong and secure rela-tionship, your baby will be able to reach his or her full potential.

DEVELOPMENT FROM BIRTH TO SIX WEEKS

At birth, babies can focus on objects which are about 20cm (9in) away, which also is the approxi-mate distance between the baby's and mother's

As early as three weeks a baby's eyes are sufficiently focused to enable him to stare fixedly at his own reflection in a mirror.

PLAYING

From birth onwards your baby will enjoy watching moving colours and shapes, and will be fascinated by a mobile strung across the cot or pram, or hung from above especially if it makes a pleasant sound as it moves. Equipment which helps to stimulate your baby's normal development is good value.

Bouncing cradle	From about one month he will have developed enough head control to be able to sit comfortably in a bouncing cradle from where to watch you and see what is going on. These chairs are light enough for you to carry your baby around the house in the chair, but never place it on a worktop or table, however tempting. Some are made of rigid plastic and can be adjusted to a reclining position. The cheaper varieties do not adjust but they are equally comfortable, and are made of cotton or soft plastic. Make sure the fabric is washable and easy to remove from the frame.	**Baby walker**	This is by no means an essential item but some babies do enjoy being able to move around in an upright position. However, a baby walker is not likely to cause a baby to learn to walk any earlier. Do not use a walker for a baby under nine months, and do not leave your baby in a walker for long periods, or unsupervised; stairs are a particular hazard. Furniture is also likely to suffer. Baby walkers do take up a lot of space, though some models are foldable.
Playpen	A playpen is not a substitute for a childproof room but it comes in useful for short periods of time, from about six months of age until your child is walking. Babies should not be left for long periods in a playpen, as they can feel confined and restricted. The square wooden playpen with bars and a built-in floor is sturdy. You can fix toys or an activity centre on to the bars, but check that the bars are close enough together to prevent the baby's head getting trapped in between. Some playpens are foldable, but those without a built-in floor are very easy for a child to drag around the room. A circular or oval 'lobster-pot' design is available which is very light and has fine mesh sides and a padded plastic top rail. This is foldable and may be useful for travelling but is very small. Since it is difficult to tell if paint is non-toxic, it may be safer only to buy a natural wood playpen if you are getting one secondhand. Check that there are no sharp fittings.	**Baby bouncer**	Many babies enjoy baby bouncers as they can swing and jump and twist and turn, or just dangle and bounce. A bouncer has no effect on walking abilities, although your baby will learn the feel of the floor under his feet. Baby bouncers are only suitable for babies over the age of four months, when they can fully support their heads. Never leave a baby in a bouncer for more than fifteen to twenty minutes, even if he still seems to be enjoying himself.
		Toys and storage	You may prefer to plan in advance where and how you will store your baby's toys and clothes. Shelves are useful for baby equipment, later for toys and books. Nursery furniture is often expensive and doesn't last too long because it is small. Wire drawers, plastic stacking boxes and drawers on rollers are all practical and reasonably cheap, or you can build your own simple shelves.

faces in the standard feeding position. Mothers automatically bend this close to their babies when talking to them. A favourite time is while changing the nappy – this is when many parents see their baby's first smile. During the next few weeks babies become able to focus on more distant objects. Watch your baby closely when he is alert and wakeful but not crying – you will be astonished at how interested he is in his surroundings and particularly in your face.

A new baby responds to loud noises by being startled and screwing up his eyes as if to withdraw. If you repeat the loud noise several times he will no longer be startled; he has learned that he will not be harmed by the noise and ignores it. Babies only several days old will turn their head in response to a rattle or to their mother's voice; however, they are easily distracted by what they can see. If your baby hears your voice and sees your face at the same time, his interest is likely to be held and he will follow you.

Young babies seem to respond more easily to high-pitched noises than to low-pitched noises; to their mother's voice rather than their father's. The reason is uncertain, but it may be partly due to the fact that they have become accustomed to hearing their mother's voice while still in the uterus.

During the first few weeks babies lie curled up with their arms and legs close to their body. A newborn baby lying on his stomach is just able to lift his head and turn it aside to avoid being suffocated by the mattress.

By six weeks however, most babies can focus on objects 45cm (18in) away, and will follow a brightly coloured ball. There is more eye-to-eye contact, and your baby will often watch you intently during feeds. Most babies will smile back in response to a smile by now, though you may have noticed your baby smiling long before six weeks. Ninety per cent of babies will be smiling by seven weeks. At this age

At birth a normal baby is usually curled up when lying on his front. Although he can move his head from side to side, he does not have the strength to lift it from the mattress.

At six weeks a baby will have begun to extend his legs and move his arms around. Although his head is still floppy, he can usually lift it up from the mattress when lying on his front.

By three months a baby can lift his head and shoulders up to look around when lying on his front supporting himself on his arms. (By four months he will be doing press-ups – pushing himself right up on his hands.)

At three months, a baby's neck and back muscles are also strong enough to begin to stop his head from falling back when pulled to sitting. By four months he will be able to keep his head in line with his back – a first stage towards sitting.

By six weeks, and often earlier, many babies smile freely when they can focus their attention on a familiar face, especially one of their parents.

you will be able to sense his pleasure at being handled and bathed, and the enjoyment he shows in faces. Even a very tiny baby will look intently at his own image in a mirror; a mirror fixed inside the cot will give interest and delight for several months.

By this age you will probably have noticed your baby 'stilling' to a sound, and turning his head towards its source. He will be starting to show his pleasure by making 'cooing' noises, as well as communicating his discomfort or displeasure by crying. Six-week-old babies are generally alert and interested in their surroundings.

Head control is beginning to develop, alongside the ability to see more clearly. When lying on his stomach, your baby will briefly lift his head and turn his face to one side. When pulled to a sitting position from lying down on his back, he will lift his head for a moment before it lags. You should not do this often, however, as his head is still very unstable. A certain amount of head roll is inevitable, for instance when passing the baby from one person to another, but you should try to support it when you pick your baby up or when holding him since a sudden jerk could be damaging.

A six-week-old baby has sufficient head control to be able to enjoy sitting in a bouncing cradle, although these do give enough support for babies from about three weeks. A row of brightly coloured toys strung across the chair will amuse him, and he will be able to see what is going on around him. A mobile hung over the cot will give him pleasure from birth, and some of these are musical. You can make your own mobile by tying bits of brightly coloured cloth or paper cut into spirals or squares on to a wire coat hanger with string. Bits of jewellery or even kitchen foil make good mobiles at least while the baby cannot reach them. With this sort of stimulation your baby may be happy for a while when awake but by himself.

When asleep on his stomach, a six-week-old baby adopts the same posture as a newborn baby – curled up with the pelvis high. When awake, he will lie flatter, with his legs outstretched and his pelvis lower.

The primitive reflexes (see p. 112) are beginning to disappear by this age. The stepping reflex disappears by six to eight weeks, the grasp reflex and Moro reflex by about three months.

DEVELOPMENT AT THREE MONTHS

By now your baby will have become more sociable, smiling spontaneously when spoken to, and will be just as ready to smile at a stranger as at his mother or father. He will also communicate his pleasure by squeals and the beginnings of repetitive babble using consonants. He sleeps less during the day and may sleep through without waking for a feed in the early hours of the morning. He will have begun to look at his hands, and will bring them together in front of his face, playing with his fingers, studying them with fascination. He is learning that his hands are a part of himself. He will pull at his clothes.

His vision is now very well developed and he will turn his head to see where people are going. He is also learning to coordinate his eyes with his hands. Soon he will be reaching out for things suspended above the cot – this starts by three to four months. Already by three months most babies will hold on to a rattle for a few moments when it is placed in one hand. The hands of a three-month-old baby are open – ready for grasping – unlike those of a newborn baby, which are closed most of the time.

Head control is much firmer, and there is very little head lag when you pull him up to a sitting position from lying down. When lying on his stomach he will stretch his legs out behind him and lift his head and shoulders off the bed, propping himself up on his forearms. It is a good idea at this stage to let him spend some time lying on a rug on the floor in this position rather than always leaving him on his back or propped in a chair, since it helps to strengthen his back and arm muscles.

Rattles and toys which can be grasped or squeezed will help him from this stage onwards, as well as things to look at and listen to. Your baby needs to spend some of his time playing alone and some of it playing with his mother and father. The

A newborn baby's hands are usually tightly clenched; the grasp reflex means that a baby will involuntarily grip a finger placed in his palm strongly enough to be lifted up.

At six weeks of age the grasp reflex has usually disappeared and the baby's hands are generally more relaxed. However he cannot hold anything or make very purposeful movements.

By three months a baby can open his palm and may start to reach for a toy. But he still has little control over whether his hand is open or clenched.

time you spend with him is an essential part of his learning and development, for he needs the security and the encouragement as well as the stimulation.

THE HEALTH VISITOR AND THE CLINIC

The health visitor is a fully qualified state registered nurse who has had some obstetric experience and extra training in the care and development of children. She does not do conventional nursing procedures but is able to advise you on all aspects of child care, from parentcraft and feeding to immunization and growth and development. Her role is to keep you and your children physically and emotionally healthy, rather than to diagnose and treat illness. However she is in a good position to pick up any problems at an early stage and to arrange further help when appropriate.

In Britain, health visitors are employed by the District Health Authority, but many are attached to GP practices and look after all the parents and children who are registered with the GP. Health visitors who are not practice attached will work in association with a child health clinic. Every district has one of these clinics, each with its own clinic

HOW WELL CAN YOUR BABY HEAR?

A parents' check-list

In the newborn baby:	Your baby should be startled by a sudden loud noise such as a hand clap or a door slamming and should blink or open his eyes widely to such sounds.
At four to five weeks:	Your baby should be beginning to notice sudden prolonged sounds like the noise of a vacuum cleaner and he should pause and listen to them when they begin.
At four months:	He should quieten or smile to the sound of your voice even when he cannot see you. He may also turn his head or eyes toward you if you come up from behind and speak to him from the side.
At seven months:	He should turn immediately to your voice across the room or to very quiet noises made on each side if he is not too occupied with other things.
At nine months:	He should listen attentively to familiar everyday sounds and search for very quiet sounds made out of sight. He should also show pleasure in babbling loudly and tunefully.
At twelve months:	He should show some response to his own name and to other familiar words. He may also respond when you say 'no' and 'bye bye' even when he cannot see any accompanying gesture.

HOW WELL CAN YOUR BABY SEE?

A parents' check-list

In the newborn baby:	The centre of the eye (pupil) should be clear. If you think that it looks white or red, then report this as soon as possible. The baby should look at your face when he is feeding and the eyes should be steady.
At six weeks:	He should look at you and also follow your face as you move from side to side. The eyes should be steady when looking at something and should move together. If the eyes are not working together, then there will be a squint. This should be reported.
At six months:	He should take great interest in looking at everything around him. He should reach out and grab small toys, for example small bricks. Any squint, however slight, must now be investigated.
At nine months:	Very small objects, the size of raisins, will be looked at and raked up. (Watch that he doesn't choke on small objects.)
At twelve months:	Neat 'pincer' grip of raisin-sized objects. Points to things across the room.

Problems with hearing and vision often run in families, so if parents or brothers and sisters have eyesight or hearing problems, then there is a higher risk of this being found in your baby. If you are worried about your baby, get advice from your doctor or health visitor.

doctor. The health visitors here will look after families who live within a defined geographical area, which will span several GP practice areas. In this situation there is less communication between the GPs and the health visitor, which is a disadvantage. On the other hand your child health clinic may be more convenient to get to than your GP, and may have more sessions per week than at a GP's surgery.

WHAT DOES THE HEALTH VISITOR OFFER?

You may have already met your health visitor during your pregnancy, when she will have given you advice and information about keeping healthy during the pregnancy and preparing for the arrival of your baby. After the birth, the health visitor has a duty to visit you at home when your baby is ten days old. This should happen automatically – you do not need to send for her. On this occasion she will be able to answer any queries you may have – and there will probably be many – and help you with any difficulties you may be having, such as with feeding, bathing or any aspects of your baby's behavioural patterns, such as sleeping or crying, or with emotional problems. She will also examine the baby to check that all is well. After this she may visit you at home several times more, especially if you live in difficult circumstances.

Afterwards the health visitor will be available (and easily accessible) on the telephone or in the clinic or surgery to help and advise you. Don't be afraid to contact her freely for any worry you may have, even if you feel it is trivial. If you think your baby is ill, you should of course contact your GP.

Well baby clinics organized by health visitors are generally informal and unhurried, whether they are held in your GP's surgery or in the child health clinic. They are held at regular times each week, but you do not need an appointment and you can go as often as you wish.

Mothers used to be advised to take their baby to the clinic weekly to be weighed; nowadays such frequent weighing is known to be unnecessary and anxiety-provoking (see p. 156). Occasional weighing – perhaps once a month – is quite sufficient if the baby is otherwise well. Satisfactory weight gain does not automatically mean there are no problems. Excessive weight gain is as much a problem as insufficient weight gain, and is more common.

The value of a well baby clinic is less to do with regular weighing than with the fact that it provides you with a link with someone experienced in baby care, whom you will get to know and trust over the first few years. It is very reassuring to know that your baby is progressing normally. If you do not feel up to going to the clinic – perhaps because you are

feeling depressed or very tired – do ring your health visitor. She will try to visit you at home.

Another benefit of going to the clinic is the opportunity to meet other parents. Many mothers feel isolated at this time, and such contact is vital. Information about various groups and facilities is usually to be found on the clinic notice board.

You will also be able to buy vitamins and baby foods at the clinic. Your health visitor will advise you on when vitamins are needed and what quantity your baby requires, and of course she will advise you about feeding and weaning.

Advice and information about immunization (see p. 251) will also come from your health visitor. She will tell you where and when it is done and give you the opportunity to discuss your feelings about it. You will usually be offered the choice of having your child immunized by your GP or by the clinic doctor.

CHILD HEALTH RECORDS

Health visitors carry out full developmental checks, together with the GP or the clinic doctor. These are usually done at six weeks (see overleaf), eighteen

The child health clinic is a source of advice on all aspects of baby care, and any problems can be discussed with a health visitor or doctor.

months, two and a half to three years (see p. 238) and just before starting school, though these ages vary from district to district and from one GP to another. Vision and hearing tests are also done at seven to eight months, and in between as well if you are worried. Extra hearing tests are usually done after a bad ear infection (see p. 266), although you may have to ask for this if your GP does not run his own well baby clinic.

The health visitor keeps a record card of your child's health, which helps her to follow your child's progress throughout childhood. The record is transferred to the school when your child enters school. The purpose of these records is to anticipate areas where problems might arise, to pick up any problems or delays in development or growth at the earliest possible moment, and where possible to prevent problems arising.

Recorded on the card are details of your pregnancy, labour and delivery, and any significant details of your medical history which could affect your child. Weight, height and head circumference are charted on centile charts kept with the card. A note is entered each time you visit the clinic, and any particular difficulties or areas of worry recorded. Dates of immunization are noted. Details of the routine developmental checks are also recorded, and any areas of delay or possible delay are noted, along with what action was taken, such as arranging another check or an appointment with a specialist.

Many districts also provide records for parents to keep, so that you can enter yourself the details of your child's growth and development. The age at which significant milestones are reached can be noted, and such details as the appearance of teeth. You can also record your child's immunizations, and any illnesses, medicines or allergies. If you are not given such a booklet, it is definitely worth making one up for yourself. It will provide you with an extremely valuable record of your child's progress as well as a reminder of when the next check or immunization is due. Moreover it can be very helpful to your doctor who may not always have access to clinic records.

There are arguments in favour of parents keeping charge of all clinic records concerning their child – this already happens in several countries, for example France. Since you are the most important people concerned with the welfare and progress of your child, it seems obvious that you should always be fully informed and therefore better able to make choices and share decisions in the management of your child. Records might be more easily available if they were kept safe by parents. Perhaps this will come about in the future.

THE SIX-WEEK CHECK

The six-week developmental check may be done by your GP or by the clinic doctor. If your baby had problems at birth, the check will probably be carried out by the paediatrician in the hospital. The six-week check is an opportunity for reassurance that your baby is healthy and to air any difficulties you may be having.

To begin with, your health visitor will see you and your baby, who will be weighed and measured. She can advise you about feeding and any other problems you wish to discuss. She will also remind you about the date of your baby's first immunization at three months.

The doctor will be interested to know how you have been feeling and what sort of difficulties you have encountered. He or she will ask how your baby has been responding – whether he has smiled, whether he seems to respond to your voice or to other sounds, whether he watches you or follows objects. The doctor will check the growth charts and enquire about feeding.

You will be asked to undress your baby (bring along a spare disposable nappy or two) and the doctor will look at his posture lying on the couch. At the same time the skin can be inspected for any marks or rashes. The doctor will pull the baby to a sitting position to observe the degree of head lag, then will hold him under his abdomen, face downwards to see how well he holds his head up.

The doctor will check the baby's reflexes (see p. 112), and will examine the baby's vision by getting him to follow a brightly coloured ball or brick from side to side. The doctor will look into the baby's eyes with an ophthalmoscope (eye torch), looking for evidence of a squint or other abnormalities such as a cataract.

The doctor will feel the fontanelles (soft spots) to make sure they are neither too tense nor sunken, and will feel inside the baby's mouth to check the sucking reflex.

The baby's heart and chest will be listened to, and the pulses of the arteries felt in the arms and the groins to ensure that the circulatory system is normal. The umbilicus will be checked to see that it is properly healed, and the abdomen felt to make sure that the internal organs are not enlarged. The doctor will look for hernias in the groin, and, in a boy, will check that both testes have descended into the scrotum.

Examination of the hips for dislocation is very important. Although this is checked by the paediatrician in the hospital or by your doctor after the birth (see p. 112), occasional babies slip through and babies are rechecked at six weeks.

At the six-week check, your baby's newborn reflexes may be tested to see if they are still present, such as the walking reflex shown here.

Clicking hips are not uncommon in babies of this age; they are usually due to loose ligaments and will disappear with a few weeks. If your baby's hips do click, your doctor will want to recheck them later. If there is any suspicion of a dislocated hip, the doctor will need to arrange an X-ray and an appointment with a specialist. The doctor will also look at your baby's feet, to exclude a club foot or any other deformity.

PROBLEMS WITH YOUNG BABIES

All parents have worries about their new babies. The problem may seem trivial, but nonetheless if it is causing anxiety it makes parenting that much more stressful. Many of the conditions listed here are common – most babies suffer from them some of the time. Many are normal, but if you are at all worried that your baby is unwell or if the suggested remedies aren't effective don't hesitate to contact your health visitor or doctor.

COLIC

Quite a number of babies have regular long crying sessions, usually in the evenings. They often draw up their knees and appear to be in pain, and are said to have colic, because it is assumed that wind in the bowel causes the pain. Although there is no good evidence of this, no-one has yet come up with a better explanation. Babies draw up their knees whenever they cry, so it is impossible to assess whether or not they actually do have pain in the abdomen.

Whatever the cause, it is undoubtedly true that a baby with what is known as colic is extremely trying for his or her parents. Evening crying is particularly wearing if you are a single parent or if one or both partners has a job, since this is usually the only time during the working week that they can be together. The parent who has been at home with the baby all day is likely to be very tired, while his or her partner will also be wanting to relax after a day at work. If both are faced with a baby that cries for two, three or even four hours with little respite, the situation can become very tense, and that tension can be transmitted to the baby, who may become even more upset.

Rocking, singing a comforting lullaby, walking about with the baby, laying him or her over your knee and rubbing the back, are all methods to soothe your baby at least temporarily. Preparations such as gripe water given in very small doses can also give relief for an hour or so. Some mothers who breastfed have found that cutting milk and milk products out of their own diet has helped. (Medicines which stop bowel spasm are no longer prescribed for babies under six months because a few babies became ill after taking them.)

Try to get out of the house and away from the problem once in a while – this is a very good way of getting the situation back into perspective (see p. 194). It is much easier for a friend or relation who understands babies to deal with a crying baby who is not his or her own. Friends who have already suffered from a colicky baby are often very sympathetic. The important thing to remember is that babies grow out of this condition and colic almost always disappears by about three or four months. But if you are worried about prolonged bouts of crying, check with your doctor (see p. 255).

REGURGITATION

Regurgitation of a small amount of milk after a feed is perfectly normal. Possetting, when a small amount of milk is brought up with a burp is also normal. Most babies will occasionally vomit an entire feed, and this is not a cause for alarm. However, repeated vomiting is a sign of illness and you should seek medical advice as soon as possible, especially if the vomit is projected forcefully in one go (see p. 262).

CONSTIPATION

The frequency of passing a stool varies from baby to baby and between breast and bottle fed babies (see p. 109). Breastfed babies pass loose stools but may do so infrequently – even once a week or less. Bottlefed babies pass harder stools more frequently. If your baby's stools are very hard as well as infrequent, he or she may be constipated. Passing a hard stool may be painful and sometimes causes a small crack to occur at the anus (anal fissure), which can bleed.

Constipation is often due to lack of fluid, and sometimes due to lack of food or to vomiting. Occasionally there are other causes. Giving more to drink may be all that is required. Some people suggest adding a little brown sugar to the feeds or giving fruit juice to drink, but this is rarely necessary; constipation should not be a cause for worry.

DIARRHOEA

Loose, green, explosive stools may be perfectly normal in a breastfed baby. Copious diarrhoea which is more frequent than normal may be due to infection (see p. 261). If your baby is not drinking very much or is vomiting, dehydration can occur very rapidly and you should call your doctor as soon as possible. Mild diarrhoea in a breastfed baby may be due to the mother taking a laxative, or may be related to her diet. Diarrhoea is treated by giving the baby clear fluids only to drink – no milk. You can give your baby boiled, cooled water in a bottle, but your doctor may prescribe an electrolyte solution which replaces the glucose and salts lost during dehydration. There are various types – the most usual come in powdered form in a sachet to be dissolved in boiled water and given in a bottle. Milk can be restarted when the diarrhoea has settled.

SPOTS AND RASHES

Up to about eight weeks, babies are often quite spotty. This may be due to the change of environment from liquid to air which occurs at birth, or to hormonal changes. Although they can be rather unsightly especially on fair-skinned babies, these 'milk rashes' are harmless and they disappear in time. They have nothing to do with milk. Heat rashes may appear on the face and neck, shoulders and chest when a baby is too hot and sweats a lot.

If your baby has a very dry skin, a little baby oil added to the bath water applied after a bath will help. If you add oil to bath water be careful when lifting your baby out as it makes the skin more slippery. Excessively dry or flaky skin requires a medical opinion. Infantile eczema does not usually appear before two to three months of age (see p. 270).

Septic spots are important to recognize as they are caused by bacteria and may require treatment with an antibiotic. They usually have a white central part with a red inflamed surround. If you have any doubt about any spots or rashes, it is best to ask the doctor or health visitor to have a look.

CRADLE CAP

Babies whose skins tend to produce a lot of grease are likely to develop cradle cap, or seborrhoeic dermatitis of the scalp. Brownish scales or crusts develop on the scalp, occasionally with very mild inflammation. The condition is harmless, and usually disappears on its own during the first few months.

Recently formed crusts can usually be washed off with a solution of one teaspoon of sodium bicarbonate to 600ml (1 pint) of water. One per cent cetrimide solution is also effective, or you can use one of several medicated shampoos which are available. Persistent crusts can be removed by softening them overnight with olive oil, then lifting them off gently with a comb. Once the crusts have been removed, regular shampooing keeps the condition under control.

NAPPY RASHES

Since it is not always possible to change a nappy as soon as it becomes wet or soiled, babies inevitably spend some time each day in a wet nappy. Not surprisingly, from time to time they will develop a sore bottom, and this can happen very early in life, if your baby has a particularly sensitive skin.

Ammonia dermatitis is the commonest form of rash. It is caused by the ammonia released when urine reacts with faeces. The longer your baby lies in a wet and soiled nappy, the more chance there is of ammonia forming. Breastfed babies produce an acid stool which discourages this chemical break-down; babies fed on cows' milk produce an alkaline stool, so are more likely to get this type of rash.

Terry nappies should be washed and rinsed very thoroughly to remove all traces of ammonia (see p. 169). Use non-biological powders; the biological ones can themselves cause irritation if any trace is left. A final rinse in diluted vinegar (acetic acid) in the proportion 25ml (1 fl oz) to 4.5 litres (1 gallon) will help to prevent ammonia forming. If your baby's bottom looks sore, wash and clean it very gently, be sure to dry thoroughly and apply a thick barrier cream. Avoid plastic pants as they prevent air from circulating around the skin and they make the nappy soggier. Use a one-way liner inside the nappy. If possible, let your baby spend a few hours each day without a nappy on, perhaps lying on a nappy or a towel on the floor, as exposure to the air helps the rash to heal. Otherwise change the nappy as frequently as possible and as soon as you are aware that it is wet or soiled.

Seborrhoeic dermatitis is an occasional cause of nappy rash, and may be extended to the armpits and the groin as well as the genitals and buttocks. Cradle cap will most probably be present as well. Treatment of the cradle cap and management of the nappy area as described above usually leads to clearance of any other areas affected.

THRUSH

Thrush (Candida albicans) is a kind of fungus which thrives in warm, moist areas. It is commonly found in the mouth as well as in the nappy area. In the nappy area, the appearance of the rash is often difficult to distinguish from ammonia dermatitis (above).

If a thrush rash in the nappy area does not respond to the measures described for ammonia dermatitis, or if you are concerned, ask your doctor to have a look. Thrush is easy to treat using an antibiotic cream which your doctor will prescribe.

Thrush in the mouth appears as little white patches inside the cheeks or on the palate and the tongue. These cannot be easily scraped off, unlike milk curds, and they make the baby's mouth sore, so that feeding becomes uncomfortable.

Mouth thrush is common in babies because they have not yet developed resistance to infection. Incompletely sterilized bottles and teats increase the risk of thrush infection, but it can occur even when sterilization is adequate. Thrush is treated using an anti-fungal preparation in liquid form, which is dropped on to the tongue after feeds.

THE UMBILICUS

A moist umbilical stump can be encouraged to heal by cleaning with spirit swabs and applying anti-septic powder (see p. 109). If there is any sign of inflammation your doctor or health visitor should have a look. Very occasionally a bright red fleshy 'polyp' forms on the stump. This can be treated by your GP or health visitor, who will touch it with a silver nitrate pencil which will make it heal.

An umbilical hernia is common in babies. It is caused by a delay in the closure of the muscles around the umbilical cord. No treatment is required and most umbilical hernias will disappear within a year or two. Unlike inguinal hernias (see p. 261) there is no danger of the bowel getting stuck inside the hernia, so an operation is not needed. Although umbilical hernias can be quite large and protrude even further when the baby cries, they are no longer strapped up as they used to be, as it makes no difference and may even delay the disappearance of the hernia.

COUGHING AND SNEEZING

Sneezing is the normal means by which a baby clears his nose, and it does not indicate that he or she is unwell. Many babies become snuffly from time to time. This is not a problem as long as it does not interfere with feeding. If it does, nose drops can be prescribed to clear the nostrils before a feed.

Babies sometimes cough a little during or after a feed, but more persistent coughing usually indicates an infection (see p. 265).

STICKY EYES

A yellowish discharge from the eyes occurs very commonly during the first few days after birth. Later this may recur and is sometimes due to a bacterial infection (conjunctivitis). This usually clears after a day or two of cleaning the eye gently with boiled water or cotton wool, wiping from inside outwards. If it does not, or if the discharge is profuse and the eye red, see your doctor (see p. 261).

A few babies have a blockage of the tear ducts, which drain tears from the eyes to the nose. This causes watering of the eyes and frequent mild attacks of conjunctivitis. Antibiotic drops or ointment may be sufficient to clear the blockage. The ducts normally reopen spontaneously within about nine months; if they do not, they can be opened by gentle probing under a general anaesthetic.

SQUINT

Many babies have squints during the first few weeks, until the muscles which move the eyes become sufficiently developed and co-ordinated to move the eyes in parallel. By three months they should have disappeared.

Squints may be divergent, when the eye looks outwards, or convergent, when it looks inwards. One or both eyes may squint. Babies whose noses have a broad flat ridge often appear to squint because the whites at the inner side of the eyeballs cannot fully be seen. Chinese babies always have this appearance. Your doctor will be able to distinguish this from any true squint. If you think your baby has a squint, all or part of the time, you should ask your doctor to see him (see p. 261).

THE EXASPERATING BABY

No babies are easy all the time, and some babies are particularly difficult most of the time. Nearly all parents, at some time, become quite desperate and feel capable of shaking or hurting their child. When you reach this stage you know that the only thing to do is to put your baby in another room for a while and make yourself a cup of tea. Parents who do batter their children react abnormally and cannot control their feelings at this dangerous stage.

If you are worried that your feelings for your baby are not normal, either because you very frequently have the feeling that you could hurt him, or because you feel you cannot love him or you dislike him intensely, do try to talk this over with your doctor or health visitor. Loving your baby does not happen immediately or automatically. There is no doubt that some babies make it easier for their parents to love them, by responding to attention and by being easily contented. Difficult babies evoke mixed feelings in parents, which in turn give rise to guilt.

You may need help to get your feelings into perspective, and to learn to understand your child's development and cope with the difficulties. There may be underlying psychological or emotional problems which need to be explored, and feelings which need to be released. A friend at the end of the telephone may be an invaluable help at a crucial moment. Even if you feel no more than a vague uneasiness, it is better to share this with someone than to keep it to yourself. Otherwise you may not recognize when the situation is getting out of hand.

LEAVING YOUR BABY

The first time you go out without your baby you will probably have very mixed feelings. On the one hand you probably need a change, may be tired, tense and generally lacking in confidence. On the other hand you feel guilty at leaving him in someone else's care when he is so tiny.

There is no good reason why a very small baby should not be left with someone else for a few hours, as long as it is someone you can trust. It is better for you to take a break from your baby than to remain constantly with him when you are too tense to enjoy him. A babysitter only has to cope for a few hours; you are with your baby 24 hours a day. You should not feel guilty about leaving your baby; the adjustment you have had to make in your life is, after all, enormous. It would be very surprising if you didn't need to take an occasional 'breather'.

MAKING CONTACTS

Many parents, especially mothers, begin to feel trapped and isolated when they realize how time-consuming looking after a baby and a home is. There seems to be no time to see friends and no free time in the day. But it is important to maintain contacts and to establish new links with mothers in a similar situation. You will feel very reassured to know that you are not alone in finding life with a new baby tough going. Your health visitor will know of local mothers' groups, or you may see notices in the library or child health clinic in your area. You may already have heard about such groups through your antenatal classes.

GOING TO WORK

There is no right or wrong time to return to work; this is a very individual decision. Some women feel the need to return to work – either full-time or part-time – soon after their baby is born, while others feel unwilling or unable to do so for a long time. You may also be obliged to go back to work for financial or other reasons.

The decision to return to work is often a very hard one, and again you will probably feel ambivalent about it. If you had a fulfilling career before your baby was born, you are likely to miss the stimulation and may feel bored at home. On the other hand, some women feel pressurized to return to work but suffer guilt at leaving their baby.

You must decide what is right for you and your family. A bored, unhappy mother at home all day with her baby but not enjoying him is worse than a happy, relaxed mother who is away from home for part of the day but has the energy to enjoy and care for her baby when she returns home. Don't feel guilty about needing stimulation outside the home. Neither should you feel guilty, if you feel wholly satisfied in your role as a mother. As jobs go this is one of the most demanding and the most rewarding.

When you do return to work, you may have the possibility of taking your baby with you if there is a workplace nursery. Otherwise, you will have to decide carefully who will look after your baby while you are away, unless in your family it is the father who is the primary caretaker.

THE FATHER AS PRIMARY CARETAKER

Women in our society are no longer limited to the roles of mother and housewife. A woman's career is just as important as a man's, and society is slowly changing to accommodate this. The father who

More and more fathers are taking on and enjoying the main responsibility for their children's care, and in running the household generally.

adopts the role of primary caretaker at home with the child, whilst his partner is out at work, has gained greater acceptability. Although still uncommon, this may well happen more often in the future.

As a father, you may have some difficulty in adjusting to this new role, just as a woman does. As a woman out at work, you need to support your partner in his role and understand his difficulties; don't underestimate just how demanding a job it is. Share the difficult times as well as the rewards.

Parenting does not come automatically for men or for women; there is no right or wrong about who should be at home with the baby. What is important is that it should feel right for both of you. If this is so, the atmosphere at home will be relaxed and loving, and your child will grow up feeling secure.

CHOOSING THE RIGHT KIND OF HELP

There are a number of options available, and it is worth considering very carefully what kind of help would suit you best, depending on your lifestyle as well as on your financial situation. Young babies are best looked after in their own home where the surroundings are familiar. This is not always possible, however, especially if your job is not well paid.

It may seem early days to be thinking about the right kind of help in the first three months of your baby's life, unless the demands of your career mean you are going back to work very early. But most women taking maternity leave will be returning to work within six to nine months of the birth, and it sometimes takes a month or two to find the right kind of help, especially if you are employing a nanny who may have to give a month's notice from her previous job. It is also worth pointing out that around six months of age babies start to cling to their mothers and be wary of strangers, so you may have difficulty if you start to leave your baby just at this time (see p. 214).

Try to introduce a new helper a little earlier than this age if you can, and spend time together so that your baby will learn to feel safe with the new person before you have to leave.

GRANDPARENTS

If you or your partner have parents of your own who are able and willing to help, you are indeed lucky. Grandparents can be a tremendous help. Your own mother may have been brought up in a different generation, but her experience and support will be invaluable.

Be careful not to take grandparents for granted, however. They will find their grandchildren very tiring after a while. They may be delighted to babysit for you quite often but might understandably resent being expected to do so on a regular basis. It would be unfair to expect a grandparent to look after your baby when you go back to work; they do still have their own lives to lead!

A sensitive grandparent can often be helpful with a difficult child. When you are caught up in a vicious cycle of tension and tiredness, they remain relatively detached emotionally, and will be able to take over for a couple of hours to relieve you.

Difficulties can arise at times, however, especially if there is disagreement about methods. Sentences beginning 'In my day . . .' are apt to be irritating. Implied or outspoken criticism can be undermining at a time when you feel the need for emotional support. Do listen, though, before you reject advice. Parentcraft hasn't changed all that much over the years, and experience still counts for a great deal. Perhaps the best approach is to talk to your health visitor or doctor, and decide for yourself what is best. Point out that there are several equally good methods of coping with a problem, and that you are choosing the one you think is best.

Having your own baby may bring you much closer to your mother. So many aspects of your upbringing and your mother's feelings become clear for the first time. Of course the difficult areas may also be reopened, but often the whole family will experience a renewed warmth and harmony.

BABYSITTERS

Babysitters can be useful from the moment you come home from hospital. Clearly, the younger your baby, the more carefully you must choose and brief a babysitter. A babysitter needs above all to be responsible and trustworthy. He or she should also have some experience of handling babies, though most have no special training. Relatives are often good and willing babysitters, but again you must be careful not to take them for granted. Agencies generally provide reliable sitters but you may find them expensive. Local groups of parents who have set up their own babysitting circles are often the best answer. Your local child health clinic will probably have information on these. It is probably best not to employ young people under sixteen to babysit for a baby under two.

If you leave your baby with a sitter when he is only a few weeks old, make sure the sitter feels comfortable with handling an unpredictable, crying, hungry baby and knows how to feed him, and change a nappy. If you are breastfeeding you can leave milk which you have expressed in a bottle. The older baby will have developed a routine; let the sitter know exactly what this is, including any rituals, for example before going to sleep.

Always leave telephone numbers, yours where you will be, and your doctor's, so that the sitter can contact you if there is any problem.

NANNIES

The advantage of a qualified nanny is that she is a trained professional whose job it is to look after children. Most nannies will have acquired the nursery nurses' qualification, the NNEB, which is the result of an intensive two-year course covering all aspects of baby and child care, child development and paediatric nursing. This is a nationally recognized qualification which is also very highly regarded in other parts of the world. A nanny with an NNEB will have had practical experience of looking after children even straight from college.

Nannies can either live in or out, and you will be responsible in most cases for their income tax and National Insurance contributions. Their rates of pay vary greatly depending on where you live. If you work part-time, you may be able to share the expense of a nanny with another family, either by having her spend part of the week with you and part with the other family, or by having her look after both sets of children together. You could advertise in a suitable magazine for a 'nanny share' or apply to an agency specializing in this type of employment. Some local branches of the National Childbirth Trust also run 'nanny share' registers, which is useful since you know the sharer lives nearby.

Nannies are not expected to do any domestic work. They are 'mother-substitutes', in that they take over the job of caring for your child, which is valuable if you are out at work all day. With two or more children they are also a great help. The disadvantage of this situation is that your child may become very attached to the nanny, and may be confused by having two mother-figures. A good nanny will be careful not to interfere with a child's relationship with his parents.

When choosing a nanny, make sure she is someone you like as a person, in addition to being properly qualified. Check that her ideas on upbringing are not too dissimilar from yours, and that she has a flexible approach.

MOTHER'S HELPS AND AU PAIR GIRLS

Mother's helps and au pair girls are not professionally trained. However they are more adaptable and will help you with housework as well as with your child. They tend to be more temporary than nannies. This may be disruptive for you and your child, but it lessens the problems of deep dependence which arise with a more permanent mother-substitute. They are probably less help when your baby is small than when he is older. They may be ideal if you are only out for a few hours each day.

Au pair girls come from abroad to learn English. They generally work for a few hours a day, attend language classes and live as part of the family. They are entitled to board and lodging and pocket money. Mother's helps are paid a wage and work full time. Some live in, some live out.

As with a nanny, it is worth interviewing an au pair or mother's help very carefully, especially if your child will be spending a lot of time in her care. Most are young girls who enjoy children and are very good with them, even if their knowledge of English is limited. A few may only be interested in social life and aim to do a minimum amount of work.

DAY NURSERIES AND BABYMINDERS

Employing a nanny, mother's help or au pair is only possible if your income and/or your accommodation is large enough. For many people the alternatives are care outside the home in the form of day nurseries and babyminders. Local authority day nurseries are usually only available to the most needy families; privately run nurseries are quite expensive. Check that a private nursery is licensed by the local authority.

Babyminders also have to be registered with the local authority and have therefore to conform to a reasonable standard of care. They may however look after several children at a time. But they are supervised to ensure that they provide adequate care for every child, which includes the provision of enough space, and the number of children in their care is restricted.

Most babyminders are good, but some are not, despite the supervision. Check that a babyminder is in fact conforming to the regulations concerning space and numbers. Courses in child care are available for babyminders; ask if yours has been to any. See that there are plenty of toys around – toy libraries run by the local authority can provide these.

The disadvantages of babyminders are that they do not provide individual care and the baby is not in his own home. An older baby will feel unhappy in strange surroundings in the absence of his parents. The presence of other children dilutes the amount of attention each child receives, and the children may not get enough stimulation. Despite these problems, many babyminders are excellent. Sometimes this may be the only option for a working mother, and is the least expensive.

CHAPTER THIRTEEN

THE GROWING BABY

Advice on the major milestones in your baby's growth
and development, from three to fifteen months

From three to fifteen months, a baby makes astonishing and rapid progress in understanding, mobility, communication, play and self-help. From being a helpless infant, he develops into a small child with a defined personality. Keeping up with his changing needs and abilities can be great fun for both you and your baby as you discover new skills, but it can also be tiring at times.

Each baby is different and it is the parents who are the experts on their individual child, rather than the professionals whose job it is to advise them and to share their knowledge of child care and development. While there are general principles, there are few hard and fast rules in baby care. However, the belief that there are rules – which are constantly being broken – is a cause of anxiety to some parents. But it is extremely difficult to do harm to something as well made as a healthy baby. Parents and other caring adults bring to the baby growing understanding of the world around him and also build trust and an understanding that this is a good place to be.

FEEDING IN THE FIRST YEAR

The young baby's life centres round food. Feeding is a pleasurable experience in its own right, as well as being a time when the baby has the full attention of the person who is feeding him. As the baby grows and becomes more curious, food becomes a fascinating plaything to experiment with, and meal-times are an excellent opportunity to exercise new skills, such as self-feeding or dropping things on the floor. The trouble is that what your baby thinks is interesting and fun may not always coincide with your thoughts on the matter. When your baby rejects some lovingly prepared meal you may feel hurt and upset; when he smears it over his high chair in a determined effort to feed himself you may feel disgusted or angry. Food and feeding can take on a disproportionate importance in the minds of some parents; like all aspects of baby care it's as well to keep things in perspective.

Parents often worry whether their child is getting enough food or not. Babies themselves are by and large able to regulate their own intakes far better than we can judge it for them. Where parents and baby disagree on this, mealtimes, far from being an enjoyable experience for both, can rapidly become a battleground in which no-one is the winner. Remembering that it is difficult to do harm by giving your baby food, and that he will generally take as much as he needs, can avoid most of these problems. To a baby and parents, giving food and giving love are often much the same thing. When problems arise, both can feel hurt and rejected. In contrast, mealtimes can also bring pleasure for everyone and should be a time in which company and attention are shared.

VARIATIONS IN INTAKE

Although there are recommended intakes of food for babies these are only guidelines. The variation within the range of normal babies may mean that one baby may be taking double, or half, what another is taking, depending on which way one looks at it. Both babies can be growing normally. Rather like the motor car, some of which do fifteen miles to the gallon and others do 30, babies may also need quite widely differing amounts of food.

MILK FEEDING

Until the age of six months the only suitable milks for babies are either breast milk or infant formula. From this age, although of course breast milk and formula can still be used, whole pasteurized cow's milk or follow-up milks can be introduced instead (see p. 158). Pasteurized milk does not have to be boiled at this age. Skimmed milk or semi-skimmed milk should not be offered to babies in the first year of life since the low fat content means they do not have enough calories (energy). From twelve months, whole pasteurized cow's milk is the most suitable one to offer to most babies.

Your growing baby is a constant source of delight as he responds more and more to the people he knows and loves best – his parents.

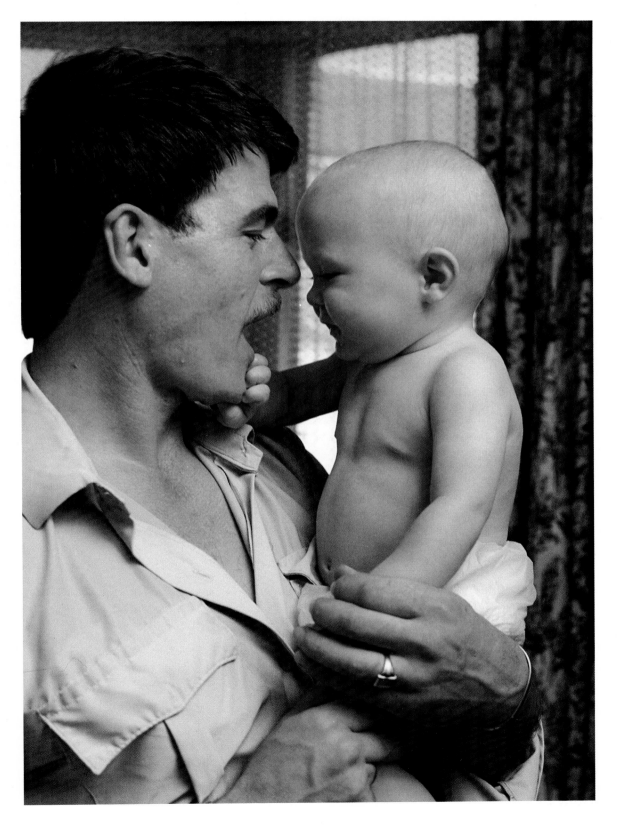

WHEN TO STOP STERILIZATION

From the age of six months it is unnecessary to sterilize everything that babies use, although bottles and teats should still be very thoroughly washed and rinsed in hot water. Of course, general aspects of hygiene are important throughout life, both for yourself and your baby. It is important from an early age to get into the habit of washing his hands before eating and letting him see you do the same, so that when he is old enough to do it himself it will happen as a matter of course. This becomes much more important than sterilizing feeding utensils: hands are the main source of food-borne infections which can be dangerous for babies and children.

INTRODUCING SOLID FOOD

Milk is the only food that babies need until the age of three to four months. Some babies are happy to continue with milk feeding until six months, but after that milk is not enough to provide all your baby's nutritional needs. If you don't introduce solid food until six months, you may also find that you are feeding more frequently in order to keep your baby satisfied.

Introducing solids can take quite a while. Babies often need time to get used to the spoon, and to the texture and taste of solid food, even though the consistency of these first meals will be similar to thin cream or soup. Baby rice is probably the best food to start with. Prepare it exactly according to the manufacturer's instructions and do not add sugar. If you are starting before six months, it is as well to sterilize the feeding spoon, so a plastic one is best.

GIVING THE FEED

Choose a time when you know your baby is usually contented and amenable – perhaps the morning feed, or in the middle of the day. Don't bother if you know your baby is tired and likely to fall asleep

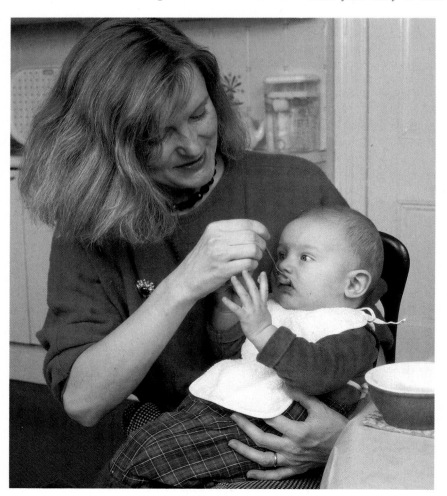

When feeding solids to your baby for the first time, sit him on your lap, holding him firmly with one hand, while you gently introduce the spoon into his mouth with the other. To start with, just stroke his upper lip and gum with the end of the spoon and let him suck the food off (it should be the consistency of thin cream). Later he will learn to open his mouth in anticipation and may try to grab your hand or the spoon, so be prepared for mess.

EQUIPMENT FOR FEEDING			
Bottle feeding equipment	Bottles, teats and sterilizing equipment are covered in Chapter 11.	**Plates, cups and bibs**	Feeding cups, plates and cutlery are to be found in abundance. Plastic bibs with a 'drip tray' are easier to keep clean than fabric or towelling.
High chair	A high chair is essential and will be used for at least two years. Choose carefully, for practicality and safety as well as for looks. The chair must be stable and have fixing points for a safety harness. Look for a chair with an easy-to-wipe surface. A lip on the tray helps to avoid spills. Some high chairs can be adapted to a low chair with a table. Wooden chairs are not always as practical as some of the simpler metal and plastic chairs – nor as cheap. One model adapts from a low reclining chair to a swing or a high chair.	**Portable chairs**	Table-mounted chairs are a simpler, less expensive alternative. Two types are available: one kind balances on the table with rubber bumpers above and below the surface, the other kind has to be clamped to the table. These chairs are reasonably stable provided that the table is too. Even simpler for travelling is a fabric support which is designed to be hung over an ordinary chair. Booster seats which strap on to an ordinary chair are useful for an older child but give insufficient support to a young baby.

straight afterwards. Trying to offer solids under these circumstances will only lead to frustration and tears.

At first simply offer a tiny amount on the tip of the teaspoon after the feed. Alternatively try offering it during a 'natural break' or rest period in the middle of the feed, when the baby's initial urgent hunger has been satisfied, but he is still interested in the idea of food.

You can either sit at a table with the baby on your lap, firmly held in the crook of your arm, or you can sit the baby in a baby chair or bouncing cradle in front of you. This latter method probably involves the least mess, but it is wise to protect your own clothes with an apron, and your baby's with a plastic-backed bib.

Don't try to force your baby's mouth open, but just stroke his upper lip with the tip of the spoon and let him suck the baby rice off the end. The first few attempts may not be very successful – the baby may spit the food out, or let it dribble out of the corners of his mouth simply because he doesn't know what to do with it. But with patience, good humour and the acceptance of a certain amount of mess on your part, your baby will soon get the hang of it.

New tastes should be introduced one at a time at intervals of several days, then if something disagrees with the baby, it is easy to identify what it is. You can always try it again at a later date. Always remember to let the food cool down to a suitable temperature before offering it to the baby. Rejection might mean that the food is too hot rather than that the taste isn't acceptable.

FOOD FOR YOUR BABY

Commercial baby foods are quite acceptable, but it is just as easy and much cheaper to make your own. Use boiled rice, lentils and beans, root and green vegetables and some fruits (avoid soft and citrus fruits to start with). Cook the food first then sieve or blend it to the right consistency, adding boiled water or a little infant formula.

The main rules are to use fresh ingredients and to ensure that everything you use to prepare them is clean, especially your own hands. Never add salt – a young baby's kidneys cannot get rid of salt, so it could build up to dangerous levels in the blood, particularly when the baby is ill with diarrhoea or vomiting. Do not add sugar to baby foods either (see p. 217). Your freezer is a very convenient place to store ready prepared baby meals. When the baby is small and taking only one or two spoonfuls at a time, freezing your home-made food in ice-cube containers allows you to prepare it in suitable quantities.

Left-over food from the baby's plate is best thrown away. Open jars or other containers from which some food has been removed should be covered and stored in the refrigerator for not more than 24 hours. If a microwave oven is used for re-heating food, remember that the inside can be very hot while the outside is still cold. Always test the temperature of food heated by this method to avoid burning his mouth. Microwaves do not sterilize food unless it is cooked for a very long time.

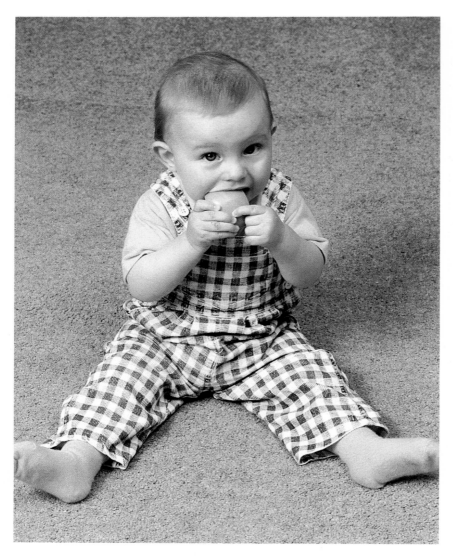

Once your baby can hold an object firmly, at seven or eight months, he will be ready to try finger foods such as pieces of carrot, toast or apple. However, never leave him alone with food as he may choke.

Once solid food has been established on a regular basis, try to aim for balance in your baby's diet. Include fruit, vegetables, cereals and dairy products such as eggs and cheese, plus meat and fish if you want. If you can introduce a wide variety of foods at this stage, you may find your child is less fussy later, although this is unfortunately not always the case.

Children, unlike motor cars, can thrive on a wide variety of fuels. Much is written about some foods being good for babies and children, and others being bad, but a course of moderation is probably the best one to steer between the various pressures which can and do cause a lot of anxiety to many parents. Food is meant to be enjoyed by everyone rather than just being a vehicle to provide for the nutritional needs of the child.

TRANSITION TO FAMILY FOOD

From six to seven months, when the baby begins to chew, you can introduce food which is more substantial, such as grated cheese, flaked fish, more coarsely mashed fruit (such as bananas), boiled eggs or yoghurt. A baby doesn't have to have teeth to be able to chew – watch your baby put a toy into his mouth to prove this – and enjoys food which can be held, such as toasted crusts, pieces of raw carrot or apple and even celery. This is often a good way to persuade a baby to eat a type of food he might otherwise reject in cooked form. However, never leave your baby alone with any food, as he may choke (see p. 274).

From now on, more and more of the family's normal diet can be introduced. Babies do differ in their ability to cope with lumps, but hopefully by the beginning of the second year, they should be sharing many of the same foods as their parents, except perhaps highly spiced food or food with lots of small bones which even some adults find difficult. There is really nothing magical about baby food apart from its consistency and the fact that it should not contain added salt or sugar.

DRINKS

Ordinary tap water is perfectly suitable for babies – and it is obviously cheap. Until the age of six months when sterilization stops, it is wise to boil the water first and then let it cool. Bottled mineral waters are not always suitable for babies; many contain high levels of sodium (salt). Too much salt can make a baby more thirsty, which will make him want to drink more, thereby setting up a vicious circle. As it is sometimes difficult to discover how much salt is contained in these waters they are best avoided altogether, unless there is no other source of safe water.

Softened water is also high in salt. If you have a water softener installed, make sure the kitchen tap (which should always be connected to the rising main) is exempt from the system and take all water for the baby from this source only.

Of course, babies can have many other types of drink, particularly fruit juices. Avoid juices with added sugar, and also bear in mind that some 'pure fruit juices' naturally contain very high amounts of sugar, so could be just as bad for teeth as those with sugar added (see p. 217). Fruit juices can be quite strong and may result in loose stools, so it is as well to dilute them at least half and half with water.

Fruit squashes are best avoided as these are often very sugary or contain artificial sweeteners and colouring (see below).

VITAMINS

A balanced diet including milk as already outlined should provide your baby with all the essential vitamins. Infant formula milks have the correct vitamins added and breast milk should supply sufficient vitamins if the mother's diet is adequate (see p. 151). In addition, nearly all commercial baby foods contain added vitamins. For this reason, vitamin supplements are not necessary for all children. Some diets may be lacking in vitamins and for these babies suitable vitamin drops are available from child health clinics. If you are worried whether your child is receiving enough vitamins there is no harm in giving them – you cannot overdose your baby by giving him the recommended daily amount.

Sweet syrups containing vitamins should not be used, however, as the sugar in them will damage developing teeth (see p. 217).

SWEETS AND CHOCOLATE

Sweets and chocolate are not appropriate to offer at this age. They encourage the habit of high sugar content which leads to early tooth decay and obesity. Young babies can also easily choke on small sweets. Never give babies and children under two years of age peanuts to eat (see p. 274).

ADDITIVES

Foods manufactured specially for babies are usually free from artificial additives such as colourings, preservatives and flavourings. By and large, however, babies moving over to the usual family diet do not seem to suffer ill effects from these substances when they come across them. In a few children, however, additives can cause problems in behaviour or allergic reactions (see p. 270).

SELF-HELP WITH FEEDING

As soon as your baby learns to grasp objects he will be transferring them to his mouth. It is not surprising therefore that babies will want to grab the spoon that you are using for feeding and will also want to feed themselves with their fingers. Some babies become very frustrated because they want to feed themselves, but are unable to do it. Having a spoon each may get round these difficulties and with practice the baby's skills will gradually improve.

Sometimes parents discourage self-help as a baby's first attempts are so messy. It is however best to persist so that by nine months he should be skilled at finger feeding and beginning to be able to handle a feeding cup or a bottle by himself. Given the opportunity, by the age of twelve months, your baby should be able to handle a cup and spoon-feed himself with only occasional adult help.

Food can be good to play with as well as eat, but adults might not share the child's delight in fingering, smearing and playing with food. To avoid the problems of playing with food it is best to remove the plate once your baby has had enough to eat. If your baby goes through a stage of throwing food about, put newspaper or plastic sheeting under his high chair to minimize the mess.

Once your baby is able to feed himself, then mealtimes at which everyone eats together become a more practical proposition. But remember that babies are not very good at waiting for their food,

When your baby wants to feed herself, the first few tries may not be very successful, so stand by with another spoon to fill in the gaps.

especially when they are hungry, and are poor respecters of other people's (usually adults') wishes to eat in peace and quiet!

DIFFICULT FEEDERS

Some babies and young children are particularly difficult at mealtimes and it is very easy for their parents to become angry and irritable. Unfortunately this type of response only conditions the baby to be even more difficult when he is being fed. Letting him feed himself, however messy, may get round some of the battles. Force feeding is never recommended as it achieves the opposite of what is intended and the baby can easily end up by eating less. There is no doubt that hungry babies *will* eat if

offered food, so your baby's appetite might not be as big as you think it is. A patient, relaxed attitude will succeed in the end.

If you are worried about your baby's behaviour at mealtimes, it is best to get help before difficult feeding patterns are established. Advice on feeding is often easier to give than to put into practice, but regular support from friends or from the health visitor can be very valuable.

VOMITING AND DIARRHOEA

Vomiting after feeds, which is fairly common in young babies, usually improves dramatically when solid food is introduced. If it does not, it is useful to discuss this with your health visitor at the clinic so that she or the doctor can check the baby is growing normally. However, it should be said that some babies, especially if they have been bottle fed, continue to vomit after meals for some time. It occurs effortlessly, and the baby is not upset, and in this type of vomiting the whole feed is never regurgitated. It usually subsides at eight or nine months when the baby can sit up properly. You may find it helps to add a little arrowroot to the milk to thicken it slightly, though not so much that it does not flow properly from the bottle (see p. 158).

Some babies who are growing perfectly normally develop persistent diarrhoea starting between the ages of six and 24 months. The stools contain undigested food such as peas and carrots. The problem ceases as the child gets older and is not due to any serious disease. However, it is wise to see the doctor or health visitor to check that the baby is growing normally and that there is no other cause for the diarrhoea. If the doctor reassures you that it is not due to illness, you might be able to reduce the problem by cutting down the fibre (roughage) in your baby's diet – don't give him such things as peas or sweetcorn for a while, and mash vegetables such as carrots and potatoes. Avoid soft fruits as well until the diarrhoea subsides.

GROWTH

Growth is a good means of checking on the baby's overall health, as has been described already in Chapter 12, but for a healthy baby who is lively and active and eating and sleeping well, frequent measurements are not needed and can be combined with the clinic visits for immunization and hearing testing (see p. 212). The variation in size at all ages is wide and comparisons with other babies can be misleading and cause unecessary worry. For instance the size of baby clothes is often recorded in months. This is a very crude guide and many babies need the size bigger or the size smaller.

Big babies are not necessarily fat or unhealthy. Some are generally big in every dimension and this reflects the body build of their parents. Others are significantly above the average weight for their length and age. It used to be believed that these would grow up to be overweight adults, but the majority will not. One of the best signs of whether a child is likely to be overweight in adult life is if the parents themselves have weight problems; where this is so, a little early caution in controlling the intake of fattening foods might be helpful.

Most small babies are also healthy. They usually take after their parents. A small lively baby is most unlikely to have any serious illness. However, a child who is growing slowly and has signs of ill health such as recurrent loose stools, vomiting, difficulty breathing and who seems lethargic or unduly irritable should be carefully examined by your doctor.

CHECKING ON DEVELOPMENT

At the clinic and at home, both you and your health visitor and doctor will want to check the baby's development. His speed and pattern of development will depend very much upon characteristics that he inherits from you, the experiences that he has in his everyday life and his general state of health.

Looking at babies' development in the clinic is not quite like doing an MOT test on a car. Although some babies might not necessarily accomplish all the tests that we might expect from their age level, this does not mean that there is something seriously wrong. In fact, eight out of ten babies whose development gives concern early in life will have no problems whatever when reviewed at an older age. What seems to be important is not looking at the baby on a single occasion but development observed over a period of time and looking at its rate. The rate may obviously vary over time, being sometimes slow, sometimes very rapid.

When you go to the clinic to have your baby's development checked, a few observations of what your baby can do combined with the doctor's or health visitor's own tests form a reliable guide that he is progressing well. If there are problems, for example in the areas of hearing or seeing, parents are usually the first to recognize them (see p. 188). So go to the clinic prepared to share the knowledge of how your child is getting on, together with any concerns you may have.

Although development over this age band from three to fifteen months is quite remarkable, it is easy sometimes to over-estimate babies' understanding and ascribe to them motives and reasoning which they could not possibly have. Although your baby may seem frustrating and difficult at times, at this age he is not doing it deliberately to irritate you – though he may well be trying to gain your attention. This is a sign of his close attachment to and need for you, so try to respond positively.

The next section summarizes development over this period, looking at ways that you can help and indicating how you can also help to pinpoint some problems early on.

PROGRESS TOWARDS WALKING

The progress from a small baby only capable of lying where he is placed by his parents to an inquisitive and mobile toddler is one of the most exciting elements of development in the first fifteen months or so. As has already been mentioned (see p. 182), this usually follows a set pattern (though *not* a set timetable).

The high chair is a favourite place to practise dropping things on purpose, a game that twelve-month-olds love, but which adults find exasperating.

'PRESS-UPS'

By the age of three months, most babies have developed strong arms and good control over the position of their head. This means that when lying on their fronts they can lift their head and upper part of the chest clear and maintain this position, both to their own delight and that of their parents.

ROLLING OVER

In learning to roll over the baby has learned to co-ordinate not only the right and left sides of the body, but also the movements of head, arms, trunk and legs. Some babies become very alarmed at the sudden changes of posture that they can now bring about, and all are now at risk of falling off surfaces on which they were previously safe.

SITTING UP

Most babies will learn to sit on their own between the ages of five and eight months. To do this the baby requires not only physical strength in the back but, just as important, the ability to balance. At first the baby needs to use his arms to secure his position on the floor and needs to make lots of rather clumsy adjustments in order to maintain this posture. Eventually he will topple over, or will not remain stable while sitting if at the same time he is using his hands to grasp a toy. By twelve months, however, the baby can sit for an indefinite period of time and does not topple when he is reaching out for objects or using his hands to play with toys. He is also easily able to get himself into the sitting position, and his view of the world for most of the day is now the same way up as it is for adults.

The development of mobility begins at five or six months with the ability to roll over (above) – a movement which often takes babies by surprise at first. The next step is to sit up unaided (left); for the first time a baby sees the world from the same angle as an adult, only usually much lower down.

Standing up and getting her balance has to precede walking; at nine to twelve months most babies will have learnt to pull themselves up in the cot or playpen, on items of furniture, or even your legs!

With crawling and standing comes the ability to climb. Stairs become a particular hazard, as babies take much longer to learn how to come down again, so it is sensible to fit a safety gate.

CRAWLING AND STANDING

A baby must learn to sit before learning to stand. Standing requires strength, balance and courage in view of the inevitable association with falling. Crawling provides a good intermediate step between sitting and standing. It also provides a rapid and convenient method of getting about before walking is established. However, not all babies crawl and those who do not, take longer to be able to stand and walk. The most common variation of crawling is bottom shuffling, in which the child bounces along on the seat of his pants. These babies also learn to stand and walk later as they are doing things the hard way. It does not indicate that anything is wrong.

At first the baby can only stand while holding on to something. Most babies will be doing this by ten months, and can pull themselves up, so that you often find your baby standing in his cot waiting to be lifted out after a sleep. But it may take a further three or more months before they can stand on their own.

WALKING

Most babies go through the sequence of crawling, standing and walking. Some, as have already been described, shuffle along on their bottoms, a few haul themselves along using their arms alone and a few creep along on their hands and feet. Some miss out all these alternatives and go straight from sitting to walking. At first a baby needs to hold on to objects when walking and cannot get across gaps where there is nothing to hold on to without going down on all fours again. Between twelve and fifteen months most children are walking on their own, though others, particularly bottom shufflers, might not walk until after the age of eighteen months. At first, walking on his own is an uncertain process consisting of wide based and unsteady movements prompted by frequent falls.

It helps to allow your baby to walk with bare feet to start off with as he will find it easier to balance, though this may not be possible if the weather is very cold. Soft shoes with non-slip soles are suitable

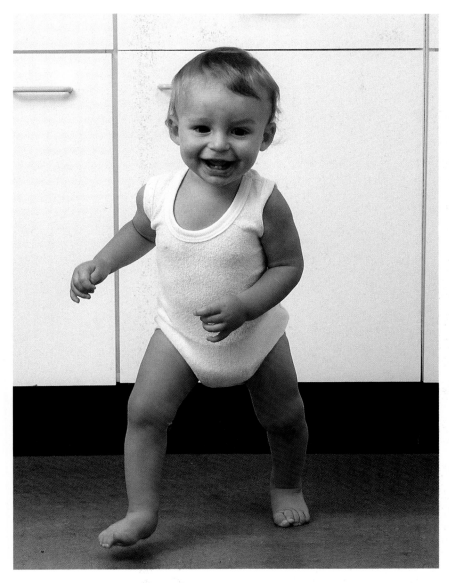

Walking is the big milestone between infancy and childhood, and is looked forward to by parents, even though it brings its own problems of safety and so on. The first steps are often very uncertain, and may be interspersed with bouts of crawling before walking is fully established. Babies learn quickest in bare feet – shoes are not necessary for the first few weeks except out of doors.

at this age. Do not let your baby walk around only in socks since he may slip on polished floors, and socks come off very easily. It is not usually necessary to buy specially fitted shoes until your baby has been walking really steadily for at least four or five weeks, or maybe more.

CLIMBING

Crawling on the horizontal soon leads to the ability to crawl upstairs and to get on and off furniture. However, children learn to climb up before they learn to climb down. Thus, like the kitten in the story, they can be 'trapped' on the object on to which they have climbed or are likely to fall when trying to get down. They, of course, are unaware of this potential hazard, so it becomes vital to keep your baby in sight at all times.

THE EFFECTS OF MOBILITY

Learning to walk and move about widens the child's horizons in terms of exploration and learning. It also vastly increases the possibilities for mischief and for danger. Try to anticipate these hazards and provide restraints in the home, the street and the car. These may take the form of gates to restrict access, particularly on stairs, guards to keep saucepans out of the way of young hands and straps for safety in chairs and cars (see p. 272).

Developing manual dexterity

Your baby will develop increasing hand control during the first year or so of life, combined with visual development.

1 At three months, your baby will make efforts to grab for toys he thinks are within reach.

2 At four to five months he can grab an object and hold it, soon learning to bring it up to his mouth for further exploration.

3 From six months, he will be transferring objects from one hand to the other.

4 From about nine months, the more efficient way he grasps an object (see opposite) enables him to shake a rattle, responding to and experimenting with the noise.

5 Being able to co-ordinate two hands at once to do different things means that around twelve months your baby may be banging one object against another.

USING THE HANDS

Learning to use the hands does not depend upon the hands alone, but the correct use of vision in locating objects and watching and directing what the hands are doing. At first this co-ordination of hand and eye requires intense concentration.

EARLY STAGES

At first the baby stares and stares at his own hands watching carefully the movements that occur, perhaps trying to work out what they do and how the movements can be controlled. This watching occurs around the age of three months, when the child will also be able to reach out and swipe nearby objects such as a row of beads across the pram. When the baby first reaches out and grasps an object he may, rather like a learner driver, 'over-steer' to both sides before grasping the required object very crudely in the palm of the hand. The baby soon lets go of the object involuntarily, and it is then forgotten.

From six months, as the baby gets better at holding on to things, these are soon transferred to the mouth for further exploration. His own feet are also objects which can be grasped and explored in the mouth. Once the grasp is secure, the next stage is to transfer the object from one hand to the other.

From the age of nine months a much more useful grasp is developed using the thumb and index finger rather than the palm. This enables the baby to manipulate smaller objects and to be more precise in his movements. The repertoire of movements increases, including shaking, banging and pulling, and toys such as an activity centre, cups and rattles provide good practice in all these movements.

At about one year the child is able to pick up small objects such as crumbs and dirt on the floor, much to his parents' disgust. Throwing things off the highchair or out of the pram or pushchair and seeing how they drop, is a favourite game known as 'casting'. Objects can be grasped in both hands at the same time and banged together.

At fifteen months most children will be quite good at using both hands together. They may be able to build a tower of two bricks and the index finger can be used for pointing to desired objects.

NEW SKILLS, NEW HAZARDS

Developing skills in hand control and in mobility means that children can get to and reach objects that previously were not a hazard for them. They can pull trailing flexes, open cupboards and gain access to household chemicals such as bleaches, medi-

Developing hand control
At about six months a baby grasps an object crudely with his whole palm and all five fingers, like a scoop.

Later on, at about nine months, he can begin to use his fingers and thumb together to grasp an object between them (human thumbs are said to be 'opposable' in this context).

By twelve months, most babies can use the index finger and thumb together in a fine pincer movement, to pick up quite small objects such as a raisin.

cines and other dangerous substances. The baby's natural desire is to explore and this is only moderated by a rudimentary sense of danger. It is therefore necessary to imagine things through a child's eyes and remove or lock away dangerous things before your baby develops the skills which would help him to gain access to them.

HEARING

Babies need perfect hearing in order to develop and understand speech. Sound also gives them lots of clues as to what is going on around them, such as hearing footsteps coming, the sound of dinner being prepared, the sound of traffic. Parents are the best people to detect hearing problems and are nearly always right (see the check-list on p. 188), but if you have doubts about your baby's hearing at any age you should contact your health visitor. Most children's hearing problems get better on their own and are often related to catarrh (see p. 266). However, all babies with suspected hearing problems must be carefully assessed, which may mean going to a special audiology unit either in a clinic or in a hospital, on referral by a doctor.

HEARING TESTS

The hearing of babies is tested by the health visitor or the doctor at your local clinic, between the ages of seven and nine months. The test used is called a distraction test, and it needs two people as well as yourself to carry it out.

The baby sits on your lap and his attention is focused on a toy held on the person sitting in front of him. When the baby is alert and his attention fully focused on the toy, this is removed from his sight and the second person makes a very soft sound about one metre from the baby's ear and outside his line of vision. The baby should turn towards the test sound. The baby's hearing is tested for both low pitched and high pitched sounds.

Babies who do not respond appropriately are usually re-tested after a short period of time. Test failures can be due to the baby being tired or irritable, having temporary hearing problems associated with a cold, or sometimes because he is too immature to localize the sound properly yet. However, if a baby fails the test twice, then referral for specialist examination is necessary. Later re-assessment may also be recommended if it is thought your baby's speech development is delayed.

VISION

Just as in the case of hearing, parents are also usually the best people to detect whether their baby has any eyesight problems (see p. 188).

Your baby's sight will be assessed by the health visitor or doctor at the clinic at around the same time as his hearing. This is usually done by observation, by seeing how alert the baby is to his surroundings and his ability to reach out for and handle fairly small objects, which indicates how well the baby can co-ordinate the movement of his arm and hand with what he can see. The doctor or health visitor may also look closely at the baby's eyes. In young children only major problems that seriously interfere with eyesight need to be detected. Such problems would include anything which prevents light getting into the eye, examples being a cataract in the lens or clouding of the pupil. Parents usually notice this and with early treatment normal development of the child's vision can be ensured. It is also important to detect squints. A squint will produce a different image in each eye and the baby can only cope with this by ignoring one image. This will eventually lead to a 'lazy eye' (see p. 261).

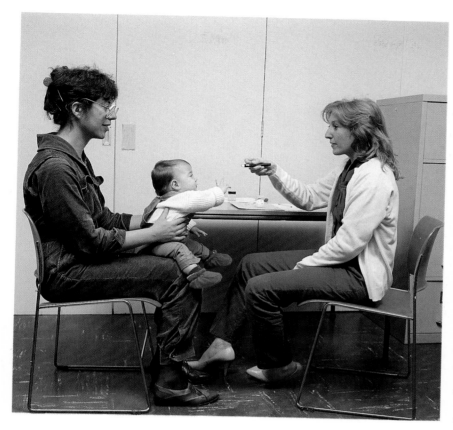

The health visitor or doctor will test your baby's sight at seven or eight months (left) by observing his general alertness and his ability to follow a moving object such as a ball or car. She may also shine a special torch into the pupil to look at the retina.

A baby's hearing is tested at seven to eight months by using the so-called distraction test (far left). Once the baby's attention is distracted by an assistant with a toy, the health visitor or doctor will make a number of different, very soft noises about a metre away and out of the baby's sight. Hearing is tested by seeing if the baby turns to the sounds.

THE DEVELOPMENT OF LANGUAGE

Language is the most complex and highly developed of human skills. It is needed to transfer thoughts and feelings, and is also used internally when we are thinking. The unfolding of child development is in itself a miracle, but the ability to acquire speech is the most amazing part. It involves skills of listening and discriminating the individual sounds in what the child hears, being able to repeat those sounds and to recognize meanings to which those patterns of sounds are attached. The child also picks up important laws of grammar in an easy and painless way, in contrast to an older child or adult's difficulty in learning other languages at a later age.

Babies begin to vocalize by making indiscriminate babbling noises at four to five months, which gradually coalesce into more recognizable consonants like 'ba', 'na' and 'ma', usually repeated. At first they learn to make and copy sounds, and then to understand that some of these sounds have a specific meaning. Your baby may be imitating words like 'mamma' and 'dadda' at nine months or so – eventually realizing that you respond to these words in a specially rewarding way. By about twelve

months your baby will probably have found at least one word that signifies 'mother' or 'father' – possibly one that is interchangeable!

Babies learn speech by hearing you speak to them. Therefore, in every day life, talking through all the daily activities will help your baby to begin to learn the meaning of words. For instance, tell your baby about his spoon, cup and plate at mealtimes, about his clothes while you are dressing him, and parts of the body whilst you are bathing. Nursery rhymes are enjoyed from a very early age and certainly do help the development of speech. Most importantly, they are fun for you and the baby. Very simple stories from simple picture books can be introduced from the end of the first year, when your baby will show genuine recognition of simple objects illustrated on the page.

It is a long journey from the first babble, to gaining understanding of simple words such as 'Mum', 'Dad', and 'no', through the copying of whole words without meaning, to the production of the first proper words used correctly, at about the age of one. It is often difficult to appreciate how few words a baby or young child actually understands. The child of one year will understand 'no' but not an explanation about 'no'. A young child will pay

Even as early as twelve months a baby will be able to recognize a simple object in a book, and to point and try to name it, even if she hasn't started speaking properly yet. Words with strong consonants, like 'cup', 'duck', 'cat', and 'car', which are also familiar everyday objects, may be the first words she says after some version of 'mummy' or 'daddy'.

attention to sound because it sounds nice, and because it is combined with loving attention from his parents. Understanding the full message comes a lot later on.

THE IMPORTANCE OF MEMORY

Memory is one of the most important developments in the first year of life. With it the child can build upon previous experience. A young baby lives very much in the immediate world and that which is not immediately visible is forgotten; a young baby forgets a toy once dropped, whereas a full-term baby of seven months will look for it. Memory develops with regard to people, events, strategies for solving problems, games and rules. For example, from about seven months of age, babies recognize which people are familiar and which people are unfamiliar and become wary of strangers, which can make babysitting difficult (see p. 196).

GROWTH OF CONFIDENCE AND TRUST

Between the ages of three and about fifteen months your baby should gain confidence in himself and trust in the world about him. He is helped in this by having his needs for both care and love met and by there being a consistency in his daily life. He will gain confidence by being successful in things he is trying to do, and by other people's appreciation of that success. Where parents' expectations are too high, putting success out of reach of the child and giving rise to what in the parents' eyes is failure, then the child may well grow up to be unsure of himself.

DIFFICULTIES WITH SLEEP

Many babies do not sleep through the night until they are eighteen months old and some even older. They come to no harm through this, but clearly their parents do. The baby has very little control consciously over when he is awake and when he is asleep and only an anaesthetist can alter this situation with any degree of certainty. As the child gets older he may no longer disturb his parents at night, but is likely to be equally wakeful but without their knowledge.

GETTING THE BABY TO SLEEP

It is unrealistic to expect that a wide-awake, active baby, or for that matter an adult, will go to sleep simply by the action of being put to bed. The first rule is not to start under these conditions. A bedtime routine is obviously of help. This may consist of a meal, followed by putting toys away, a bath and finishing off with a bedtime story or lullaby depending upon the baby's age and preference. It is important to make sure that the baby does realize that the night is different from the day by making the room dark, though obviously not so dark that the child cannot see. A room of his own is often very helpful if this can be arranged. If a baby wakes up and immediately sees his parents, he will obviously demand attention. In the case of a breastfed baby, the smell of mother's milk may act to stimulate his appetite.

IF YOUR BABY WAKES

Don't rush in immediately your baby wakes at night, unless the cry is obviously an unusual one. Waiting five to ten minutes and then being comforting is much more effective than responding straight away but being irritable. Because breastfed babies may have their appetite stimulated by the smell of mother's milk, it may be easier for the father or someone else to go to an older baby at night. It is often useful to leave a night light on and some safe toys in the cot for the baby to play with if he awakes. These simple manoeuvres will help with quite a lot of children. However for some, only patience and the child growing older will solve the problem.

Where regular night waking is becoming an exhausting problem for the parents, seek advice from your doctor, who may suggest trying a medicine for a trial period to help the baby to sleep.

DAYTIME NAPS

The amount of sleep the older baby needs over 24 hours is incredibly variable. Some parents find that their baby may get up at eight in the morning after twelve or fourteen hours' sleep, have breakfast and be ready to sleep again almost immediately for another two hours! Another baby may be wakeful most of the day, perhaps 'catnapping' for half an hour or so. Both these examples are normal – though the latter may be more inconvenient for some parents.

You will soon recognize the signs which let you know that your baby is tired during the day. At this age, babies will always sleep if they are tired, although it is not surprising that a lively baby will cry when you leave him, as you are the best source of interest to him. It is reasonable to expect that your baby will want a nap in the morning and afternoon, but for how long varies enormously. If your baby is alert and happy while awake there is no need to worry about the length of time actually spent asleep.

CRYING

Babies cry for many reasons. They may be hungry, they may be uncomfortable, they may need changing, they may also be bored or unwell or sense you are not at ease or are worried. Prolonged crying causes stress in the adult and the reaction to this, far from relieving the baby's distress, may actually serve to enhance it. Parents can become extremely tired due to the amount of attention the baby needs and as a response to the constant loud noise. You may also become emotionally strained due to the frustration at being unable to soothe your baby, or from a sense of failure. The response may also be anger, which all parents feel at some time because of the baby's incessant demands and their own apparent inability to fulfil them.

When the baby is crying, look for a physical cause, such as hunger, discomfort or fatigue. If you feel that the baby is unwell or not his normal self, see your doctor. Your baby may be bored, or frustrated by being unable to do something either because he is too small or because you have prevented him. In this case you might find a break from routine, such as a walk outside, or changing to a new activity may well benefit both you and the baby. Unfortunately at this age babies cannot wait to have their demands fulfilled however much we would like them to.

At times it is very easy to feel that everything is getting on top of you. It is essential at these times to share the load by getting help from your partner, from relatives or from neighbours. You need a break to sort yourself out. Looking after a young baby is the only job that lasts 24 hours, seven days a week, with no holidays. It is therefore not surprising that parents as well as their children can often feel angry and frustrated. You should see your health visitor or doctor if you feel that things are getting on top of you and that you are losing your temper too easily.

AIDS TO GETTING THROUGH THE DAY

As your baby gets older and sleeps less during the daytime, your daily activities need to be planned to ensure that both your needs and his are met. A little forward planning can resolve a lot of troubles. If he is hungry he cannot wait, so planning meals in terms of timing and preparation is very important. Planning of activities both indoors and out will give a variety of experience and stimulation, relieves boredom and keeps the baby happy and contented.

Along with the baby's needs, of course, your own needs must also be met. It is hitting the right balance that is important to ensure that you are both contented. Where life seems frustrating and difficult

Babies often enjoy swimming from quite an early age, although it is advisable not to take them before the age of nine months.

it is often useful to write down your day's activities to see how your own and your baby's needs are being met. There can also be conflicts between time given to your baby and time given to your partner. The best solution is for you to share the load as far as possible between you and try to get some time together on your own occasionally (see p. 194).

TEETH AND TEETHING

The ages at which teeth first appear are very variable. Some babies are born with teeth, though this is rare, and others do not cut their first teeth until they are twelve months old. However, on average, the bottom two teeth in the middle, known as incisors, appear at around the age of six months.

These are soon followed by the appearance of the two upper teeth. By ten to fourteen months the four top and bottom incisors have come through and usually the first of the molar teeth at the side of them are also seen.

The appearance of teeth is said to give rise to lots of other complaints. There is no doubt that it can be painful, is associated with excessive salivation (enough to soak many bibs) and the baby indicates the site of his discomfort with his fingers. Babies who are teething often appear to have a cough. This is usually due to large pools of saliva, which, instead of dripping out of the front of the mouth, accumulate at the back. The baby may then cough, though this is not usually due to infection. It is possible that when babies are teething, they might be more susceptible to other problems such as skin rashes, diarrhoea and colds. However, it is dangerous to dismiss such symptoms as simply 'due to teething' and it is wiser to consult the doctor.

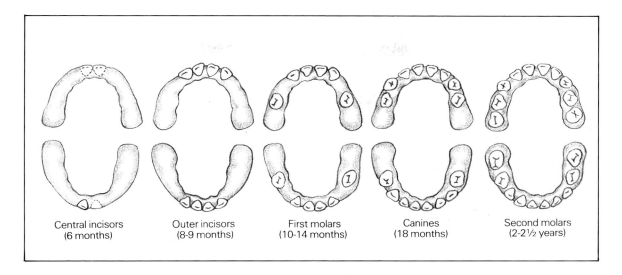

Central incisors (6 months)   Outer incisors (8-9 months)   First molars (10-14 months)   Canines (18 months)   Second molars (2-2½ years)

A baby's first teeth usually appear in the order given above, although there is enormous variation in the age at which the first tooth breaks through. This can range from about four to twelve months.

DENTAL HYGIENE

Once teeth come through, to start with clean them gently with a small piece of gauze or a cotton bud. Introduce a tiny toothbrush and fluoride toothpaste at twelve to fifteen months or when your baby has at least six teeth. The importance of avoiding sugar (see p. 201) cannot be over-emphasized – sugary foods and drinks can damage the teeth even before they erupt through the gum. Sugar is broken down by bacteria in the mouth, forming acid which attacks teeth, causing them to decay. Cleaning the teeth properly should remove the acid, but avoiding sugar and introducing fluoride (see below) help to avoid the problem in the first place.

THE USE OF FLUORIDE

The addition of fluoride to water supplies in many areas has dramatically reduced the amount of dental decay seen in children living in these areas. Your health visitor should know if the water contains an adequate amount of fluoride or not. You should also be able to obtain this information from the water authority or from the local dental officer. Fluoride drops are available for babies living in areas with low levels in the supply; the amount needed depends upon the age of the baby and the level of fluoride in the water. Your health visitor or dentist should be able to tell you the right dose for your area. The drops can conveniently be added to your baby's bottle or drinking cup.

KEEPING YOUR BABY CLEAN

As your child gets more mobile, day-to-day tasks of washing and nappy changing might become more difficult, and the opportunities for getting dirty become infinitely greater. The most important parts to keep clean are of course the hands and face as stomach upsets, especially diarrhoea, can be caused by the introduction of germs into the mouth. A little dirt elsewhere is not such a big problem. Babies generally enjoy a bath, which can be a time for play as well as for washing, as long as an adult is always with them. Babies often enjoy swimming too, as long as you are close at hand, although it is wise not to take a baby under nine months.

Some babies dislike having their hair washed, probably because of the sensation of water going into their eyes. If your baby wriggles and gets soap in his eyes, it may also make him apprehensive in the future. Lying the baby down, well-supported, on his back in the bath can avoid this, or you could use a special cap which prevents water running down over the face. However this is not always successful and it is probably best then to wash the hair no more than once a week and get it over with as quickly as possible.

An active wriggling baby who has learnt to roll over may be extremely difficult when nappies need changing, and terry nappies and pins may present hazards under these conditions. A switch to disposable nappies may ease the situation considerably. Children are not usually ready for toilet training until at least the age of two years, so don't try to introduce it as a way to get round the difficulties associated with nappy changing. It will only serve to increase tension between you since your baby is being asked to do something which he is not yet able to carry out.

EXPLORING THE WORLD

How to cope with the joys and frustrations of the toddler years, from fifteen months to two and a half

From the age of fifteen months, your child will become more and more mobile and the clinginess and separation anxiety of the one-year-old will decrease. With intellectual and language development allowing a better understanding of the world, there is an increasing need to explore. Exploration takes place from a safe base, usually with frequent retreats to a parent to check that all is well. A child of fifteen months will be climbing stairs, climbing on to low stools and chairs, and showing great delight in her new abilities. To start with she will not be able to get back down, and you may have to show her how to turn round and climb down backwards. She'll be falling over a lot too, so she needs to be watched closely at most times. There is an urge for new discoveries, and cupboards will be turned out, baskets emptied, and possibly even the contents of the refrigerator pulled on to the floor, given the opportunity!

FROM BABY TO CHILD

Although children of this age may play with something that interests them for as long as 20 minutes, mostly they have a constant urge to go from one thing to something else. An active toddler has a short concentration span, toys get rapidly thrown to one side, and a great deal of imagination is needed to keep her occupied. On the other hand, when something does interest her she will examine it minutely and will try to see how it works. For instance, instead of examining things with hands and mouth, she will use her fingers with more precision: a small car will be turned upside down and the wheels pushed round with one finger.

However tiring, this period can be rewarding since you can share the excitement as she acquires new skills literally every day. As young children often enjoy activities which involve imitating their parents, your child may happily push a toy vacuum cleaner around, make attempts at sweeping with a dustpan and brush, bang with a toy hammer or splash in washing-up water with a cloth and plastic dishes while you get on with the chores yourself. She may even enjoy actively helping, with varying degrees of success!

Because of the child's natural curiosity and interest in discovering what is inside and on top of things, this is the period when you have to give your home a hard look to make sure that it is child-proof – a little forethought about safety and about the whereabouts of your own treasured belongings will save battles and breakages later. For instance, make sure equipment like the telephone and the hifi are placed well out of reach – and bear in mind that a piece of furniture will often be used by a curious eighteen-month-old to push up against a wall or chest, in order to climb up and get to something which looks interesting. Don't let wires trail where inquisitive hands might try to pull them, either.

If you don't want books pulled out of the bottom shelf of the bookcase, empty it for the time being or put books or other objects there which don't matter. Fix safety catches to kitchen cupboards where breakables or dangerous household cleaning substances are kept. You could keep one cupboard accessible with pots, pans, wooden spoons and other interesting items in it so that she can explore there without causing damage to herself or anything else. Keep medicines locked away and use child-resistant containers – her new manual skills mean that she will try her best to open a tempting looking pill bottle and she may still want to put the contents in her mouth. Eighteen months to two and a half is a peak period for accidents in the home involving the swallowing of things like tablets, bleach, paraffin or weedkiller, and can be avoided by taking a few simple precautions (see also p. 272).

PHYSICAL GROWTH

Growth during this time begins to slow down, the rate of weight gain becoming very much slower than in the first year. The proportions of the body gradually change so that the head is less large in

Small children are extremely imitative and enjoy being allowed to join in with household chores and other tasks which older children – and many adults – find boring!

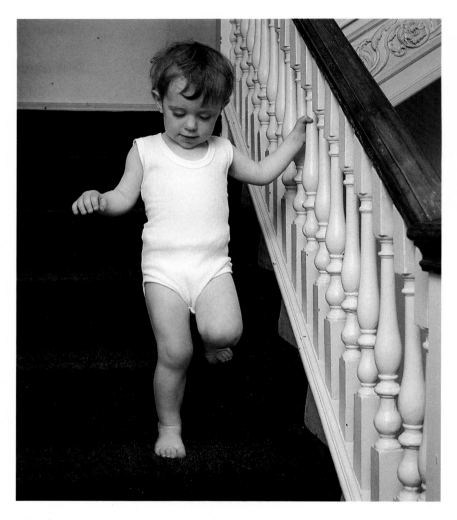

Negotiating stairs can be hazardous, even when your child is walking steadily, and at first she should be encouraged to turn round and climb down backwards. But by 22 to 24 months she may have gained the confidence to come down forwards, a step at a time, and usually with the help of a steadying hand on the wall or bannister.

relation to the rest of the child's body. A glance at the growth charts on page 180 and 181 will show you that in the second half of the second year (from eighteen months to two years) average weight gain is around 170g (6.5 oz) per month, with average weight at two years being 12kg (28 lb) and average height 86cm (34 in). Of course, this varies a lot from child to child and depends on such factors as birth weight, how active the child is, the sort of family the child comes from, the child's diet, illness and stress, race and social class. For instance, a Chinese baby is, on average, smaller than a European baby coming from families with similar living standards.

A child's activity level will influence body weight at this age, as at any other, with the active toddler who is never still for a moment likely to be lighter than a more placid, less mobile child who does not burn up as many calories in spontaneous exercise. Hence there is no 'correct' weight for a child of, say,

eighteen months, but plotting weight and height on the chart should indicate that all is going well. A falling off of weight across percentiles can indicate that a child is not eating enough, or can sometimes be an indication of illness (see p. 261). If there is any concern about your child's weight or height, it is sensible to consult your doctor or health visitor.

LEARNING TO SPEAK

At fifteen months, your child will have already started to say one or two words (see p. 213). The first words are usually naming words, most often 'Mummy' and 'Daddy' or some equivalent. Quite often, the recognizable name of a sibling or grandparent may be used at the same time, or another familiar person such as a nanny or childminder, or even a family pet. People are of most importance in the child's world, so naming them usually comes a month or two before naming objects.

The first objects to be named are familiar everyday items which are talked about often, such as 'shoe', 'drink', 'ball', 'teddy', 'car', and by eighteen months the average vocabulary is six to 20 words, as well as a lot of unrecognizable chatter. Sometimes quite difficult words are acquired by a child early on if they are important in that child's world. For instance, apart from 'Mummy' and 'Daddy', the first word a little boy who lived on a farm could say was 'tractor'. Other early words which are commonly used are those which produce an effect when used, such as 'up' when wanting to be picked up or placed on a chair, or 'more' for more milk, and so on.

Words expressing feelings and descriptive words come soon after and by the age of two, words such as 'no', 'naughty' and 'cross' are often used, and it is remarkable how early a small child can perceive the feelings of others and put them into words, often accompanied by gesture. Well before developing a vocabulary, the child has learned a lot about the meanings of tone of voice and inflections, and will use speech sounds in a musical way to ask questions, or make disapproving or demanding noises. Turn taking in speech, as when you hold a conversation with someone, is also an early part of language development, which is established long before words are used with meaning. Vocabulary rapidly increases during the second half of the first year and thereafter, and by two-and-a-half most children have a vocabulary of around 200 to 300 words.

USING SENTENCES

While vocabulary increases rapidly, developing the use of sentences is a much slower process. This starts by the child putting two words together to make a short phrase, such as 'Daddy gone', 'more drink', 'baby cry'; by two years most children are using these sort of two-word utterances. By three years, sentences of three and four words are being

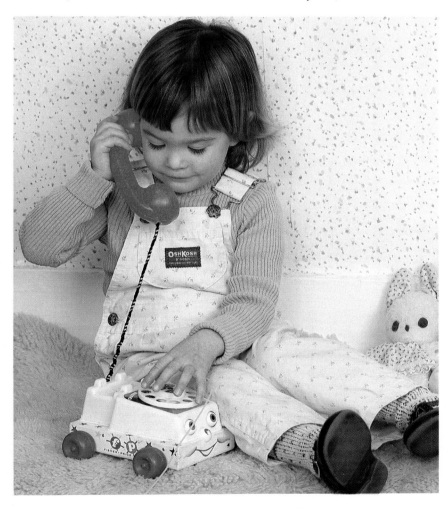

As children's language develops during the third year, they often use imaginary conversations, perhaps on a toy telephone or to their toys and pets, to experiment with this new skill.

used, although the grammar is often incorrect. It is interesting that children do not imitate the 'correct' sentences that they hear adults using, but first develop their own sort of 'telegrammatic' speech.

Alongside the use of words to communicate, the child is learning to understand the meaning of other people's speech, and an understanding of speech develops before the child can use the same words herself. So a child of eighteen months, when asked to go and close the door, will understand and do so, although she cannot yet say the words 'door' and 'close'. She will also, by two, be able to understand a more complicated request such as 'can you fetch your shoes, which are on my bed?', again long before being able to say this herself. Also, she will know the names of parts of her body and be able to point to eyes, nose, mouth, tummy and so on when asked, particularly if you play such naming games regularly when dressing and at bath time.

TALKING TO YOUR CHILD

There is quite wide variation in the ages at which children start to speak, and on the whole, girls are somewhat ahead of boys, just as they are in some other aspects of early development, such as gaining bladder control. Many factors can interfere with the process of language development, but the most important influence is the amount that the child is spoken to. So, talking a lot to a child right from the early weeks is important, and even children as young as one year will enjoy looking at picture books and magazines with their parents and pointing out well-known objects. Playing games like pat-a-cake and other rhyming games, singing songs and nursery rhymes are very much a part of childhood experience in almost all societies; they are fun for parents and children, and there is no doubt that they encourage language development. Reading stories, too, encourages speech and, later reading skills; it is sad, but probably true, that parents read to their children less since the introduction of television sets into most homes. While taped stories and music or nursery rhymes are no substitute for mother, they are also much enjoyed, encourage listening, and are useful on car journeys and for times when one is busy, or perhaps occasionally at bed time, if it is difficult for you or your partner to read a story yourselves.

DELAYS IN SPEECH DEVELOPMENT

Apart from the amount of stimulation in the child's home as outlined above, there are other factors which affect the rate of speech development. Children mature at different rates, and just as some children walk a lot later than others, so some will begin to talk later. Many children who appear to have slow speech development are simply 'late talkers' with no other problems. Others may be generally a little slower in all aspects of their development. A doctor who is asked to see a child where there is concern about slow speech will want to find out how much the child can understand, how her overall development is progressing, and of crucial importance, whether her hearing is normal.

Hearing loss will obviously affect speech development, and one type of hearing loss ('glue ear', which is due to fluid in the middle ear, behind the ear drum) can appear gradually. It can also vary, depending on whether or not the child has a cold, so may not be detected by parents. It is not always accompanied by ear ache, but can be detected by careful testing of a child's hearing and examination of the ears (see p. 266).

OUT OF NAPPIES

In the early months, babies pass urine fairly frequently with dry periods, but are certainly not in control of either bladder or bowels. It used to be thought that babies could be 'trained' to open their bowels when a few months old, and if put on a pot after a feed some babies will 'perform'. However, this is due to a reflex opening of the bowels, not due to the baby controlling the situation and responding to a cue. Toilet training is not normally started until well into the third year of life, when children are really able to understand what is happening, rather than having it forced onto them.

At around the age of sixteen months, some (but not all) children may be aware of being wet, and may cry to have their nappy changed. At some point after this (around eighteen months to two years) they may indicate that they are passing urine, and may even acquire a word for it, such as 'pee-pee'. At this stage, they do not have control over their bladders, but recognition of passing urine is a first stage. Soon after this they may recognize the feeling of having a full bladder and may tell someone before passing urine. When this stage is reached it is a good time to start toilet training; trying before this will probably result in frustration. Bowel control is a similar process, but is usually acquired a little earlier than bladder control. The urge to open the bowels is a more recognizable feeling and is usually slower to build up, so less urgent. However some young children seem to prefer to continue using a nappy for this purpose even though they may be dry in other respects, perhaps only opening their bowels once the nappy is put on at night. This is inconvenient, but you should try not to make an

*While your child is
learning to use the pot,
it is a good idea to keep
it near where she is
playing, so you can
respond immediately
when she asks for it.*

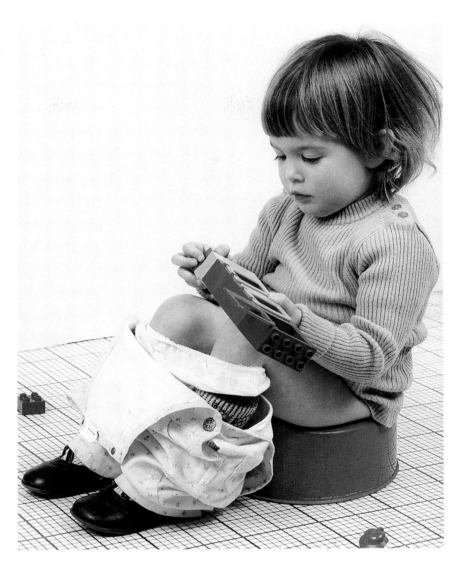

issue of it. The two skills match up in the end.

By about two-and-a-half, most children are able to tell their parents (by gesture if not words) that they need to pass urine, and some may be completely dry during the day at this age. However, many children are not reliably dry during the day until around three years, and even then are likely to have accidents, and may be forgetful when they are involved in interesting play.

TAKING YOUR TIME

Different children gain bladder and bowel control at different ages, and like speech, this depends on a process of maturation. Girls tend to develop control earlier than boys. There will always be somebody down the road whose child is dry several months

before your own! What is important about toilet training, whenever you decide to start, is to be relaxed about it. Tension and anxiety over toilet training is usually counter-productive, with a child becoming resistant, and it is an area where conflict should be avoided.

The approach that seems to work best is plenty of praise and encouragement for dry pants and using a pot or toilet appropriately, with no fuss when accidents occur. It helps to let your child go around without nappies, pants or trousers some of the time, so that it is easy to use a pot. If you want your child to use a toilet, it helps to have a child's toilet seat (sitting on a large toilet can be scary!) and something to stand on, unless the toilet is low. Because behaviour at this age is often imitative, seeing other children, as well as their parents, using

223

VITAMINS AND NUTRITION		
VITAMINS	FOOD SOURCE	FUNCTION IN DIET
A & Carotene	Carrots or any green vegetable. Fruits, liver, butter and fortified margarine, fortified bread, fat fish such as herrings, sardines and tuna fish	Normal vision, growth, healthy skin and nails
B1 (Thiamin)	Offal, pork, nuts, potatoes, whole grains, peas, beans, lentils	Helps the body to utilize carbohydrates
B2 (Riboflavin)	Liver, meat, eggs, milk, green vegetables	Helps the body to utilize carbohydrates, protein, fat
Niacin	Liver, poultry, meat, fish, whole grains, peas, beans, lentils	Helps the body to utilize carbohydrates, protein, fat
Pantothenic Acid	Liver, poultry, meat, fish, whole grains, peas, beans, lentils	Helps the body to utilize carbohydrates, protein, fat
Pyridoxine	Liver, poultry, meat, fish, whole grains, peas, beans, lentils, bananas	Helps the body to utilize amino acids. Assists in blood formation
Folic Acid	Green leafy vegetables, eggs, liver	Assists in blood formation and growth. Gives resistance to infection
B12	Meat, especially liver. Dairy products. (Absent from plants)	Formation of new red blood cells
Biotin	Offal, peanuts, mushrooms	Helps body use fats
C (Ascorbic acid)	Citrus fruits, cabbage, parsley, sprouts, tomatoes	Helps to keep the body cells healthy; gives resistance to infection
D	Fish liver oils, egg yolk, butter, margarine, liver. (Sunlight is another important source of this vitamin.)	Healthy bones and teeth. Regulates calcium and phosphorus usage in the body, particularly the bones

a toilet or pot encourages a small child to want to do the same. Children will soon want to be independent over wiping their own bottoms – so teaching a child to do this for herself is a good idea. (And even if they prefer a parent to do it, they will need to be able to manage by themselves by the time they start school.) Little girls' bottoms should be wiped from front to back, to avoid spreading germs from faeces into the vagina and urinary tract. Children don't usually wipe themselves completely clean to start with, but this is not important, and dirty marks on pants are to be expected until a child is quite a bit older. It is a good idea to encourage and teach children to wash their hands after using the toilet to reduce the risk of infection.

BECOMING DRY AT NIGHT

For some children, bladder control at night happens at around the same age that they become reliably dry during the day. More usually, however, night time dryness takes longer; the child has to maintain control for ten to twelve hours, and during a period of deep sleep. This requires a considerable degree of maturation, and like any other aspect of development some children get there earlier than others. Although the majority of children are dry at night by three-and-a-half to four years, around one in ten will still wet the bed most nights at five years. This may be inconvenient for the parents and unpleasant for the child, but it is not necessarily abnormal.

When your child shows signs of being able to be dry all night, perhaps by having a dry nappy in the morning, or only wetting it when she wakes, you can try leaving the nappy off. Expect to have some wet beds at first, but reward the dry nights with praise and don't fuss over the wet ones. If it is obvious that she is not capable of staying dry all night, and is wetting the bed every time, then return to nappies for a while. Don't try to get your child out of nappies too soon or both you and your child will become disheartened.

FOOD AND NUTRITION

At this age children will usually be eating more or less the same as the rest of the family, although without added salt and spices. A healthy diet is a balanced diet, with a variety of food providing all the nutritional requirements. If left to select from a variety of foods, on the whole, children will end up eating a reasonably balanced diet with all the vitamins, protein and minerals they need, and nutritional deficiencies are uncommon. It does help to understand about the sources of essential nutrients, and child health clinics are a good source of information and leaflets on diet for toddlers.

Vegetarian diets are perfectly healthy for growing children, with protein requirements being provided by milk, yoghurt, cheese, pulses (beans, peas and lentils) and nuts, instead of meat and fish. With

If your child's timetable can be fitted in with yours, mealtimes can be more interesting for everyone if she is able to join the family at the table, rather than being isolated elsewhere.

increasing evidence that excess animal fat is a cause of raised cholesterol (linked to later heart disease) more people are cutting down the amount of meat they eat, as well as limiting high fat foods like butter and cream, and the same principles are recommended for children. Since milk and cheese are the main sources of vitamin D, which is essential, together with calcium, for healthy teeth and bones, it is important not to omit them altogether from a child's diet. Most nutritionists and doctors now also recommend a diet which is high in fibre. Fresh fruit and vegetables, wholemeal bread, chappatis, pulses, brown rice, muesli, dried fruits, are all high in fibre and also contain vitamins and other nutrients. (See the table, opposite.) A diet which is high in fibre will prevent constipation, and is also thought to prevent some of the bowel disorders which can occur in adulthood. Added vitamins are not normally necessary at this age, although some Asian diets are low in vitamin D and vitamin supplements are then recommended. Talk to the health visitor at the clinic about whether she thinks vitamin supplements are necessary.

MAKING MEALTIMES INTERESTING

If they have been encouraged to do so, children are usually feeding themselves with a spoon by the age of eighteen months. In fact, they are often extremely reluctant to let anyone else feed them and inventive games may be needed to help the lunch down if there is limited time!

Mealtimes are often messy occasions, for food is interesting to explore with the fingers, as well as to taste, and some small people always seem to end up with mashed potato in their hair and peas all over the floor. If this becomes irritating, remember it is only a stage, and placing newspaper or a plastic sheet on the floor under the high chair can make cleaning up a bit easier. Learning to feed by oneself is part of learning independence, and exploring the texture of foods is a necessary stage of development which does not persist for many months. Gentle correction in holding a spoon and fork can help, but don't make an issue of it.

THE FUSSY CHILD

The child who is fussy about certain foods is sometimes more of a problem, but it is very rare for a child to develop unhealthy preferences. Preferences tend to go in phases too so that after a month or two of eating what seems like only sausages and peas, the favourite food will probably change, and your child will surprise you by finishing every mouthful of something she has been refusing for weeks. Even a little bit of variety helps, and small pieces of fruit or raw vegetables are often eaten, even if the more usual vegetables are consistently refused. It helps to be a little inventive, and to present food in an interesting way; also remember that fish fingers and baked beans do make quite a good diet. Sometimes, eating with other children is helpful – a child will sometimes try something that she sees other children eating.

It is important to avoid giving snacks and drinks between meals to fussy children, or children who refuse to eat much at mealtimes. It is often tempting to give a child who has refused breakfast a few biscuits and a glass of milk to 'keep her going' until lunchtime, but this only increases the likelihood that lunch, too, will be refused. Snacks are also often sugary, and sugar is best avoided for two reasons: first, it is bad for children's health and increases the risk of tooth decay, and secondly, it is habit forming. Children who are brought up not having sugar on cereal and avoiding sweet puddings, do not miss it, do not need sugar, and are less likely to spend their pocket money on sweets when they are older!

PROBLEMS WITH EATING

Children who refuse to eat, or eat very little, usually make their parents very anxious. Part of everyone's idea of good parentcraft is providing nutritious meals to build your child into a healthy young person, and it is very frustrating if your child blocks your best attempts to do this. When carefully prepared and cooked delicacies are spat out, thrown on the floor, or ignored, this provokes even the calmest of parents to anger. If this is happening, it is tempting to try and force your child to eat – but this should be avoided at all costs! The battle is inevitably won by the child, but in any case, mealtimes should never become battle grounds. The child will begin to associate cooking and mealtimes with negative feelings, whereas meals should be a time for relaxing, talking, and enjoyment.

If your child refuses to eat what is on her plate, at the end of the meal simply take it away. Try not then to give chocolate pudding, or she will think this always happens if she refuses a meal! Sometimes, putting very small amounts on the plate helps, sometimes things which can be eaten with fingers are preferred to those needing a spoon, and sometimes distractions, or games, can help over a difficult period. Remember that if your child is looking healthy and is active and gaining weight then there is no real cause for worry. It is often helpful to discuss these sort of problems with your health visitor, and checking your child's weight periodically (but not every week) can be reassuring. If you continue to be worried, talk to your doctor – also talk to lots of other parents and you will probably find that other people have gone through similar experiences.

THE FAT CHILD

Some children go the other way; they have large appetites, eat everything put in front of them and always seem to want more, as well as drinks and snacks between meals. Such children can become overweight, and there are a number of reasons for this. Mostly, they are just eating more calories than they need for normal healthy growth. Some children are less active and burn up less calories than others, so tend to put on weight easily. This tendency often runs in the family, but eating habits also run in families, and overweight children are quite likely to have overweight parents. As any overweight parent knows, dieting is difficult – so it is worth keeping an eye on the weight of a small child who seems to eat a lot. It is much easier to alter and cut down on a two-year-old's diet than a six-year-old's. Again, ask

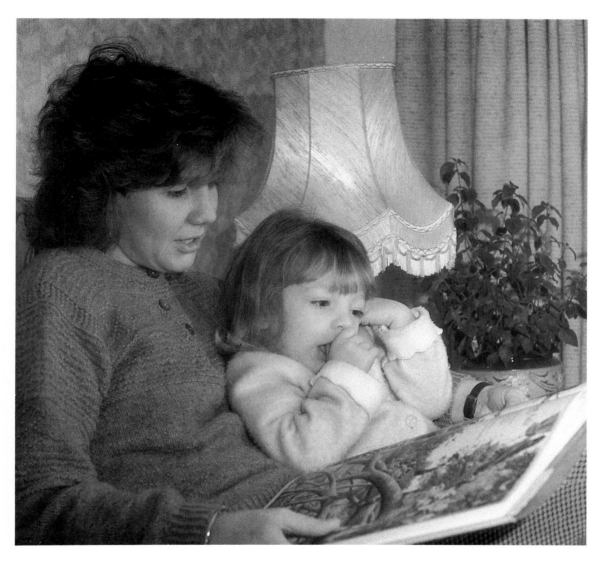

Bedtime need not be a problem if you try to establish a simple routine for your child, such as a bath, teeth cleaning and a bedtime story, which you can stick to night after night.

your health visitor or doctor for advice, and get your child's weight plotted on a growth chart if you think there is cause for concern.

SLEEPING PATTERNS AND PROBLEMS

Parents of young children have to cope with all sorts of problems and worries in the first few years, of which sleep problems are one of the most common and certainly the most exhausting. Children do not always need as much sleep as their parents do, although many people think that all children need twelve hours' sleep each night. In fact, the amount of sleep needed by each child is very variable – one child may regularly sleep eleven or twelve hours each night while another needs only nine hours' sleep. There are some children, usually the very active, alert sort of child, who need much less sleep than this, which can put enormous strain on their parents.

The most common sleep problems in the age group one to two-and-a-half years are difficulties in settling to sleep at night, and waking during the night. Many children who have difficulty getting off to sleep, and go to sleep late, will then sleep soundly until morning. Others will be difficult to settle *and* wake again in the night. Parents need time to relax and at the end of a busy day it is good to get children to bed and then sit down for some peaceful moments. It is understandable then that having a two year old underfoot and wanting to play until eleven o'clock causes irritation and frayed tempers.

SETTLING TO SLEEP

It helps to establish a bedtime routine from early on – perhaps supper, bathtime, then story – always allowing time to quieten down and unwind after the day's activities. Many children need special routines to help them settle to sleep – some will only sleep if a parent stays with them, others fall asleep on a sofa, others need the same song or story every night. These routines are hard to alter, so it is good, if possible, to find one which suits you as well as your child. A dim light, a musical box or cassette, favourite toys in bed, all help to make bedtime comforting and falling asleep easier. It helps to make your child's cot or bed a special place with favourite pictures and toys around, and perhaps a familiar mobile hung overhead. Although the house does not need to be quiet, it is more difficult for a child to stay in bed if there is a lot of noise and activity going on that she feels she is missing out on. Perhaps the most difficult situation is where there is only one room for living and sleeping, and it is clearly hard to settle a child to sleep in a corner with the light on and activities continuing.

NIGHT WAKING

Night waking, either every night or most nights, occurs very commonly in children under two, with about one in every four children waking frequently. It tends to occur less often as the child gets older, but in around one in ten children it is still a problem at the age of four years. It is also often a persistent problem: about half the eighteen month olds who regularly wake at night will still be doing so six months later. It helps to know that children themselves very rarely suffer from lack of sleep, but their parents certainly can! It is perhaps our expectations that a child should sleep through the night that are wrong, for in cultures where children sleep in the same room or bed as their parents it does not seem to be a problem.

Sometimes, waking at night can be triggered off by an illness (such as an ear infection, or whooping cough), sometimes by a major change, such as moving house, or going into hospital. Other children may show night waking, or difficulty settling to sleep, as a symptom of anxiety, such as a separation anxiety. It is often difficult for a child to express the cause of her anxiety, but time spent trying to understand it is helpful. You may then be able to reassure the child that all is well, and helping her express her fears and anxieties can help the sleep problem. Where family rows or tensions are contributing, clearly these need attention before tackling the sleep problem. Ways of coping with sleep problems vary from family to family, and no one solution will suit everyone. If you are happy with your own way of coping, then do not listen to someone else's advice to try a different strategy. Perhaps the most important thing is to be consistent; if you leave your child alone to cry one night, then take her into your bed the next night, you are giving conflicting messages which will confuse her and the problem will continue. Where there are two parents, it is sensible to discuss the issue and agree between you how to manage it. If the father wants to do one thing and the mother the opposite, again the child will get conflicting messages. Sometimes, simple manoeuvres will help, such as cutting down on daytime sleep, and giving warm milky drinks at bedtime.

It is worth stopping to think about what happens, and how you react, when your child wakes up. If she is picked up, cuddled, talked to and given a bottle, this is all rather nice and will probably encourage her to wake again as it reinforces the habit. Of course, you will do this if your child is ill or distressed about something, but on the whole the less you interact with a child that wakes, the sooner she will learn that it is not worth waking you. Try keeping talking to a minimum, and don't pick her up or play, but gently and firmly tuck the child up and settle her back to sleep. You need to make it clear that night time is for sleeping and not for games and company. If your child has been used to being picked up, you may need to withdraw gradually – say by sitting beside the cot for a night or two holding hands or stroking her, then moving further away for a few nights until, finally, you do not need to stay with your child until she is asleep.

Some parents prefer to take their child into bed with them, but others cannot sleep and find this very irritating, in which case it is not the solution. However, if everyone manages to sleep well it is one of the simplest solutions. It can become a habit which is hard to break, but you can sometimes move your child back into her own bed or cot once she is asleep. If you do this, it is a good idea to have a warm bed to put the child in, as cold sheets may wake a sleeping child. A hot water bottle in the child's bed may be a practical solution. One problem about having your child in your own bed is that it is bound to interfere with your sex life, so it can become a cause for resentment if it goes on for long. Sometimes one partner minds this more than the other, so it is best to discuss this.

HELP AND ADVICE

Other people do understand the strain and exhaustion of having a child who has sleeping problems, so if it is getting you down it is worth discussing with your health visitor and doctor, and also with other parents. On the whole, drugs are not the answer – they usually only provide short term relief, can be habit forming, and may have side effects. They may occasionally be prescribed by your doctor for very specific situations. Time off from a persistently waking child is important when you are exhausted – sometimes sending her for a night or two with a grandparent or friend is helpful. If your child sleeps through the night at a grandparent's house, you may well feel guilty and wonder if it is your fault the child is waking – the answer is no, parents are *not* responsible for children waking, but a child may not cry out if she knows her parents are not there to come to her!

FROM COT TO BED

At around the age of eighteen months some children will get fed up with their cots, resenting the restriction of the bars, and will increasingly demand to be lifted out, or may even learn to climb out. If this is happening, a low bed or mattress on the floor will be safer, and usually results in a better night's sleep for everyone. By around two to two-and-a-half, most children will prefer to be moved from a cot to a bed, and as with a cot, it helps to make the bed a special place with favourite things around.

FEARS AND HABITS

One of the earliest fears is of strange people, and is shown as 'separation anxiety' – the nine month old who gets very upset and anxious on being taken away from her mother. This is a developmental stage, which all infants go through, starting around seven months (see p. 214), peaking around fifteen to eighteen months, then gradually getting less. Many two year olds are still upset and distressed when separating from their parents, but by three years very few are. This sort of anxiety is to be expected, and reflects the personality of the child and her previous experience, as well as her developmental age. A few children are very clingy and will not let you out of their sight – even to go to the toilet. They are often children who also demand a lot of attention and can leave you feeling drained and exhausted with no space to yourself. However, lots of support and reassurance for these children during this stage is important and will help them to be independent later. You cannot force independence on children, and they have to be the ones who decides when they can cope without you. It may help to find a small playgroup or crèche where you can be in the same room as your child, while they play, meet other children, and learn to socialize in the safe knowledge that you are there if needed.

Other common fears in the second year are fears of noises, of falling and of strange objects. Fears about animals may start around two years, but fear of the dark usually only occurs later in the third or fourth years. Mostly, these sort of early childhood fears are not too distressing, and with reassurance and kind handling they do not persist long. Some people feel that children must be made to confront fears by deliberate exposure, but this is a misguided punitive approach and will make matters worse. Some fears are learned from other people – so if you yourself are terrified of spiders, or large dogs, it can easily be transmitted to your child. Although it is not always easy to avoid sharing your fears with your children, if possible you should avoid letting them know about them until they are older when they are less likely to be influenced by them. If your child shows fears that are very distressing, or longlasting, or you are worried about how to handle these, it is usually helpful to talk to someone like a health visitor or playgroup leader about your worries.

DUMMIES AND COMFORTERS

During the first year, many babies have bottles and often a dummy as a comforter, and if not weaned off these at the end of the first year they can become a habit. A lot of children need some comfort object to help them fall asleep and when they are upset, and some children use their thumbs or a corner of a blanket, while others like the teat of a dummy or bottle. There is nothing wrong with this, and no point in distressing a child by removing the favourite object. Using a dummy constantly during the day tends to discourage the child from speaking and, if possible, the use of dummy or bottle should be reserved for bedtimes and perhaps when the child is upset. The main worry is tooth decay – sweet drinks in a bottle or honey on a dummy should be avoided. If you think your child is *never* going to give up that bedtime bottle, just remember that one never sees 10 year olds going to bed with bottles!

OTHER HABITS

Apart from dummies or comforters, young children sometimes develop other habits, such as hair twiddling, or stroking, or perhaps finger sucking. Nail biting is uncommon at this age. Most of these

Many children form a special attachment to a particular object, such as a blanket or a soft toy, which forms part of the ritual of bedtimes and rests.

habits are similar to using comforters, and will diminish over a period of time. Getting cross about these does not usually work, but distraction to other things sometimes does. If it becomes a serious problem, such as hair being pulled out, see your doctor, who may refer you to a child psychologist who will suggest ways of helping to break the habit.

Head banging or rocking may occur in babies, often when tired, and sometimes appears to be a soothing mechanism for getting off to sleep. Head banging can be quite alarming, especially in a hard cot, and although babies do not injure themselves they can sometimes get bruises. It is wise to pad the cot with foam or rubber pads covered in cotton. Too much attention paid to the banging or rocking may increase the problem; it tends to diminish in the second year without anyone interfering. Very occasionally, a child who persists with rocking or banging may have an underlying emotional problem; it is more commonly seen in children, for instance, who have been separated from their parents. Habits of this sort are a little more common among children with developmental problems, and

in such children habits like head banging may persist for quite long periods. If you are at all worried about your child's habits, then do talk to your doctor or health visitor for reassurance.

CHILDREN'S SEXUALITY

From a very early age, children learn that it is pleasurable to touch their genitals, and one study of one-year-olds found that genital play occurred in over a third of children. Baby boys get erections even earlier than this – this is not due to anything sexual, but is a reflex associated at first with a full bladder or bowels. Masturbation is common at all ages, but much more common in boys than girls. It need not be discouraged, but should be accepted as a normal part of children's sexual development. As your child grows they should be advised that masturbation is a private activity and not to be done publicly. Very occasionally a child masturbates frequently and compulsively, although this is pretty unusual below the age of three. This may be due to anxiety or an escape from some stress in the child's world, and if you are concerned you should discuss this with your doctor or health visitor.

Interest in the opposite sex usually occurs when children discover that there are physical differences between boys and girls. Often this occurs after starting at playgroup or nursery, and exploratory games out of curiosity are then common; adult over-reaction should be avoided.

TEMPER TANTRUMS

When temper tantrums start, often around the age of eighteen months, many parents are unprepared and begin to think they have done something wrong. However, tantrums are so common that they can be considered a normal part of development. Small children do not have the same control over their emotions as older children and adults, and do not understand their own feelings of frustration. If they are upset and angry, or unable to do something at the stage before they can express their feelings in

Temper tantrums can be so overwhelming that they can frighten the child, so parents need to combine firmness with comfort.

words they will react with a tantrum. Two is the peak age for tantrums, and at that age around one in four children have tantrums at least once a day; some have three or four a day. The frequency of tantrums tends to decrease with age, although a small proportion of children will still be having them by school age.

Tantrums are more likely to occur when children are tired, hungry or unwell, and if tantrums are regularly occurring just before lunch or dinner, it often helps to bring mealtimes forward by half an hour or so.

The world of a two-year-old is full of intense feelings about what is happening *now*, with very little understanding of time. If a child of that age wants something, she wants it now and not when Mummy comes home, or after tea, as she cannot think that far ahead. Also she is becoming increasingly independent and wants to control the world around her (which she sometimes seems to be able to do!). When things go wrong, or she does

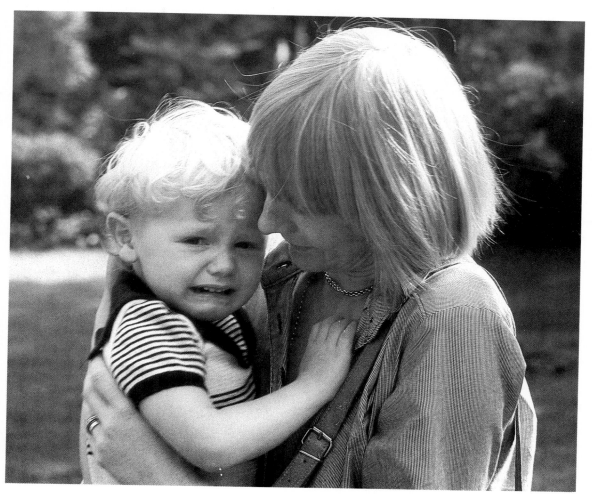

not get what she wants, then anger can explode as a temper tantrum. This is often provoked by something very simple, like being unable to reach a toy or book from a shelf; often, too, by being refused something such as a tantalizing packet of sweets at the supermarket check-out. However, most tantrums at this age arise because of some conflict between child and parent, usually because the child has been prevented from doing something. Because your child's anger seems to be directed against you, it can often make you feel angry too. But responding with anger by smacking or shouting back only makes things worse and tends to prolong the outburst. If you feel angry with your child try to walk away, and calm down, and understand that your child really cannot control all those powerful feelings inside her.

Because you know your own child best, you are likely to know what will trigger a tantrum, and can handle each tantrum sensitively. Sometimes you can distract a child and stop one happening, which needs imagination and humour. If you can pull a funny face or find something else interesting for the child to do, or spot something outside the window, you may be able to prevent a full-blown tantrum.

HANDLING A TANTRUM

If a tantrum has been caused by your refusal to give your child something, or let her have her own way, then don't give in – if you do, she will learn that by having a tantrum she gets what she wants, so you would, in fact, be encouraging her to have more in future. Probably the best way to deal with a tantrum is to keep cool and try to ignore it. Either walk away and get on with something else until it all subsides, or take the child quietly to another room. If the child appears very deeply upset you may prefer just to hold her gently and talk quietly – but it is no good holding a child if you feel really tense and upset yourself. It sometimes helps later on to have a quiet talk and a hug to show you are not cross, and perhaps to discuss what caused the upset.

When a tantrum occurs in a public place, such as a supermarket, it can be extremely embarrassing. Everyone around will be staring, and making judgmental remarks. In these circumstances, it is often best just to pick up the child and carry her out firmly, even if kicking and screaming, and let it blow over away from public view.

Tantrums occur much more commonly in children who are late to talk, and tend to lessen as communication with words becomes easier. Tantrums are more likely too if you are forever saying 'no' to your child. If everything is forbidden and every exploration results in a restriction, or a 'don't

do that', it is bound to cause frustration. Some children are endlessly on the go and into everything and will be helped by going to larger spaces, like playgrounds or parks as much as possible, where they are less restricted. Perhaps one of the biggest problems of bringing up young children in cities is the lack of safe play space nearby. You may have to travel some distance to a park or playground, although most local authorities are recognizing the need for more of these facilities.

WHEN TO SAY NO

Sometimes days may go by when you seem to be saying 'no' and 'don't do that' all the time. If this happens, stop and think about what is really important. It is not worth having battles over every little thing; your child will win many of the battles and you will feel exhausted and demoralized. It is easier for everyone to have fewer rules and fewer arguments, and only say 'no' about the more important things, particularly those that involve safety: for instance, playing with electric plugs.

It may be easier sometimes to let your child choose what clothes to wear, and when you are not in a hurry, which way to go to the shops. Children need to feel that some of the time they do have a choice – remembering that you will be making the decisions 90 per cent of the time. It helps to avoid fuss and pressure if you give your child a few minutes' warning before you need to do something. Tell her 'it's time to start clearing up, because we're going out in a few minutes', rather than 'stop that now and put your coat on, because we're going out now'. Remember to encourage and praise your child for trying, even if she hasn't quite managed or finished something. If it has been a difficult day and you have been tired and cross, it's good to sit down for a cuddle and to say sorry – if you can apologise to your child, you are teaching her to be able to apologise to you.

Try not to have unrealistic expectations of your child, and not to be unduly upset when she is unco-operative or does just what you have asked her not to do. Children are at times overcome by their own curiosity and desire to do something, which may be a stronger urge than needing to please you. It helps if you are firm and reasonable (even when your child isn't!), but stay calm; shouting at your child is only effective if you don't shout often.

Again, an occasional smack does no harm, but repeated smacking is not only unhelpful but can get out of hand. The use of physical punishment such as smacking will often result in the child becoming aggressive, as children learn from the behaviour of adults. Many parents decide they will never smack

Toddlers don't always need to play with conventional toys: household objects like pots, pans and wooden spoons provide plenty of interest.

their child, but then will do so in a tense moment, and feel very guilty about it afterwards. Most parents have done this at some point and it certainly does no long term damage. But if you feel yourself getting tense and angry, it is sensible to try to walk away from the situation – breathe deeply and count to twenty, or go next door and make a cup of tea – just to give yourself time to calm down before going back to talk to your child.

LEARNING AND LIMITS

Sometimes life can seem one long battle with an active two-year-old – not for nothing is this period of life sometimes referred to as the 'terrible twos'. This

is a time for exploration; the child is learning what she is capable of doing and trying out new skills, as well as learning what the limits are, and what is acceptable behaviour to the adults who care for her. It can be a confusing world for the child, and it may help to think about what children of this age need, to plan ahead, and perhaps to anticipate some of the difficulties.

As well as having their physical needs met, children need love and security, and praise and encouragement for their achievements. Without this they cannot develop self-confidence and a positive view of themselves. They need stability in their relationships with adults, and consistency in the way their behaviour is dealt with, so they can recognize the adult 'rules' of their world. If one day a child is allowed to pull out the contents of her mother's handbag and play with them, and the next day is told off for doing so, she cannot learn what is expected of her. If she is allowed to fall asleep on the sofa in the living room for a few nights, then the next night put in her own bed to fall asleep, she will be confused about the rules of bedtime and will, understandably, protest.

THE NEED FOR PLAY

Children also need to play – a lot of learning in the pre-school years happens through play – and this does not mean expensive toys. With imagination, and a little thought, many things around the home are good play material. Cardboard boxes and an old sheet can make a play-house, plastic bowls and wooden spoons are good for cooking meals for dolls, and dried food, such as pasta, beans or lentils, makes 'real' food. You cannot spend all your day involved in playing with your child, but setting up an activity for her just takes a little thought and time and may even mean you can get on with something else.

Try and give your child, whichever sex, a range of playthings. Dolls are not just for girls. Girls, too, enjoy playing with cars and garages and tool kits. It is wiser to offer a choice, so that children are brought up without sexual stereotyping. They will, of course, imitate the behaviour of the parent they most closely identify with, so girls often want to use their mother's lipstick, or put on scarves and beads. But given the chance, both girls and boys love to play football, and to cook and wash up.

WIDENING THE HORIZON

Every child is different, with different needs and different personality. You will know your own child best and will learn that some children need much more structured boundaries than others. While some children are content and enjoy playing at home for long periods, others are more restless and active and need to be watched every minute. Activities outside the home can provide fun and stimulation and be more relaxing for you. As well as parks and playgrounds, in many areas there are places that welcome parents and young children. Libraries have a children's section, and many recreational centres and swimming pools now cater for toddlers.

Creches or mother and toddler groups pave the way for nursery school or playgroup later, so ask your health visitor what is available in your neighbourhood. Many local authorities produce a booklet on facilities and services for under fives and this is normally obtainable from public libraries or the local child health clinic. As well as providing facilities which can be difficult to organize at home

– such as sand and water play – these activities will help your child to socialize with other children, and are good places to meet other parents of young children. It can be extremely lonely and isolating to be with a small child, or children, at home all day, and although going out can seem a big effort it usually makes everyone feel better. You, too, need people to talk to and meeting other parents can be a real tonic. You may feel able to invite them to your home, too, providing a new interest for you and your child, and probably leading to further invitations out in return.

LEARNING TO SHARE

Although children from eighteen months to two and a half years enjoy being with other children, they are not ready yet really to play with another child. They will play alongside, but have not yet learned about

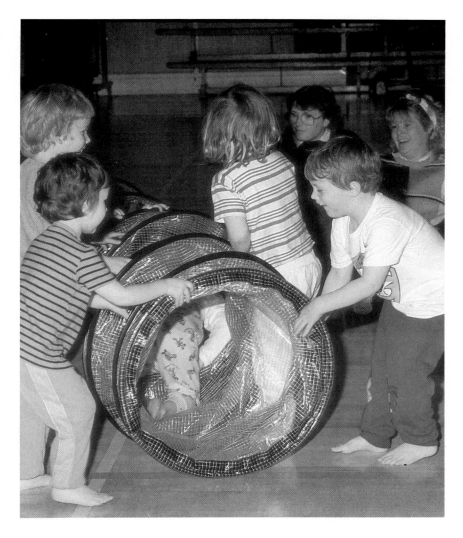

Physical development is just as important as intellectual growth for the pre-school child, and there are now a range of activities available for this age group, such as toddlers' gym clubs, or inflatable 'bouncing' apparatus which vary the routine of park or playground.

turn-taking in games, and so on, and can find sharing very difficult. Hence, there is often some aggression – fighting over toys, pushing another child off the tricycle, which will need gentle handling and an explanation about turn-taking from an adult. With time, children learn all these things, but it may seem a slow process.

TRAVELLING WITH CHILDREN

Planning ahead is essential if you are travelling with small children. Think about exercise, games and entertainment, and food and drink. Children cannot be expected to sit still for long periods, so it is best to plan a few short stops, unless, of course, you are travelling by air. Ask your travel agent what facilities are available for young children on your airline – package tour charters are usually rather basic, but some airlines can be helpful on scheduled flights.

If you are in a car, stop and let them run around for five or ten minutes every hour or so. In a train, take them for walks down the corridor and to look out of a different window for a bit. Taped music and stories on cassettes are useful in cars, but might annoy other passengers in a coach or train. Games and drawing materials do not take up much space and will help pass the time. A supply of fruit and crisps (less harmful than sweets!) and small drinks is useful – somehow children are always hungry or thirsty the moment they are settled in a car and off on the road. Travel sick pills, taken a half hour before the journey, will help if your child gets sick – check the dose with your chemist. A packet of tissues, and a damp flannel in a plastic bag are always useful for sticky fingers, or emergencies. If your child is hooked on using her own potty, take it with you – it could save a scene over using an unfamiliar toilet, or peeing on the grass.

CHAPTER FIFTEEN

TOWARDS SCHOOL

The transition from toddler to school child through your child's developing independence

The years from two until school age are a time of increasing independence and socialization, and for most children this period passes smoothly. In Britain the majority of children experience some form of pre-school provision before starting compulsory education at the age of five years, and over 40 per cent of children (in 1985) will have attended either nursery schools or nursery classes in primary schools before starting 'real' school, in addition to those who have attended playgroups, etc. A child's main security and support remains her home, with the love and affection given there ensuring the confidence to enter the wider world and explore relationships with other adults and children. For many children, going to some sort of pre-school provision at around the age of three may be their first experience of relating to other children, or having a significant relationship with an adult other than their parents. It is an important time for a child, both for intellectual development, and for learning to inter-relate with other people.

DEVELOPING INDEPENDENCE

In these years many new skills are mastered, children's conversation becomes more interesting as their vocabulary and experience widens, and questions are increasingly asked from the age of three. This is the age when you will forever be answering the question 'Why?', and you will probably find that you are asked the same question several times in one day. It can sometimes be exasperating, but it is evidence of your child's natural curiosity, which is the basis of learning. If you get fed up explaining why the bus is red for the seventh time, try to distract your child's attention with another topic or by singing a song. It won't be long before the next 'Why?' comes along, but it will give you a little respite!

Your child's increasingly complex language development involves recognition of rules of grammar now, and the way she can use speech to communicate a wide range of ideas reflects both her growing understanding of the world and her own intellectual development. This is the age when adults are being constantly surprised and delighted by a child's original view of the way things work both physically and socially, and listening to two three and a half or four year olds playing a game of make believe can be hilarious.

Children at this age master skills which increase their independence, such as going to the toilet on their own and making pretty good attempts at dressing and undressing. This often goes along with strong views on what to wear and what not to wear! This can lead to the occasional tantrum in the particularly obstinate child, but on the whole temper tantrums tend to occur much less frequently. Most of the earlier feeding problems resolve themselves, too, although again a minority of children may still be fussy about certain things and can articulate their dislike more forcefully now.

Difficulties over settling to sleep and waking in the night are much less common over the age of three, although this is cold comfort to those whose children are still waking. However, older children who do wake at night will often not need their parents to get up to them as they are more likely to be prepared to play on their own by finding a favourite book or toy before falling back to sleep again.

The imaginative child may still have worries and fears especially at night which need reassurance, but children at this age are capable of listening to reason and accepting explanations which younger children could not. As with younger children, however, praise and encouragement and simple rewards will reinforce good behaviour. However, there are still likely to be occasional conflicts, and many parents still find their children difficult to manage between the ages of two and a half and three and a half. The advice given in the previous chapter will still be relevant for this period.

BEDWETTING

Children from families where one parent wet the bed after the age of five, or children who have perhaps been a little delayed in some other aspect of their development, often take longer to be reliably

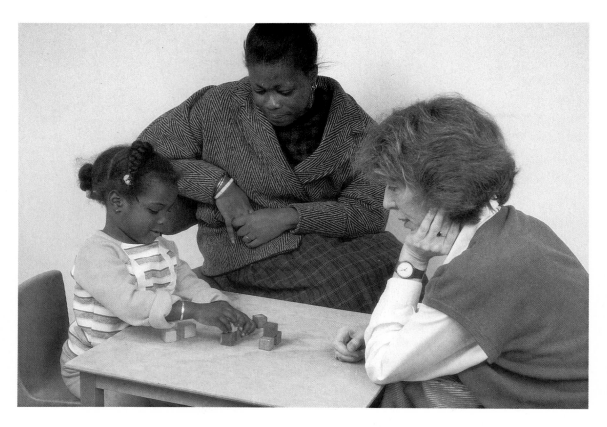

Pre-school developmental checks use simple but effective techniques in an informal atmosphere to test a wide range of skills.

dry at night (see p. 224). Any child may wet the bed in response to stress or during an episode of illness, and children who have an unhappy experience during the time when they would normally become dry (such as separation of their parents, starting school or a stay in hospital), may go on bedwetting longer than others.

Bedwetting is not a deliberate act, and some children become extremely upset when it happens. Try to avoid telling your child off or punishing her if she wets the bed – it makes matters worse as the child then becomes anxious. Lots of praise and encouragement for dry nights and a gentle 'never mind' approach to wet beds is best. You can avoid the problem to some extent by lifting your child on to the pot at the time you go to bed yourself. Most children will urinate in this situation without really waking or protesting. However, if you find this wakes your child and she has difficulty in going back to sleep, or if it upsets her at all, it is probably best not to pursue it as it could again be counter-productive and actually delay the slow but steady transition to dry nights.

DEVELOPMENTAL CHECKS

Most health districts in Britain offer developmental checks to all children living in the district during the pre-school years. Some areas will check children at eighteen months and three and a half to four, others at around two years and three and a half. These checks are part of the regular assessment begun when your baby was six weeks old (see p. 189).

You will probably be offered an appointment either at the local child health clinic or your doctor's surgery, and your child will be seen either by the health visitor or the doctor, or possibly both. The aim of such examinations is to check that each child is developing to his or her full potential, and to spot any problems as early as possible. This child will usually have height and weight checked, and there will be a physical examination including looking at the teeth and inspection of the ears. Some assessment is made of the child's overall development and of her sight and hearing.

THE THREE-YEAR CHECK

A check at three years old is particularly important, since a child's speech and understanding should normally be such that a quite detailed examination

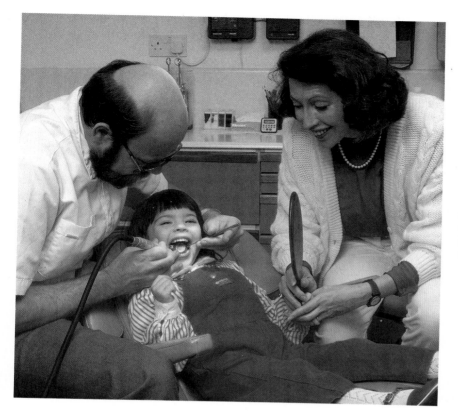

Dental check-ups can be fun for your child with a dentist who has a special interest in caring for children's teeth. Start six-monthly visits at the age of about two-and-a-half, and if these are combined with the prevention of tooth decay by regular brushing and avoiding too much sugar, your child need never be frightened of going to the dentist.

of such things as sight and hearing can be done reasonably accurately. It includes looking at the way your child uses her hands (fine motor abilities), by such activities as brick building, drawing and bead threading; and the use of her body and limbs (gross motor abilities), such as running, jumping and kicking or throwing a ball. Her language development will be assessed as well. Hearing is tested, and the eyes examined for a squint (by now this would be obvious and should be treated without delay). At three and a half to four sight can usually be successfully tested by matching the shape of letters on a card, even if your child isn't able to name them yet.

Use the check-up to spend time talking to the health visitor or doctor about your child's development and behaviour, and discuss any worries or problems that may be brought to light. Quite a number of children may refuse to co-operate or do things in a clinic that they are quite capable of doing at home, although if you don't make too much of the check-up to your child beforehand and let her think of it simply as a special series of games with the doctor, you will probably avoid trouble. However, as parents are the people who see most of their children and usually know exactly what their capabilities are, don't be afraid to tell the doctor or

health visitor of any skills which your child is unwilling to display to order!

If there is even a slight doubt about some aspect of your child's development, the doctor may refer you to a specialist. If this happens at the clinic, the doctor will probably want to arrange this through your GP. For instance, if it is felt that your child's speech development is slow, she may be referred to a speech therapist. Sometimes the doctor or health visitor will just want to keep an eye on your child, after discussion with you.

Although the check-up is one particular opportunity for you to discuss your child, you do not have to wait for an appointment if you have any worries. Your health visitor or doctor are available at any time to discuss your anxieties, just as they were when your child was a baby, and often by raising things early on you can stop minor worries from becoming major ones.

CARE OF THE TEETH

Encouraging brushing of teeth after meals and particularly before bed is good practice, and sensible from around the age of eighteen months. Regular visits to the dentist should be encouraged from two and a half years onwards, as initially the idea is to get the child used to opening her mouth and having her teeth examined. Not all dentists are skilled at communicating with young children, but many health centres and clinics offer a dental service which is particularly aimed at children. If a child does require dental treatment, such as a filling, at any age, it is clearly an easier experience if the child is already used to the dentist and to being examined. Most dentists recommend check-ups at approximately six monthly intervals.

A NEW BABY

The decision when to have another baby is a very personal one, which varies with individual families. The decision may well depend on such factors as housing and income, as well as the age of the mother, and of course even the most careful plans don't always work out as expected. Babies are not always conceived when you hope for them, and miscarriages can occur. While some families choose a small gap between children of two years or less, others prefer to wait until the first child is three or older. The advantage of having two small children close together is that the years of nappy changing and broken nights are got over consecutively, and with luck the two children will get on well without fighting constantly.

Many people feel that two is an age of extreme jealousies, but this depends more on the child's personality than her age, something that may be difficult to predict when you are contemplating whether to try for another baby. An older child is able to understand and communicate more about a new baby's arrival, and will participate actively in the baby's care if given a chance.

THE EFFECT ON THE OLDER CHILD

The birth of a younger sibling can be both an exciting and a worrying time in a young child's life. Inevitably, there will be anxiety about being displaced from the parents' love and affection, as well as some jealousy of a new baby. It helps to give a lot of thought to preparing your child for the arrival of a new baby, and to encourage her to participate both during the pregnancy and after the baby is born. Talk to your child about the baby, how it grows inside and moves around, and answer any questions as honestly as you can.

Try and involve your child in practical preparations, like choosing baby clothes and toys, and try to make her feel it is her baby too (not just yours). Stories and picture books about babies are helpful to read to your child, and if you are not having a home birth, she will need to know that her mother will go into hospital for a few days, but that she can visit. Reassurance about little things is important – and the maintenance of the usual routine even while you are in hospital. The more both parents are involved in the care of the child the easier it all is – there is some evidence that children who are close to their fathers and used to being looked after by them are less adversely affected by the birth of a new baby.

NORMAL REACTIONS

You can expect jealous and angry reactions, which are quite normal, and commonly some regression to an earlier stage of development. Some children may start wetting the bed again, having been previously dry; others may want to go back to having a bottle or dummy 'like the baby'. There is no need to discourage this – the child needs to be able to work through jealousies of this sort before becoming more mature. Some children react the opposite way and decide, now they are the older brother or sister, they will behave in a very 'grown up' way – perhaps by giving up an earlier habit, or starting to do something for themselves which you previously had to be involved in.

Jealous and angry reactions to a new baby brother or sister are by no means inevitable, and even when they do occur there will also be very positive reactions. Children, even as young as two, can be clearly upset when a baby cries, and will often try and comfort the baby; they will also enjoy making the baby laugh and chuckle, showing that even at this young age they are sensitive to a younger child's expression of feelings.

GIVING YOUR CHILD ATTENTION

How a child reacts to a new baby depends as much on their own individual personality as on how the situation is handled by the parents. Inevitably, the new baby will need a lot of attention, and time to spend alone with an older child will be difficult to find. It does help if you can organize some time alone with the older child, even if briefly. But grandparents and friends can help too – by giving special attention to the older one and going out for walks and expeditions so that she does receive the undivided attention of one adult for a time. Interestingly, children who seem to show no jealous feelings about their own baby sibling are quite capable of showing marked anger and resentment when one of their parents cuddles someone else's baby. It is almost as if they understand the need to love and care for the baby in their own family, but an outsider's baby may be the last straw!

Learning to work together as a group is one of the most important aspects of nursery education. Children particularly enjoy singing and counting games which also help speech and co-ordination.

The time of arrival of a sibling is not the appropriate time to start a child at nursery or other form of pre-school provision. The child may then feel she is being pushed out of the way so that you can be alone with the baby. Plan it so that a child is already happily settled in before the baby arrives – or wait three or four months until she has adjusted to the reality of life in a larger family before planning to start at a nursery.

PRE-SCHOOL PROVISION

There is a range of provision in this country for pre-school children, although there is enormous variation from area to area in the amount and type of provision available. Handbooks which list the local facilities and services for under fives are produced in many areas. They can be obtained by asking at your local library, citizens advice bureau, social services department or health clinic. Nursery schools and classes may be run by the local education authority, and have a specifically stated educational purpose. The ratio of staff to children is quite high compared to infant school, and the staff will have professional teaching qualifications. While in some areas nursery schools will admit children as young as three, in other areas they will only take children of four plus. There is often considerable demand for places, and, whether privately or local authority run, many nursery schools have quite long waiting lists, with priority given to brothers and sisters and families living close to the school. Nursery schools are also run by many independent bodies (such as Montessori nurseries) and private individuals.

Playgroups exist in many parts of the country, but more particularly in towns and cities. They are usually run by the parents themselves, and a key feature is that parents are expected to be involved in

Experimenting with the colour and texture of paint is just one of a number of 'messy' activities which a nursery school or playgroup can offer.

helping in the organization. Many playgroup leaders have been on courses or taken qualifications in this field. They usually cater for children over the age of two and a half and are often run in a local church hall or similar facility. If there is no playgroup in your area, it might be worth getting together with other parents to start one up – help can be obtained from the Pre-school Playgroups Association.

Mother and toddler groups are run at some clinics, health centres and community centres, and some of these places also run creches where your child can be left for short periods. However, mostly parents are expected to stay with their children, and they are usually organized so that play materials and often a playleader are available to the children, with an opportunity for parents to talk to each other. Often simple catering facilities exist so that cups of tea and orange juice, etc. are available.

Nursery schools and playgroups are not really designed as childcare facilities for working parents; most operate on a part-time basis with quite short morning or afternoon sessions, although a few will take priority children for two sessions with lunch. Even then, the afternoon session generally finishes

at or before 3.30 pm, and nurseries will have normal school holidays. If you want or need to go back to work once your child reaches this age, you may be able to get a day nursery place; otherwise you will need to look at the childcare options already discussed on page 196.

PLAYGROUPS AND NURSERY SCHOOLS

Places at playgroups or nursery schools are usually available either on a daily or half-daily basis, for a limited number of days a week, or a five day week. Clearly, your own needs in terms of hours must be considered when making your choice, and practical factors, such as the distance from your home and travel arrangements, will need to be taken into account. A playgroup or nursery close to your home makes it easier for your child to have local friends, and is a good way to meet other parents who can often become quite a supportive network both to you and your child.

The aim of playgroups and nurseries is implicitly educational – not just in the field of encouraging the child's intellectual development but also enlarging the child's social skills in relating to other children and adults, and encouraging independence. Children at play need time to run around and let off steam, as well as time for constructive play, and a

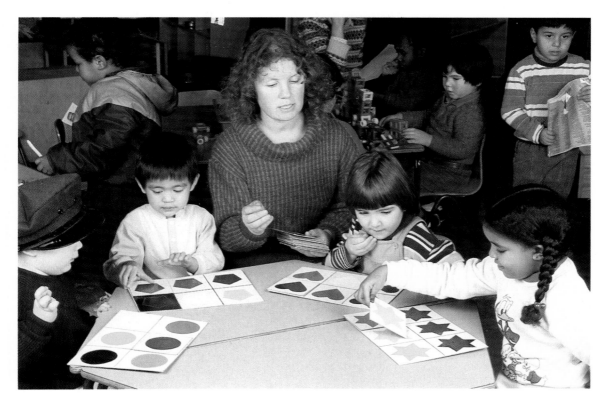

Matching shapes and colours in a simple game supervised by an adult helps pre-school children to begin to think mathematically.

good nursery or playgroup will offer a healthy balance between free and structured times of the day. It is important to have some structured activity in each play session, as this encourages concentration and task-solving, hence encouraging intellectual development. Typical activities of this sort which children enjoy are all types of art work (you will be presented with armfuls of drawings, paintings and collages every week!), colour matching games, construction materials, puzzles and make-believe sessions, such as dressing up, doll's houses, hospital corners, and so on.

Three-year-olds onward particularly enjoy periods of make-believe and will develop complex imaginative games and conversations, particularly if left alone without adults to inhibit their imagination. In these imaginary games at this age children often play best in pairs, and most often seem to choose friends of their own sex. By three, children are well aware of whether they are boys or girls, and may already be developing stereotyped ideas of how each sex should behave in response to adult and environmental conditioning. One hopes to find nurseries which employ staff of both sexes, and

where children are encouraged to play within a wide range of activities, such as woodwork, cooking, and so on in a way which does not encourage sex stereotyping.

Although at times liking to play with one special friend, for much of the time children also enjoy playing in groups, particularly for singing and dancing games, and stories. Being with other children encourages learning to co-operate with others, to respect other children, and to listen to and help others. All this increases a child's self-confidence as well as helping their social development, and helps to make the transition from home to school an easier process.

CHOOSING A PLAYGROUP OR NURSERY

Selecting any form of pre-school provision may seem rather daunting, particularly if you are lucky enough in your own area to have considerable choice. It is very much an individual decision, based on your own needs and what you feel is most appropriate for your own child. Do not be too influenced by other people's opinions, but go and see for yourself and trust your own intuitive feelings. It is important to find somewhere that seems truly to like and value children, and that is warm and welcoming to both parents and children. Beware of

POINTS TO LOOK FOR WHEN SELECTING A PRE- SCHOOL GROUP.

☐ Is there a warm, welcoming atmosphere?

☐ Is there parental involvement?

☐ What variety of activities are available?

☐ What is the staff/child ratio?

☐ How do the staff interact with the children – are there plenty of hugs and humour, or are attitudes authoritarian and judgmental?

☐ Do the adults talk to the children, or to each other?

☐ Is the group (including staff) multi-cultural, and what are attitudes towards sexism and racism?

☐ Are children adequately supervised, and what safety precautions are taken?

☐ How is a distressed or angry child handled and how is aggression coped with?

☐ What is the policy of settling in new children?

☐ Do relationships between the staff seem good?

☐ What is the level of communication between playleaders and parents?

☐ Do kitchen areas and toilets appear clean?

the too-tidy nursery, and be sure to ask about the aims and philosophies of the place in order to find out if your ideas are similar to theirs. This is particularly important in respect of discipline, competitiveness, attitudes to toileting and meal-times. Don't be afraid to ask questions about aspects you find worrying, and look for open, frank answers. Good nursery teachers and playgroup leaders will welcome parental interest and constructive criticism, and will be happy for parents to become involved in nursery activities.

Some nursery schools stress the educational nature of the activities offered to children and may even encourage early reading. Although some children will enjoy these, those who aren't ready for reading (the majority of four-year-olds) will be put off or discouraged by these activities, especially if they are forced to join in. There is no evidence to suggest that it is helpful for children to learn to read before starting school at five, and for many children it is an unnecessary pressure which can undermine self-confidence. Education is far broader than learning to read and write, and all the 'play' activities in pre-school groups are in themselves educational (see above).

SETTLING IN

When considering any change of environment for your pre-school child, try and plan it carefully. Small children do not respond well to sudden changes although there can obviously be circumstances that cannot be planned for, such as a parent becoming ill and having to go to hospital. But with most arrangements for childcare there is time to think about it well in advance and to plan settling-in time in a way which will least upset your child. Some children are sociable and extrovert and will cheerfully wave goodbye on their first day at a new nursery; others are perhaps more apprehensive and anxious about separation from a parent and will need a few weeks of settling.

Many children's centres have a policy that a parent is expected to plan for a six week settling-in time, during which they will be around as much as necessary – this is because they recognize that a considerable number of children do find the transition from home to another environment quite difficult. It depends not only on your child's personality but her age, and also her previous experiences. At three and older it is very much easier for a child to cope with new adults and children and playthings than at two – a two-year-old may well be a bit bewildered, but a three-year-old has had more experience and is better able to understand that if you go away you are coming back again later.

Children who are used to playing in other people's homes, have extensive networks of family or friends and are used to relating to other adults, have no difficulty in adjusting on the whole. For children who have previously always been at home with their parents the settling-in period will almost certainly be longer. Talk to the nursery or playgroup staff about what they expect, try and visit a few times with your child before it is time to start, and be a bit wary if the staff try to tell you that you need not stay on the first day! Any pre-school centre that understands parents and children will know that you both need to come to start with. It is reassuring for you as well as your child to meet the other children and experience the morning routine and see perhaps how another child who is upset is handled by the staff.

If your child finds it hard to leave you she will need one special adult to relate to and make a friend of – so that if necessary you can physically hand your child to that person when you have to leave.

Depending on your child, you should plan to spend several sessions at the centre, not always directly with your child but just being around for reassurance, before going away for short periods. Be prepared to be flexible – but don't try and go away for hours until you and the staff feel your child is reasonably happy and secure in the centre. Even after a long period, some children will always cry on saying goodbye – but usually they are cheerfully playing ten minutes later. A phone call to check can be reassuring for you. A favourite toy or something of yours, like a scarf, can be reassuring for a child to have with her until it is time to go home again. If you have a child who is clearly unhappy after three or four months, then it is important to discuss this with someone, perhaps your health visitor, as you may need to re-think and have your child back at home until she is a bit older.

PROBLEMS WITH BEHAVIOUR

It is not unusual for a child to show some change in behaviour after starting at a playgroup or nursery. Some children become a bit quiet and withdrawn until they have made friends and become confident in their new setting; others may be quite boisterous and bossy with other children. Sometimes the behaviour can be distressing for you and other parents, if your child starts to be aggressive towards other children, or is at the receiving end of this sort of behaviour.

Biting, kicking or hair pulling are not uncommon, and may simply be a reaction to a new environment and learning to share with other children. Sometimes biting happens in response to aggression in a different form – perhaps being pushed by another child – or if a child is angry and upset about something she finds hard to talk about. With careful handling by the staff and parents this behaviour usually stops fairly soon. It must be made clear that the biting is unacceptable, but punishment by smacking or biting back should be avoided as this will make matters worse. If such behaviour persists, do discuss it with the staff and your doctor or health visitor – other parents are understandably protective of their own children and may not be too tolerant.

STARTING SCHOOL

The transition to school is a big step, which on the whole is easier for children who have experienced some sort of pre-school group. Even so, the school environment is very different, there are perhaps different expectations of behaviour, a lot more children, and certainly far fewer adults around to give individual attention. Most five-year-olds cope well after the first few days, and it will be easier for them if they have visited the school beforehand. Some schools arrange for a 'staggered' intake at the beginning of term, so children can be settled in a few at a time with plenty of attention on the first day.

Generally, children enjoy the stimulation of school, but are likely to be very tired after school and may be irritable for the first few weeks. It is after all an effort to cope with all those other children and another new environment. For the majority it all quickly settles down, but around one in ten will still have some difficulties with coping after the first term. It is important to discuss with the child's teacher how she is coping in class – sometimes a child who appears upset and clingy and demanding at home will be fine at school, and just needs extra reassurance from you. But any anxiety should be discussed with your child's teacher, and parents are now normally welcome in the classroom in most infant schools.

Your child needs you to take an interest in the work (and play) she is involved in at school, and as at playgroup, you should expect to come home with armfuls of paintings from time to time.

ANXIETIES ABOUT SCHOOL

Common dislikes and complaints in the first year or so are often about intimidation in the playground, teasing by other children, school meals, changes in friendship, and so on. Toilets, too, can be a cause of anxiety. Sometimes the cause of a worry is obvious – such as custard poured all over the pudding – and a note to the teacher about a hatred of custard will cure the problem! However, some children find it hard to tell their parents what is worrying them and subtle questioning may be needed.

If you continue to be anxious about your child after discussion with the teacher there are other sources of help – the school doctor or nurse can be contacted, and when appropriate the school's educational psychologist can often help sort out your child's difficulties.

SCHOOL PHOBIA

Occasionally anxiety over some aspect of school will cause a child to refuse to go to school (school phobia) – she may even develop the symptoms of an illness. This is fairly uncommon in the first years at primary school but can occur at any age. It is important to find out what is the cause of the problem, which will usually mean a visit to the school. Your child will need a lot of reassurance but you need to be quite firm about the fact that she does have to go to school. Visiting the classroom with your child and encouraging her to tell you all about her day at school will usually identify the source of the problem.

Sometimes school phobia is not due to a problem at school at all, but may occur if a child is worried about leaving home for any reason. This can happen if one parent is ill or has perhaps been in hospital, a situation which can make a child very anxious and reluctant to be separated again. Discussion and reassurance will again be needed; if you can anticipate a possible time of difficulty, such as a time when one parent has to go into hospital, tell your child's teacher so that he or she can keep a special eye on the child during this period.

SLOW LEARNERS

There are two or three children in every class who are not really ready for formal schooling at the age of five and may experience considerable difficulty

The age at which a pre-school child can produce even a crude human face varies enormously, as can be seen from the drawings reproduced below, by a two-and-a-half-year-old (below – a remarkably early example) and a four-year-old (bottom).

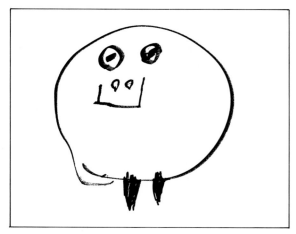

with mastering early reading and writing skills. Children develop and mature at different rates and need to be allowed to go at their own pace without being made to feel they are failing to keep up with others. In many countries formal schooling does not start until the age of six, since it is recognized that many childen are too immature at five to cope with some of the classroom demands. Some British schools mix five- and six-year-olds in groups, which benefits both slow learners and early developers.

If your child seems slow to learn, don't apply pressure but encourage by reading stories and looking at books together. Find out what reading scheme is used in the class, and talk to the teacher about how you can help. Trying to force the pace is counter-productive, and pressure can put a child off attempting to tackle any new task for fear of failing. If both you and the teacher continue to be concerned about slow progress then the school may feel it is appropriate to consult the educational psychologist.

THE SCHOOL MEDICAL EXAMINATION

Although some districts have a policy of offering a pre-school health check at around four and a half years, the majority of health districts in Britain now arrange for the check to take place once the child has started school, between the ages of five and five and a half years. The aim of such an examination is to ensure that each child is going to get the most from their schooling, and to identify any medical or developmental problems that might interfere with the child's education. None of these examinations involve tests which will be 'passed' or 'failed', nor do they involve producing a score or IQ for each child. It is recognized that different children develop and mature at different rates, and that children's development is often uneven.

Children differ in the things they enjoy doing and in the things they are good at. Special skills may exist in one area, perhaps drawing and creative skills, while the same child might lag behind others of the same age in another area. The aim of any assessment of a child is to offer help if it is needed in any particular area, and to discuss with parents and teachers the best way to ensure a child's optimal development. Some children may need help with concentration, and be better in small groups for teaching, while those who are very active may not be able to cope with too structured a day and will need time to let off steam. Some may need extra help with copying and writing skills; children who perhaps have had some hearing loss in the past may need help to develop listening skills.

A school medical examination should not take

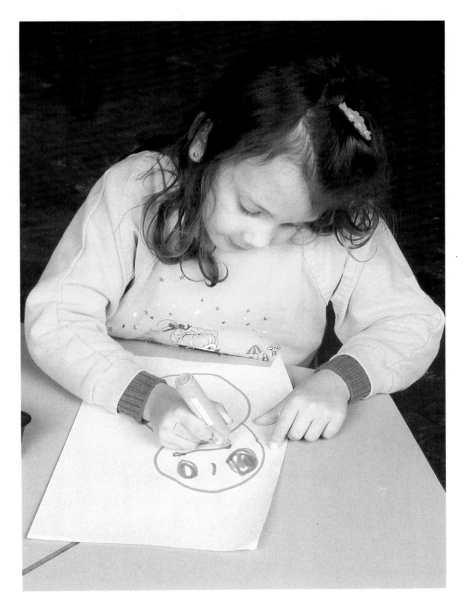

Drawing helps children to express themselves while learning the control of a pen or pencil eventually needed for writing.

place without the parents, as it is an opportunity for discussion with those who know the child best. A check of both eyesight and hearing will be done, as clearly any defect in either of these areas (which may be unsuspected by parents) can interfere with optimal learning.

Sometimes stress at home, such as illness in a family member, or separation of the parents, can helpfully be discussed – teachers too need to know of such events. If a child is anxious or worried about something going on at home he may be quite unable to relax and concentrate at school, and family stress is not an uncommon cause of learning difficulties.

PRIVATE SCHOOLS

Some private schools do not have a school doctor or nurse, and parents are expected to consult their general practitioner over any medical or developmental problem. There will not be any routine checks of your child's eyesight or hearing, so subtle defects can go unnoticed, possibly leading teachers to think your child is lazy or slow. If you have any cause for concern, and particularly if your child's learning seems to be suffering, make sure you seek your doctor's advice and arrange for your child to have hearing and vision checks to be done in the surgery or elsewhere.

Chapter Sixteen

THE SICK CHILD

Understanding the pattern of your child's health, and preventing or coping with illness or accident

Children in our society enjoy a very high standard of health. Medical advice, at varying levels of expertise, is widely available in the media and books, and everyone has access to a general practitioner who aims to look after the whole family, including children. However, the breadth of advice may be bewildering and is often conflicting. Furthermore, many parents are interested in caring for their children and making their own decisions about coping with childhood illnesses.

Unfortunately there is an assumption by many patients and doctors, that illness, even relatively trivial, requires medication. This is not always necessary, particularly for children. It is essential therefore that parents should be familiar with the common illnesses of childhood to understand, not only when formal medical advice is needed, but also when they should be able to manage the problem themselves, particularly when there is no specific treatment and general supportive measures alone are appropriate.

Understanding the patterns of illness and treatment will allow both parent and doctor to discuss the management of each problem and appreciate each other's viewpoint. In the past doctors were accustomed to dictating to patients, and their advice was usually followed without discussion. Fortunately this situation is rapidly changing so that parents, and indeed children themselves, are now readily involved in the process of health care.

THE SICK CHILD AND YOUR DOCTOR

The general practitioner (your family doctor) is a vital source of information and advice about illness. His knowledge of disease as it relates to individuals within a family, particularly when he is familiar with the family, will enable him to work out the most appropriate treatment of a condition. He also can co-ordinate other expertise, both medical (such as hospital-based paediatrics) and para-medical (such as physiotherapists or community nurses), for diagnosis and treatment of serious illness, and provide guidance for more minor difficulties.

Although Accident and Emergency Departments in a hospital may seem more accessible, especially during the night and at weekends, the value of the general practitioner's knowledge of your family should not be underestimated. It is more appropriate to use the hospital only in case of genuine accidents or emergencies, or when the general practitioner has requested a referral.

CHOOSING YOUR DOCTOR

It is important that the family and general practitioner have established a relationship before illness arises. Trust and confidence will improve the value of future consultations, particularly as some problems may require only telephone advice.

General practitioners with paediatric expertise will feel comfortable discussing problems this way, and parents who know the general practitioner will accept the advice more readily. Some general practitioners are especially interested in children and many will have worked in hospital paediatric departments.

It is therefore worth choosing your general practitioner carefully. Ask friends in your neighbourhood and, indeed, the general practitioners themselves about their facilities and their attitude to children's health. Many general practitioners arrange 'Well Baby' clinics from their surgeries. These are useful for the doctor to get to know the children registered with him when they are well, so that when a child isn't well it is easier to see the difference. These clinics also allow regular checks of a child's physical and intellectual development, and are useful for the discussion of common anxieties such as feeding practice, immunization, and minor ailments. Health visitors often play an integral role and contact with them and other parents either informally or in discussion groups may be very supportive (see p. 188).

If your child has a particular condition which your general practitioner feels needs more specialized attention, you may be referred to a paediatrician in a hospital. A paediatrician is a doctor who is generally concerned with the care of ill children, or children with problems.

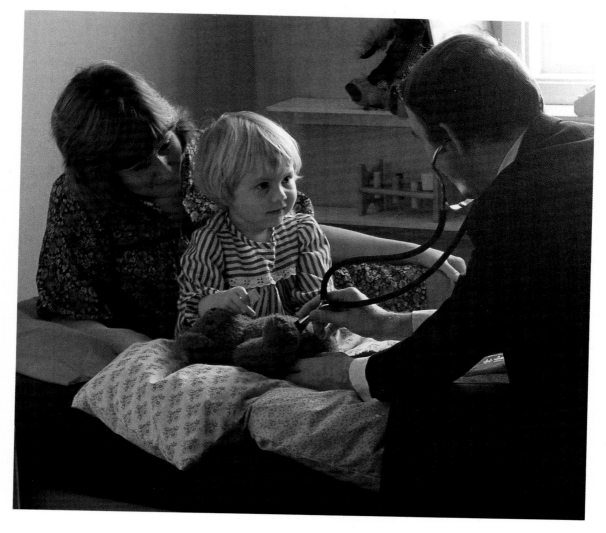

The relationship between you and your family doctor is a partnership based on the shared desire to care for your child's health.

CALLING THE DOCTOR OUT

General practitioners have varying attitudes to visiting patients at home, and it may be useful to have previously established the reasons for which he feels a home visit is appropriate. From the point of view of the general practitioner, home visits are time-consuming and may not be strictly necessary, but all general practitioners appreciate that there are occasions when a child might be best seen at home.

Similarly, direct contact with the doctor by telephone is often difficult. Some general practitioners make themselves more accessible than others, and it is useful to find out policy before joining a doctor's list. Situations when a home visit is important include high fever, severe pain, potentially infectious disease, acute lethargy and obvious illness, persistent vomiting and diarrhoea. A home visit is also advisable when the family has great difficulty in visiting the surgery, perhaps because of other young children.

There may be some delay between calling the doctor and his arrival, depending on his other commitments. At night, many general practitioners arrange to have a doctors' deputizing service make the visit. In this situation, you lose the advantage of seeing a doctor who knows the family, and if the problem is not serious or acute, an early consultation the following day is often more suitable. But delaying advice too long may be harmful to the child's well-being, and if you are seriously concerned or uncertain about the nature of the problem, call the doctor anyway.

Some emergencies might be better managed by taking the child directly to hospital, although this may depend on whether your home is near a hospital, or in the country, where general practitioners are often happy to cope with a wide variety of problems. Accidents such as deep cuts or fractures, or head injuries, should be taken to hospital. Any situation where there is very severe pain or some change in the level of consciousness, may require calling an ambulance directly. It is useful to inform the GP first as he may be able to warn the hospital more directly that a sick child is about to arrive.

CHILDREN IN THE SURGERY

If possible children are best seen early in the day, or at least early in an afternoon surgery. Children get irritable when waiting and disturb other patients, as well as distressing themselves and their parents, and the time spent waiting should be short. Well equipped surgeries will have toys and books, and one advantage of a large health centre, shared by several general practices, is the provision of a play area. Parents should be prepared for some wait, however, both for their general practitioner and for hospital clinics, and should bring favourite toys, a bottle of milk or fruit juice, and, if appropriate, an extra nappy and changing equipment.

It is also useful for parents to come prepared with one or two points about their child's illness which they have already noticed; for instance, the period of the illness, the appearance of specific symptoms and any particular concerns that they may have.

The success of a consultation with a doctor depends very much on the co-operation of the child. This requires both a gentle and unhurried approach by the doctor, and also the preparedness of the child. If he is old enough to understand, the child should have the purpose of the visit explained to him, and the possible use of any equipment, such as a stethoscope or a torch for examining the ears. False reassurance isn't helpful, but you can reinforce the idea of the doctor's good nature. It is in everyone's interest that the child be relaxed and as unthreatened as possible.

The possibility of any painful procedures should be explained but this is perhaps best left until very soon before the event. However, children who are forewarned about these procedures very often tolerate them well. Doctors, dentists, hospitals and 'unpleasant' medical events should never be used as threats, as this ultimately undermines the confidence of the child in the doctor as someone who cares and helps.

When your child's ears are examined, hold her gently but firmly on your lap and rest the side of her head against you (right), holding it steady with a hand on her forehead if necessary. You may find it easier to grip a wriggling baby's legs between your thighs.

To have your child's eyes or throat examined, position her on your lap as for examination of the ear, but hold her head forward (left). A young baby may be wrapped in a towel or blanket to control the arms and hands.

Parents should make themselves familiar with the standard procedure for holding a child being examined. This is not only useful to comfort the child and reassure him, but also allows the doctor to examine the child safely and without causing undue force. Although inevitably some procedures, such as examining the throat, do cause some slight distress, most doctors are expert in obtaining information as quickly as possible.

IMMUNIZATION

The elimination or limitation of several fatal infectious diseases during the twentieth century has been a major contribution to the improvement of health care. Poliomyelitis and diphtheria now occur very rarely in the developed world, smallpox has been eradicated, and many other conditions such as tetanus, typhoid fever, yellow fever and hepatitis can now be controlled by immunization. Unfortunately there is a tendency to forget that there is still the potential for these dangerous conditions to return, and it is essential that routine immunization of everyone in the community continues, to maintain a high level of general immunity, so it is important to ensure your child has the full schedule of immunizations.

HOW IMMUNIZATION WORKS

The body's immune system responds to a foreign organism (or germ) by producing antibodies to neutralize or kill that germ. The immune system can 'remember', for a varying period of months or years, how to produce more specific antibodies if someone again comes into contact with the same organism. An artificial challenge to the immune system is provided in essentially two ways.

Dead organisms, or a portion of dead organisms, may be injected on several occasions over a period of months. This is the basis for immunization against pertussis (whooping cough) and typhoid fever. The 'memory' against these infections usually only lasts a few years. Periodically a reminder or booster injection is required. An alternative form of providing immunity is to inject a harmless live organism, similar to that causing the disease, but without producing symptoms. Vaccines against measles, rubella, yellow fever, smallpox, tuberculosis and poliomyelitis use this principle.

Some infections need to be protected against for life (TB, smallpox, poliomyelitis), but others, such as whooping cough and measles, have their most serious effects on children, and so protection is needed only during this period of life.

MINIMIZING SIDE EFFECTS

Most immunizations produce some side effects, but in the vast majority of children these symptoms are mild such as slight fever, minor irritability, redness and a lump (which may persist for several weeks) at the site of the infection, and in older patients a general feeling of being off colour. However, the inconvenience of these symptoms is far outweighed by the advantages of immunity.

Nevertheless many parents will be concerned about possible adverse effects and it is sensible to minimize the likelihood of their occurring. Injections should be given only when the baby or child is well, without fever or severe illness, but should not be postponed just for a runny nose or mild cold. Paracetamol in syrup or tablet form (available under a variety of brand names) is useful for fever if this occurs after the injection.

Most injections are given into a muscle or under the skin. The usual sites are the upper arm, buttock or front of the thigh. Oral vaccine is taken by mouth; a few drops of liquid are placed on the tongue and the baby or child will swallow this without difficulty although it does taste bitter and is therefore sometimes placed on a sugar cube.

TIMING OF IMMUNIZATION

The timing of the immunization is important. Babies are protected from many infections by the mother's own antibodies transferred across the placenta before birth. These antibodies lasts for about six months; after this time young infants are particularly at risk from the common infectious diseases. It is for this reason that the programme of routine immunization starts at three months. Immunization against tuberculosis (BCG) is often given to newborn babies from families where there is an increased risk of contracting tuberculosis (such as a recent family history of TB or in immigrant families who have come from countries where the disease is still widespread). This practice does vary throughout the UK, however.

Routine immunization includes protection against poliomyelitis, measles, tetanus, diphtheria, and rubella. Mumps is also being added to this list. The table on this page gives the commonly accepted immunization schedule.

If a course of vaccination is interrupted for any length of time, there seems to be no need to start again and the course should simply be completed. Babies born prematurely should be immunized at the same age as other babies – in this case no allowances are made for their prematurity.

These vaccines do not guarantee total immunity

IMMUNIZATION SCHEDULE	
AGE	**VACCINE**
Newborn	BCG for babies at risk from TB
3 months	Diphtheria, tetanus, pertussis (known collectively as DTP or Triple Vaccine) and poliomyelitis
5 months	DTP; polio
9 months	DTP; polio
15 months	Measles (being replaced by combined measles, mumps and rubella – MMR).
School entry	Diphtheria; tetanus; poliomyelitis; measles (if not given previously)
10-13 years	BCG (if there is no immunity to tuberculosis)
11-14 years	Rubella (all girls, if not given previously)
School leaving	Tetanus, poliomyelitis

against these infections, but the illness, if it does occur, is usually mild. It is very useful for parents to keep a record of those immunizations given and to note themselves when the next dose of vaccine is required.

PERTUSSIS (WHOOPING COUGH)

Considerable controversy has arisen about the use of this vaccine because of the possible link between vaccination and neurological (brain) damage. Unfortunately this has led to relatively small numbers of children being vaccinated. Although it does not eliminate the possibility of contracting whooping cough completely, vaccination does lessen the severity of the disease if it does occur. The low percentage (31 per cent in 1979) of children immunized has led to a very large increase in the number of reported cases during epidemics in subsequent years.

It is difficult to answer the question 'Does vaccine cause brain damage?'. The apparent effects of vaccine are extremely rare and in 1981 a national study suggested one in about 300,000 injections was *associated* with, but did not necessarily directly cause, long-term neurological damage. To put these statistics in perspective, your child has the same risk of suffering brain damage from pertussis vaccine as from being taken on a car journey of 500 miles or more. On the other hand, neurological damage occurs with the disease whooping cough itself, and there is evidence that serious side-effects such as severe effects on breathing and seizures are probably more common than previously recognized. So it is important to maintain a high rate of vaccination because a high level of immunity within the population tends to protect those who have not or cannot be immunized by preventing epidemics.

Immunity against pertussis is not transferred from mother to baby in the uterus and the baby is theoretically at risk of contracting it from birth. Immunization, however, needs to be delayed until three months of age, as the baby's immune system is not able to respond appropriately to immunization until that time. Minor side effects are common, as mentioned previously, but severe reactions such as prolonged, inconsolable crying or a very high temperature are very rare. When these very serious reactions occur, further vaccination against pertussis should not be carried out but diphtheria, tetanus and polio should still be given.

Some groups of children require special consideration: if parents or siblings have epilepsy, or the child has a continuing disease of the nervous system, the risk from immunization may be slightly higher. But the benefits of vaccination may still outweigh this increased risk, and the doctor may still advise immunization. If there is doubt about the advisability of immunization, the issue should be discussed with your general practitioner or a paediatrician. Newer vaccines are being developed which may provoke even fewer reactions.

It is commonly believed that children with asthma, eczema or allergy should not be immunized. This is not so, and in fact such children need the protection of vaccination. If immunization has been missed or parents have reconsidered an earlier decision, it can be given until six years.

DIPHTHERIA

This serious and usually lethal illness is now very rare in the UK, largely as a result of the effect of the vaccine. But it is important that diphtheria immunization should be given to everyone, for there is the risk that the disease could return if a high level of immunity in the community is not maintained. Serious reactions to the vaccine are very rare, and there are no medical conditions which should prevent immunization.

TETANUS

The germs for this dangerous illness are present in the earth and dust. Both children and adults are susceptible and repeated immunization is important throughout life. Following the initial course, booster injections should be given every five years. Generally, if an open injury occurs and immunization is known to be up to date, an additional injection is not required. In non-immunized children, however, a booster should be given at the time of injury and possibly an injection of anti-tetanus immunoglobulin to provide immediate protection.

MEASLES

Measles is commonly thought not to be a serious illness, but it can frequently cause considerable distress to the child and may lead to pneumonia, encephalitis (inflammation of the brain) and ear and throat infections. One injection at about fifteen months provides immunity, although a mild attack of measles may still occur in those immunized. A slight fever and rash often occur about a week following the injection, and very rarely a febrile convulsion may occur. However, the incidence of this is far less than a convulsion occurring with measles itself. If the child has had convulsions previously, or parents or brothers or sisters have had convulsions, an injection of immunoglobulin should be given at the same time. A new triple vaccine, combining measles, mumps and rubella (MMR) in one dose, is replacing traditional measles vaccine in the UK.

POLIOMYELITIS

The widespread use of a very effective live vaccine against poliomyelitis has led to the virtual disappearance of this disease in the UK, but it is still common in some parts of the world. The vaccine is given by mouth and three doses are required to provide full immunity. It should not be given during an acute illness, particularly gastroenteritis. Parents who are not themselves immunized should also receive a course of vaccine. Side effects are mild and very rare.

RUBELLA (GERMAN MEASLES)

This mild illness causes few problems to a child or adult. It may however produce very serious congenital abnormalities in an unborn baby if the mother becomes infected during pregnancy (see p. 13), so vaccination is highly recommended for all pre-pubertal girls between ten and fourteen years, whether or not they are thought to have had rubella already. One injection produces immunity for many years, although older women may need re-immunization.

It is essential that women given vaccine should

not become pregnant for three months and women contemplating pregnancy should, if they are unsure about their own immunity, discuss their plans with their GP. A blood test can confirm if a woman is already immune to rubella. A mild fever might occur after immunization. Boys have not until now been immunized routinely against rubella, although there are advantages in doing this to increase the immunity of the general population and therefore prevent further transmission of the disease. The new triple vaccine, MMR, should help this situation.

TUBERCULOSIS

Immunization against tuberculosis (BCG) is usually offered to children between their tenth and fourteenth birthday. Before immunization is performed, a screening test (Mantoux test) identifies those children who require full immunization. A small injection is given on the forearm and the reaction noted two days later. If no reaction occurs, the BCG is necessary. The BCG itself is injected under the skin on the upper arm and usually produces a small swelling about three weeks afterwards. This is sometimes tender but usually heals within six to twelve weeks. No dressing is necessary unless an ulcer develops over the swelling. This, too, usually heals. Occasional mild general symptoms occur at the same time. BCG vaccination is also strongly recommended to newborn babies of families from countries outside Europe, including North America, Australasia and Japan, and also to babies of families where there is a recent case of TB.

OTHER VACCINATIONS

Immunization against other common illnesses is available, but, in the UK, is usually reserved for those patients with other medical problems or who are at special risk. Immunization is possible against hepatitis B, influenza, pneumococcal disease and meningococcus. Mumps vaccine is available but, unlike in North America, it has not previously been given routinely in the UK. It will now be included in the new triple vaccine, MMR, along with measles and rubella.

TRAVEL VACCINATION

Many illnesses, such as poliomyelitis and diphtheria, which have almost ceased to exist in the UK, are still prevalent in many countries and it is essential that parents should check that their children are up to date with all the routine immunization. In some countries, immunization against other infections is compulsory, although for others, immunization is advisable but not a prerequisite for entry. Immunization against yellow fever, cholera, typhoid fever are commonly given, and immunoglobulin for hepatitis A, while not giving complete immunity, may help prevent infection. Smallpox vaccination is no longer required anywhere.

The recommendations vary widely and parents should check the requirements for each individual country. A helpful booklet (SA35) available from the DHSS (see page 297) gives guidelines on immunization and, just as important, general information on other aspects of health care abroad including health insurance, health precautions, protection against AIDS, malaria prevention, rabies and other more general advice.

SYMPTOMS AND SIGNS OF ILLNESS

All children will become ill a number of times during childhood and the vast majority of these episodes will be because of common minor infections, most of which do not require specific medication or medical advice. However, parents may worry that a symptom may be a signal that something more serious is going on with their child, so it is important to gain some familiarity with the various signs and symptoms of illness in children. Inevitably some of these will be the same for both simple and more serious infection or illness. As a general rule, a symptom which becomes gradually worse or which goes on over a long period of time, perhaps more than a day or two, often points to something serious occurring. Parents who are coping with their first child will find the decision between a minor or serious problem more difficult to make since, as with all things medical, experience counts considerably in making the right decision.

SYMPTOMS NEEDING MEDICAL ADVICE

There are several common signs and symptoms which may guide parents in their decision. These are often non-specific and may be related to a number of different disorders. Where there is a clear connection between a specific symptom and a disease the decision is easy; if not, medical advice may be required. Certainly if you are at all anxious or undecided a phone call or visit to the general practitioner may be very valuable.

APPEARANCE

Most parents are able to judge when their child looks ill, and there is usually an obvious difference between the child who feels just 'off-colour', and one who is seriously ill. Particular signs to look for are dry mouth and sunken eyes, which are a sign of dehydration; pale, mottled or blueish coloration of the skin, which may indicate a serious infection; most rashes are usually obvious. Many rashes start behind the ears or on the face, but in some serious infections, the rash may start elsewhere on the body and not be obvious in the early stages.

The child who is unwell will often be apathetic and uninterested in what is going on around him and may not be comforted in the usual way by his parents. In particular, an ill baby may pass rapidly through a phase of crying frequently to one where even this is too much effort. It is worthwhile noting unusual smells from a child. Drug ingestion such as alcohol or paraffin will often leave a characteristic smell. An ill child who has not been eating well will also produce substances called ketones which can be smelt on the breath. These smell like pear drops or acetone (nail polish remover!).

BREATHING DIFFICULTIES

Different respiratory problems may produce a different sign or change in the breathing (see also Emergencies, p. 258). A particular sound produced during abnormal breathing often indicates the physical site of the problem. A blocked nose or pharynx (back of the throat) from mucus produced during a cold will produce a characteristic nasal voice and obviously stuffy nose. In particular, a baby may not be able to feed normally as he relies particularly on nose breathing during the feeding process. Babies or young children may also find it difficult to sleep if their noses are blocked.

An inflammation or swelling of the throat around the vocal chords will produce a characteristic croupy cough which is harsh, dry and rather brassy. Breathing will be obviously noisy, often sounding worse when the child breathes in. Croup is usually caused by a virus infection of the throat, often during the winter months. If it occurs very suddenly, particularly during the day, it may be due to an inhaled foreign body such as a peanut or a bead. The noisy breathing may also be associated with choking and a cough.

Inflammation or blockage of the airways in the lungs themselves, will produce a characteristic wheeze such as that produced during an asthma attack. In this case the noise is more marked where the child breathes out. If the breathing problem is marked, young babies may be seen to breathe very fast. This usually means a rate of over fifty breaths per minute. They may make a grunting sound with each expiration. Older children who are having breathing difficulties may prefer to sit up and lean forward, supporting themselves on their extended arms. Sometimes leaning over a pillow or a cushion during an asthma attack may be helpful. If the child has a bluish colour medical help needs to be sought immediately, because this means he is not getting enough oxygen.

CRYING

All children cry and parents soon become used to the nature of the different types of their children's crying, which varies depending on the problem. Most babies and young children cry because of simple needs, for example hunger, need for affection, or because of discomfort (see p. 166). However prolonged crying may indicate pain or distress. If there is obvious illness the cause of the cry will be quite clear. However, if the child starts crying unusually, once the basic needs have been attended to, a possible illness should be looked for. It is often difficult to assess the cause of the cry and in this situation medical advice may be useful.

Many children and babies may readily be comforted if the illness is not serious. However, if a young baby or infant screams or cries continuously and is not readily consoled, the underlying problem may well be serious. Older children can frequently indicate, even in simple terms, where they have their discomfort. Note that very ill babies or children may be too ill to cry at all and may lie apathetically, despite being in pain or discomfort.

FEVER

Children very frequently develop a raised temperature, but it is quite frequently an indicator of only a minor illness. Most common virus infections such as colds or 'flu, ear infections or tonsillitis, may produce a raised temperature. Furthermore, many serious illnesses may occur without a fever. If the cause for fever is straightforward, such as a cold, then medical advice need not necessarily be sought, even if the fever persists for several days. Provided that the fever is controllable and the child is not deteriorating, then simple measures at home are usually sufficient. However, if the temperature rises rapidly and remains very high (above 39.4°C or 103°F) medical advice may be useful.

LOSS OF APPETITE

This is often the first symptom of a child being unwell and is particularly so in a very young baby. Parents know the eating habits of their children very well and are frequently aware that a change in the feeding pattern is the first sign that all is not well. In association with a change of appetite, diarrhoea or vomiting may occur, and it is important to remember that these symptoms do not necessarily indicate a disturbance of the stomach or bowel; these symptoms frequently occur with other infections such as tonsillitis, ear infection or other general illness.

Over a longer period of time a child who fails to gain weight, or in fact loses weight quickly, will also need further advice and perhaps investigation unless there is a clear reason for the weight loss. Even straightforward common ailments may stop the child from eating normally for long enough, perhaps only a few days, for some weight loss to occur, but provided the appetite returns at the end of the illness this should not cause concern.

PAIN

Pain may be very difficult to assess, particularly in the young baby. Although crying can be a symptom of pain, it may be a more general indicator of a general feeling of being unwell. A doctor, however, may be able to find the cause of the pain during a physical examination. Younger children have difficulty in localizing pain and frequently a sore throat or painful ear may produce apparent pain in the abdomen or neck.

Pain originating in the abdomen may seem always to be near the navel in a child, when in fact it is occurring elsewhere in the abdomen. Here again a doctor may gain valuable information from examination of the abdomen. Older children may readily localize pain in the appropriate part of the body, as well as being able to give more sophisticated information such as time of onset, frequency and possible factors which produce the pain or relieve it.

POSTURE AND MOVEMENT

Further information about the site of pain or discomfort may be gained from observing the child's movements. For example, if a limb is damaged or affected by a disease then the child will be reluctant to use it or will find it distressing to have it moved or touched. It is important to take seriously a symptom of limping or non-use of a limb. Once again, however, children have some difficulty in localizing pain, and very often a pain in the hip in a young child may be described as a painful knee.

As in adults, a certain posture may be taken up by a child which gives him greatest relief. Abdominal pain is sometimes relieved by drawing the knees up to the abdomen and the child will be very reluctant to straighten out. Similarly, pain in the back of the neck, which is sometimes a symptom of meningitis, may be made worse by moving the legs. From a general point of view a very ill child or baby may remain unusually still and appear floppy. They may seem indifferent to their surroundings or people who are with them. Such stillness or lack of movement should be treated seriously and medical advice sought urgently.

CARING FOR THE SICK CHILD AT HOME

Parents vary in their attitude to illness and while some would prefer to look after their children at home, others would have them cared for in hospital. Most common illnesses do not need hospital admission and it is certainly preferable that convalescence from a more serious illness, which has required admission, be done at home. Although children's hospital wards are now much more welcoming and pleasant, most children would prefer to remain at home with their toys, family and familiar surroundings. Admission to hospital involves considerable disruption of the family routine, and parents often feel that the care of their child is taken out of their own hands, although nowadays parents are encouraged as much as possible to be involved in the needs of their child while on the ward.

The early stages of an illness may be very worrying for parents, particularly when the nature of the problem is unclear. It is important to observe the child closely and note any changes, as an illness may progress quite rapidly. Advice from a doctor, and perhaps a home visit can be very reassuring, and may well be adequate to keep the child out of hospital. Infection, particularly respiratory and bowel, and the common childhood ailments (such as chicken pox) are the most common cause of illness in children. Although the specific medical treatment for these problems may vary, there are practical considerations common to them all.

STAYING IN BED

The child will probably choose himself whether he wants to be in bed. There is usually no need to go to bed if the child feels well enough to be up, and the temperature has come down. During the day he may prefer to lie on the sofa in the living room rather than feeling isolated in the bedroom. He can still feel part of the family and watch them working and playing. There are also other distractions such as the television. But a child who is particularly miserable may want the peace and quiet of his own bed, where he may well sleep for long periods.

While it is wise to have familiar toys and possessions in the room, the bed itself should be uncluttered. Early in the illness children will often prefer books or quiet toys, but as they feel better they will want to be more active. A child confined to bed for a time will enjoy the novelty of something new each day, even if it is a cheap book or novelty, and they will also love to have their parents spend some extra time talking, playing or reading to them. Visitors from school or other friends should be allowed if the child is well enough and not infectious, particularly if he is missing school.

TREATING FEVER

Fever is a very common accompaniment to illness, particularly in childen. They often produce surprisingly high temperatures, which do not necessarily reflect the severity of the illness. Infection by both bacteria (which may require antibiotics) and viruses (which do not) may produce the same degree of fever, but attempts should not be made to reduce it completely to normal. On the other hand it is important not to encourage a high temperature by wrapping up the child. The myth of 'keeping warm' should be re-read as 'keeping comfortable'. Often light bedclothes are enough, and if the temperature is very high, specific measures should be used to reduce it. As a response to the high temperature, the body may sweat naturally which helps the loss of heat by evaporation. Shivering may be a sign of a very high temperature and is often seen as 'rigors'.

A thermometer at home is a useful guide to when to treat a fever, but it is important not to concentrate on actual temperature without taking into account the appearance and degree of discomfort of the child. Nowadays, normal temperature is usually given as 37.5°C rectally, and perhaps 37.2°C from an external site, such as the armpit, or mouth (under the tongue) in the older child. For most home situations, a rectal temperature is unnecessary, and children often object to it being taken. Commercially available temperature strips which are placed on the forehead are useful.

There are several procedures which help to bring the temperature down. Provided the bedroom itself is not cold the upper clothing may be removed and the child's trunk sponged with lukewarm water and allowed to dry in the air. This may be repeated several times. Do not use cold water or place the child in a cold bath, as this may in fact make the temperature worse by reducing the flow of blood through the skin, so that heat cannot escape. Paracetamol either in liquid or tablet form is a useful medication for reducing the temperature and

can be given four to six times during the day in a dose suggested on the packet. Aspirin is now not recommended for children because of the possible risk of a very rare illness, Reye's syndrome, which can occur in children after taking aspirin. If the temperature remains very high or the child develops unusual behaviour such as confusion or delirium, then medical advice should be sought.

FOOD AND DRINK

Many children will not feel like eating solid food when they are unwell. However it is very important that they be allowed to drink plenty of fluids, particularly if a fever is also present or the weather is warm. Fluids are also very important if the child has diarrhoea or vomiting. When vomiting and diarrhoea are the major symptoms of the illness, it is best to stop all solid food and milk and give just clear fluids. In childen under three or four this fluid is best given in the form of commercially available rehydration solutions, which are available at the chemist and simply need to be dissolved in water. Older children may manage on diluted orange juice or flat lemonade. Do not try to make up a rehydration solution at home.

Clear fluids should be continued for a day or two and then a normal diet gradually re-introduced over the next few days. For younger children this should include gradually increasing the strength of milk over two days, and for the older child a bland diet may be introduced after a day or so. Do not worry if the child has not taken solid food for several days. Most children can tolerate many days without food, provided they are drinking adequately. In the convalescent phase some children will remain rather difficult about eating. If this occurs some attempt should be made to choose particularly appetizing or interesting food, provided it is appropriate and sensible.

MEDICINES

Apart from paracetamol, your doctor may prescribe a specific medication such as an antibiotic. Most of these medicines are available in a form appropriate for children, either in a flavoured syrup or in small tablets. Fortunately there are now a number of sugar-free preparations available which are more appropriate. Generally it does not matter whether the child takes tablet or syrup; it will depend on the child's preference and ability to swallow. Many children dislike taking medication, and it may be necessary to either disguise a crushed tablet, or perhaps make a game of the procedure, such as 'Some for dolly and some for you'.

ISOLATION

In theory childen with an infectious illness should be kept out of the way of other children so as to prevent them passing it on. In practice, this is difficult to do, and often an illness is at its most infectious before anybody realizes that it is more than just a simple cold or flu. Many infections, such as chicken pox, are very readily caught in a family; this is often inevitable, and should be anticipated. However, if there are very young children in a household it is sensible to keep them out of the way of a child who is obviously unwell until it is clear that the child is improving. Similarly, if a child is taken to the doctor's surgery, it is sensible to arrange with the doctor beforehand so that he can either be taken straight into the surgery and not come into contact with with other children who may be there, or he could attend at a time when no-one else is waiting.

A child should probably not be taken outside until the infection is improving and the child feels better. It is difficult to give advice about the timing of return to school, but in general since most infections are spread by droplets from the nose or throat, it seems sensible to ensure that the child no longer has a productive cough or runny nose, that he feels better and the fever has subsided, and that any previous rash has faded or completely disappeared.

GOING TO HOSPITAL

The number of children with conditions or diseases which require hospital treatment are, relatively, few – but most parents will at some time find themselves facing an emergency.

Not all emergencies will need hospital admission but it is important to call the doctor straightaway, or if the emergency seems very serious, call an ambulance by dialling 999.

Another main reason for going to hospital is for investigations. Some investigations require admission to hospital for a day or two or a prolonged stay during the day in one of the hospital wards. Investigations may need to be performed over a period of time, and they are often done for a number of reasons, such as severe weight loss, prolonged diarrhoea, investigation of growth disorders, or investigation of breathing problems. The reasons for these investigations should be explained to you by the general practitioner or the hospital paediatrician.

Finally, your child may have to go to hospital for an operation. These can either be 'acute', such as appendicitis, requiring immediate treatment, or

'routine', such as repairing a hernia, a tonsillectomy, adenoidectomy, or insertion of grommets in the ears to treat serous otitis media (see p. 266).

PREPARING FOR HOSPITAL

It is very important to take some time to explain to a child why he is going to hospital either for a short stay, for investigation, or for an operation, or because he is unwell. Even if the admission is unexpected, spend a few moments explaining simply to the child what is going to happen and why. Children are able to understand a great deal, and it is important not to talk to others in front of them without explaining what is going on. Their fantasies, worries and misconceptions are often far worse than the reality and they are usually reassured by a factual explanation. This may need to be repeated but it is important to be clear and tell them that hospitals are to help them get well. They should be reassured that it is not a form of punishment (they are prone to irrational feelings of guilt), and that they will soon be well and coming home again.

Children going into hospital for operations are fortunately given more time. Parents are able to explain in more detail, perhaps by using play, what

EMERGENCIES	
Take your child to hospital or dial 999 for an ambulance in any of the following situations.	
Looks very ill	Very weak or floppy, or even semi-conscious. Very pale or bluish (cyanosis)
Convulsion	May be obvious with shaking limbs, or may be just stiffening of the body. May not need admission, but if a new event for that child, should be examined by a doctor
Severe pain	Sometimes difficult to be sure if pain is the problem. If in doubt, ask for advice
Persistent diarrhoea and vomiting	Signs of dehydration such as a dry mouth, fast heart beat, poor urine output, lethargy
Persistant bleeding from injury	See first aid section, p. 276
Accidents	eg: burns, scalds, head injuries (see first aid section) or ingestion of poisons, pills or solid objects
Breathing difficulties	eg: choking, obvious breathlessness, asthma or croup

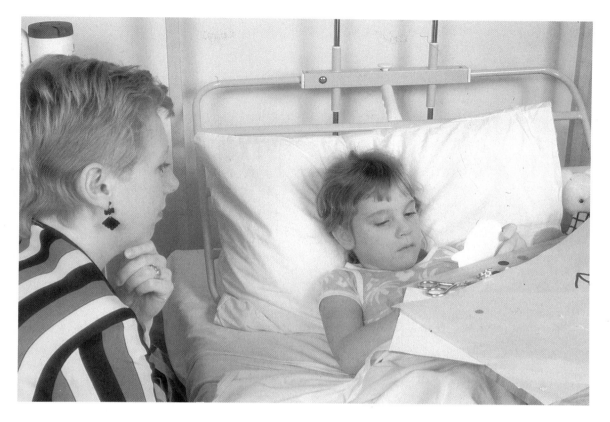

Even though your child may be bedridden in hospital, there are still interesting things to do, such as cutting out and gluing.

is going to happen to them, what an operation is in general terms, and who is in hospital to help look after them. Many hospitals have arrangements where children may visit the ward before going into hospital in order to become familiar with the surroundings. Wards may also provide booklets explaining practical details regarding clothing, food, etc. and more specific advice regarding preparing the child for admission.

IN THE WARD

It is important to take some favourite toys, games and books along to the hospital, as children get considerable reassurance by having familiar objects around them. Childen's wards should provide sleeping facilities for at least one parent. It is often possible to put a bed next to the child's own bed on the ward. Single rooms are unusual in most children's wards, and are often used for isolating infectious cases rather than to provide private accommodation for children or parents. You should always ask for accommodation and expect to stay

with your child for the whole of his hospital visit. This is particularly important for children under five, who can be very upset by the experience if they are separated from their parents even for a few days.

During the early stages of the hospital stay, it is important for parents to explain again what is going on and to point out the various activities going on around them, which may be unusual to the child. It is important to maintain a sense of normality, and it is nice for parents to wear their usual day clothing, bring photos and other familiar objects, and perhaps to bring other relatives if the stay is to be prolonged. One or other parent should try and stay with the child for as long as possible both day and night. This is not only to provide reassurance and a familiar presence for the child, but parents are extremely useful in the day-to-day care of their child. By doing this you yourselves are better able to understand what is happening to your child medically.

Nevertheless parents may find it difficult to be with their children 24 hours a day and they need a break. You should not feel guilty about leaving your child for short periods provided you explain to the child that you will come back and give him a reasonably accurate prediction of the time of your return.

Many paediatric wards now have separate supervised playrooms, where mobile children can play with a variety of toys and join in activities such as painting and modelling.

OPERATIONS

It is very nice if you can accompany your child to the operating theatre, so it is worth asking if this is possible. Hospitals vary in their policy here. While in principle it is desirable for parents always to go with their child to the anaesthetic, there are sometimes practical difficulties with this. It is useful for parents to discuss the policy in their local hospital before the child is admitted.

A simple explanation of what will happen in the operation is important for the child. Children have many fantasies about which parts of their anatomy they may lose while they are asleep and it is often very important to reassure them that they will not lose anything essential. Operations on the genitalia in boys (such as circumcision) often provoke such anxiety, and they will need to be reassured that their penis will remain behind! It is useful to describe the 'special sleep' of the anaesthetic, so that the child understands he will not feel anything during the procedure. It is also important that the parents are there to comfort the child when he wakes from the operation.

PLAY AND EDUCATION

Most paediatric wards are now equipped with play areas, teachers and various equipment. This means that most children enjoy their hospital experience. Play workers have special training so that they can find the most enjoyable activities for children to do, in spite of any possible restrictions due to the child's condition. Every child of school age in hospital needs continuing education, and it is the duty of the local education authority to provide this. Hospital teachers are specially trained in the problems of handling children's education while on a hospital ward.

GOING HOME

Parents should remember that the child may be difficult when he returns home. He is often demanding, irritable and clinging, and may often regress to a more babyish stage. For instance, it is very common for children to start wetting the bed again. How long this stage lasts varies, but it makes it easier to cope with if you expect it.

Common ailments in young babies

It is always distressing when a young baby is ill, but fortunately, with careful treatment, the common ailments of infancy can pass fairly rapidly with no long-lasting effects. However if you are at all worried about your baby's condition, telephone your doctor for advice.

Diarrhoea

The frequency of bowel action in babies varies a great deal (see p. 109), but diarrhoea is usually very watery, almost like urine, and is usually foul smelling and very frequent – much more frequent than your baby's normal pattern. Watery diarrhoea is very serious in babies under twelve months, especially if accompanied by vomiting, and you should consult your doctor immediately.

If accompanied by vomiting, the most common cause of diarrhoea is gastroenteritis, or infection of the bowel. If the baby is not unwell and vomiting and diarrhoea is not serious, then stopping the normal milk feeds in a bottle fed baby for a day or so, is usually enough. Substitute one of the commercially available rehydration mixtures (see earlier). Breastfed babies may usually continue their normal feeding pattern.

If there is blood or mucus present in the stool, it may be a form of dysentery, often caused by a particular bacterium. However, your doctor may not prescribe an antibiotic for this, as it can prolong the illness. There are also other less common causes of diarrhoea such as blockage of the bowel, appendicitis, food intolerance or other serious infection.

Eye problems

The commonest problem in a young baby is a sticky eye (see p. 193). This usually responds to frequent cleaning with sterile water, and sometimes the use of antibiotic drops or ointment obtained from the doctor. A rare cause of a persistent sticky eye is due to a blocked tear duct which may need further medical attention.

A squint sometimes causes parents concern. This is a problem of development of the muscles of the eye and may eventually require treatment. However many babies do not align their eyes and may appear to squint for the first few months of life; in most cases this will have corrected by the age of six months. However, if parents are still concerned at this stage then medical opinion is essential because sometimes an operation is necessary. Some babies do appear to have a squint because of an extra thickness of skin at the corner of their eye, but the eyes themselves are normal.

Failure to gain weight or weight loss

There are many causes of a baby failing to gain weight appropriately, although it is uncommon. The usual cause is difficulty in establishing a normal feeding pattern, and you can get very good advice from your doctor, health visitor or the local baby clinic. However, if the problem persists or there are other symptoms of illness, there may well be other medical problems causing the weight loss, and these may require investigation in hospital. Serious problems may be associated with a change in well-being and slowing of development.

Hernias

Organs inside the abdomen, such as the bowel, sometimes bulge through a weakness in the abdominal wall. This is called a hernia. In babies, a hernia usually occurs in one or two places. The commonest is at the navel (umbilical), and the other is in the groin (inguinal). An umbilical hernia appears a week or two after birth, and in some parts of the world, such as Africa, it occurs in almost every baby. The swelling is more noticeable when the baby cries, but it is quite soft and can be flattened completely with a little pressure. It usually enlarges over the first few months, then gradually disappears.

No treatment is needed as it cures itself. The small hole in the abdominal wall, which allows the gut to escape under the skin, gets smaller with age and eventually closes. Strapping the hernia does not make it disappear earlier; in fact there is some evidence that it slows things down. An occasional child needs an operation at six years or later if the hernia has not gone.

Inguinal hernias produce a swelling in the groin which often extends down into the scrotum around the testicle. The swelling comes and goes with crying. These hernias occur more often in preterm babies; in them the hernia may disappear spontaneously, but in all other circumstances an operation is needed.

A worrying complication of an inguinal hernia is strangulation, when a piece of bowel may become trapped. The hernia then becomes hard and tender, and there is often vomiting. If this happens, you must contact a doctor urgently.

Common ailments in young babies

Infantile eczema

This is a common skin disease which occurs in children of all ages although usually it begins about three to six months after birth. It is commoner in families who have a history of allergy (see p. 270). The skin, usually in the elbows, behind the knees, the nappy area, and sometimes over the face and behind the ears, is red and sometimes weeping but may also become dry and cracked. The site of the eczematous skin may become infected. Eczema is usually managed by simple moisturizing creams but may require treatment by a gentle steroid cream or anti-infectious cream, which should be prescribed by the doctor.

Infections

Early signs of infection in a young baby are often vague. They include loss of appetite, vomiting, fever and irritability or lethargy. The commonest problems in this age group include respiratory infection, gastroenteritis, an infectious rash and occasionally a urine infection. Most infections are caused by viruses and are not helped by antibiotics. However if the infection is bacterial, your doctor will choose an appropriate antibiotic to clear it.

If the cause of the baby's illness is unclear, your doctor's advice is necessary, particularly for the diagnosis of a urine infection. However if the cause is obviously an upper respiratory infection, then the baby can be looked after quite easily at home. This infection is, of course, a simple cold. But the problem for young babies particularly is difficulty with breathing and feeding because of a blocked nose. Coughing or sneezing may develop during this infection, which is the normal response for clearing the airway of mucus. Decongestants and nose drops may help but should not be used for more than a few days. Simple saline nose drops can be obtained from the chemist and given just before feeding to make breathing easier for the baby.

Bronchiolitis is a relatively common viral infection of babies under twelve months of age. The symptoms may start with a mild cold, but the baby rapidly goes on to have marked breathing difficulty, poor feeding and a cough. If there are feeding difficulties and the baby is having difficulty in breathing, admission to hospital may be necessary.

Neonatal urticaria

This is a very common rash which occurs usually in newborn babies. There are small red spots with a white or yellowy raised centre to them. They appear on the face or trunk and may be few in number, or rarely may be quite extensive. They usually fade over a few weeks and are entirely harmless.

Septic spots

These infective spots occur from time to time in young babies. They usually require antibiotics given by mouth to clear them up. However on occasion, if severe, they may mean the baby has to be admitted to hospital.

Thrush

Thrush may occur in the mouth as a white coating to the tongue, and in the nappy area as a red, weeping rash which is sometimes confused with simple nappy rash (see p. 193). If normal treatment for nappy rash does not help and it gets worse, then thrush may well be responsible. Both mouth thrush and thrush in the nappy area require treatment from your doctor, who will prescribe a special antibiotic called nystatin.

Vomiting

Vomiting has many causes in young babies and many are harmless if the vomiting is not prolonged (see p. 192). There are, however, other more serious causes of vomiting. The vomiting is usually obvious – large amounts of milk will come back, often projected several feet in front of the baby. Serious causes of vomiting include obstruction to the bowel or infection such as gastroenteritis, always consult a doctor.

Another cause may be the relatively common problem of pyloric stenosis, which usually affects babies between two and four months. This is an abnormality of the muscle which controls the exit of milk from the stomach into the intestines. Over a period of weeks the muscle becomes thickened and blocks the outlet of the stomach. Vomiting occurs during a feed or just afterwards, is often profuse and, rarely, will have a small amount of blood mixed with it. The baby is often well, although hungry and may lose weight. It is important that a doctor is consulted as this condition requires admission to hospital and probably an operation. Any cause of vomiting which is unexplained and worrying should of course be discussed with your doctor.

Common ailments in children

Older children are in a way easier to deal with when ill – they can explain reasonably accurately how they feel or where they may have a pain, and it is also easier for them to understand the necessity for treatment, even if it is only to take a regular dose of medicine. If children feel ill, they generally go to bed when they need to; the most taxing time for parents is usually the recovery period when boredom is the worst symptom!

It is sometimes rather more difficult to get the co-operation of a toddler, who may not have the intellectual development to understand what is happening to him, and may also be very resistant to treatment. Young children especially may be wary or even frightened of medical personnel, and most doctors and others who regularly care for children will dispense with their white coats and will have developed strategies to put children at their ease. It is undoubtedly true however that children's fears have to be taken seriously and it can involve a great deal of patience and tact on the part of both parents and doctors.

If your child develops one of the common infectious diseases of childhood, such as whooping cough, measles or rubella (German measles), you should always contact your general practitioner to confirm the diagnosis, even if he doesn't need to prescribe any medicine or suggest any specific treatment. This is because all general practitioners have a general obligation to notify some of these infectious diseases to the public health authorities, in order to provide them with a record of their frequency in the community.

Appendicitis

This relatively common serious abdominal problem usually occurs over the age of five. A child often complains of feeling generally unwell and slowly abdominal pain develops around the navel. Over a period of hours the pain gradually seems to move to the right lower side of the abdomen. The child may vomit, have a fever, and may also have constipation although diarrhoea can also be present.

These symptoms may also be found in other conditions such as mesenteric adenitis (see under sore throats and tonsillitis, above). If you suspect appendicitis, and your general practitioner agrees, your child will usually be referred to hospital for an opinion by a surgeon. Treatment is, of course, by surgical removal of the appendix.

Other conditions which may be confused with appendicitis include urinary tract infection, recurrent abdominal pain (see p. 268), and gynaecological problems in older girls.

Bone and joint disorders

There are a great many minor variations of anatomy which occur in children. Most of these are self-correcting as the child gets older and include bow legs, knock knees, flat feet, in-toeing and bent toes. A general practitioner or school doctor will advise on these minor abnormalities if the parents are concerned. More serious is a bent spine (scoliosis) which will need hospital advice. Other conditions which require treatment in hospital include arthritis, broken bones, and rare diseases which cause bending of the bones.

Breath-holding attacks

These are also common in young children. They are similarly frightening to parents but in general are completely harmless. A child who has a tantrum or cries or becomes upset, often when being scolded or thwarted in some activity, will suddenly stop breathing and go blue or red in the face. He may become briefly unconscious but usually wakes up without any effects. Breath-holding attacks are sometimes used manipulatively by children, and parents should do their best to keep calm during one. You will need to comfort your child afterwards as it is frightening for the child as well. However, try also not to allow your child to get his own way unreasonably. The advice on handling tantrums on page 231 may be helpful here.

Common ailments in children

Chest infections

Three types of chest infection are common in children. Bronchitis and pneumonia are caused usually by a bacterial infection of the airways or lungs. The child is usually breathless, sometimes with a wheeze and chest discomfort. The cough is marked and may be productive, although most children swallow their sputum rather than coughing it out. Antibiotics are usually required. Sometimes the infection may be particularly severe, in which case admission to hospital for a few days of antibiotic therapy and physiotherapy may be necessary to loosen the accumulation of fluid in the lungs.

Chicken pox

This very common infection of children is particularly contagious and often spreads through the family. Before the rash appears, there is a period of fever, headache and sore throat. The rash is characteristic: there is a red raised spot with a clear vesicle (small blister) on the top. The spots are very irritating. Several batches of these spots will appear over a period of a few days – perhaps three or four batches.

The vesicles will usually heal to scabs and disappear by themselves, although unfortunately they often become infected often because of scratching. The child may feel happier in bed, and the itchiness can be relieved at least temporarily by calamine lotion. Paracetamol is useful for the temperature. If infection does occur on the spots and the child remains unwell, ask a doctor's advice.

Constipation

Constipation may occasionally be part of another illness. However, generally it is due to difficulty with toilet training or a diet deficient in high fibre. Occasionally it may be associated with a small tear (anal fissure) at the outlet of the bowel (anus). This causes pain at the moment of opening the bowels, so the child may resist doing this in order to avoid the pain.

It is worth trying to resolve the constipation at home by increasing roughage in the diet by introducing high-fibre cereals, wholewheat bread, plenty of fresh fruit and vegetables, and avoiding highly refined convenience foods. A gentle laxative may be tried but this should not go on for longer than a few days. If this fails and the child continues to have symptoms, ask your doctor's advice.

Convulsions (fits)

For parents to see their own child having a convulsion is very disturbing, particularly if they have never seen one before. However fits are fairly common under the age of five years, especially in association with a high fever. Most of these so-called febrile convulsions are usually harmless and very rarely cause any damage.

Often the child will have been feverish with a cold or other illness just prior to the fit and will frequently have seemed quite well otherwise. Suddenly he may go rigid, stop breathing, perhaps go blue or red in the face and sometimes pass urine or have his bowels open. After this rigid phase the child may then shake one or all of his limbs for a few minutes. It is rare for a febrile convulsion to last more than ten minutes.

While the fit is in progress the parents should try to keep calm, turn the child on to his side to the recovery position (see p. 279), in order to prevent inhaling vomit, and perhaps loosen the clothing. It is probably unnecessary to try and open the mouth or attempt to stop the child biting on his tongue. If the fit continues beyond ten minutes then call an ambulance.

Once the fit has stopped then the temperature should be lowered as mentioned on page 00. If this is the first convulsion the child should probably be taken to hospital so that the cause of the infection can be determined. Sometimes a convulsion may be due to a serious infection such as meningitis or encephalitis and these conditions will need treatment in hospital.

About 30 per cent of children who have one febrile convulsion will go on to have further fits in association with fever during the first five years of life. Sometimes it is recommended that such children are given anti-convulsant drugs on a regular basis to prevent these attacks from happening. However, this treatment should be discussed with a hospital paediatrician or your general practitioner.

An even smaller proportion of such children will go on to have true epileptic attacks during childhood and adult life. Children who are epileptic can lead very normal lives provided they are given regular anti-convulsant medication. The side effects of these medications are generally minor and often the medication need only be continued until puberty. A discussion of these medications again should be undertaken with your general practitioner or the hospital paediatrician.

Common ailments in children

Coughs and colds

Colds are common and most children will expect to have several in a year. The severity of illness in children is often made worse by living in a smoky city, or in families where the parents smoke.

The vast majority of these respiratory infections are caused by viruses, so antibiotics are not indicated, at least in the initial stages. Some colds which persist or seem to get worse may be due to a new infection by a bacterium, and in this situation antibiotics prescribed by your doctor may be necessary.

Coughing and sneezing are normal responses to blockages of the airway. It is important therefore, that during the early stages of the cold, when sputum and mucus are present, that the normal cough is *not* prevented by cough medicines. Most colds will resolve themselves in a week or so, going through the normal sequence of events: sore throat, runny nose, fever, and productive cough which may last for several days, followed by a gradual drying up of the runny nose, and eventually a dry non-productive cough which may last for a week or so.

In the early stages, the blocked nose may be treated by simple saline nose drops, which are useful particularly in young children. Decongestant nose drops, such as Otrivine or Ephedrine, can be helpful temporarily when a baby's nose is very blocked. They should not be used for more than a day or two as they can make the obstruction worse. Steam inhalations, perhaps with the addition of menthol and eucalyptus, maybe helpful in a blocked nose and accompanying painful ears. Soothing drinks and lozenges containing lemon or glycerine may be helpful, particularly in the stages of a dry cough. Only in very rare situations should a cough suppressant be used, and only on the advice of your doctor.

A child who coughs persistently, particularly at night, without other signs or symptoms of a cold, may in fact have underlying asthma, or perhaps have mucus in the back of the throat from enlarged adenoids. A doctor's opinion may be useful in this case.

Croup

This condition is caused by an infection of the upper throat causing swelling and narrowing of the airway. It produces a characteristic harsh barking cough, and some difficulty with breathing, usually on the intake of breath. It may occur more than once in the same child.

Croup can be worrying to parents the first time they experience it in a child, but parents who have seen it before know that placing the child in a humid room, such as running the hot tap in the bathroom to make steam, or in the kitchen with the kettle boiling, produces some relief. If this does not help, and the child seems to deteriorate, it is important that a doctor sees the child quickly. This could either be your GP, or if symptoms develop suddenly, it may be necessary to take the child directly to hospital.

There is no specific treatment other than humidity apart from managing the temperature and discomfort. A child admitted to hospital will usually spend a day or two there, in a tent filled with steam.

Diarrhoea and vomiting

There are a great many causes of diarrhoea and vomiting in children. Often the symptoms are a reaction to a more generalized illness, and are not necessarily related to infection or other upset of the bowel itself. But gastroenteritis, caused by either a viral or a bacterial infection, could occur in any home, although family hygiene does play a part in its spread. Vomiting usually precedes the diarrhoea by a day or so and is often settling down when the diarrhoea is at its worst. The diarrhoea may be just like water and can be green, yellow or clear. Occasionally there is blood or mucus also present.

The treatment, as mentioned in the section on young babies, involves stopping solid food and taking clear fluids only for a day or so, gradually re-introducing a normal diet. If abdominal pain is present, or blood is profuse, then it is important to consult your doctor. Only in rare occasions are antibiotics or other antidiarrhoeal medicines prescribed.

Food poisoning, which usually means eating food contaminated by bacteria, may produce similar symptoms as for gastroenteritis. These may come on quite rapidly after the ingestion of the food. The vomiting, diarrhoea and abdominal pain can be quite severe. The treatment is the same as for gastroenteritis.

Common ailments in children

Ear infections

Infections of the middle ear (otitis media) are common in children. They produce ear pain, temperature and irritability in younger children. Ear infections often follow a previous upper respiratory infection such as a cold. It is important that the child is seen soon by a doctor who will examine the ear and usually prescribe an antibiotic. It is important that the ear is rechecked by the doctor a week or so later and the hearing reassessed, as persisting fluid in the middle ear may interfere with hearing over a long period of time. 'Glue ear', or serous otitis media, is the name given to this situation. If you feel that your child's hearing is affected after a respiratory infection, or over a longer period of time, it is important to have it checked formally. Occasionally an operation to insert small drainage tubes (grommets) in the eardrum will be necessary.

Infection of the outer ear (otitis externa), may also produce pain. It is common in children who swim regularly, play with their ears, or insert foreign bodies into the external ear, although it may occur spontaneously. The ear will require antibiotic drops for correct treatment.

Ear infections are sometimes aggravated by large adenoids which prevent drainage of fluid from the internal ear. If the child is having frequent ear infections or has poor hearing then removal of the adenoids may be necessary.

Eye problems

The eyes may become inflamed as part of general illness, for example, in measles or as part of hay fever. However infection of the eye itself is also common. Conjunctivitis may be due to bacteria or viruses. In general it is usually assumed that a bacterium is responsible and antibiotics are prescribed either as drops or as an ointment. If the inflammation does not settle down after a few days of treatment the doctor may suggest a change of antibiotic.

Infection of the base of the eyelashes (a stye) is common in children. Local treatment such as a warm compress may be helpful to ease the discomfort, but antibiotic ointment is also usually necessary. Sometimes styes occur in several crops, and it is important that the child be encouraged to wash his hands thoroughly and not touch the infected eye. Children who get recurrent styes over a period of time may be carriers of a certain germ in the nose, so antibiotic cream up the nostrils may help.

Hepatitis

There are two varieties of hepatitis. The commonest is infectious hepatitis (hepatitis A), caused by eating food contaminated with infected faeces. Although thought to be more common in other countries, it is nevertheless present throughout the UK. Symptoms include a long period of general aches and pains, headache, nausea and vomiting, and aching limbs. After this period a yellow colour or jaundice is noted in the eyes and skin. The urine may appear very dark, and occasionally the faeces may be lighter than usual. The illness is often prolonged and treatment includes temperature control, providing an appetizing diet, preferably high in carbohydrate and low in fat, and during the vomiting period, plenty of fluids are important. Only rarely is admission to hospital necessary.

The other form of hepatitis, known as hepatitis B, is carried in the bloodstream. Pregnant women who may be at risk of carrying the disease can have their blood tested to see if they are 'surface antigen positive' (HBsAg). There is a vaccine available in the UK which can be given to any baby at risk of infection from the mother at birth.

Infestations

Infestations with parasites are also common, and are not just associated with poor hygiene in the home. They are usually easy to treat and include scabies, headlice and fleas. A school nurse or doctor may provide useful information or you can ask your own general practitioner. Headlice (nits), which occur frequently in school-age children, are eradicated by washing the hair with special shampoo.

There are many worm infections which occur throughout the world, but the commonest in the UK are threadworms. These are harmless, although they produce symptoms such as anal irritation and itching and may keep the child awake at night. The diagnosis is made by examining the child's anus, underwear or faeces, when the worms will be seen as small, white, wriggling threads. A doctor may prove the diagnosis by obtaining some eggs from the anal area and examining them under a microscope. They are easily treated with oral medication.

Common ailments in children

Influenza

Several virus infections may be responsible for the symptoms of influenza. These are similar to those in adults, including fever, aching joints and limbs, headache, nausea and a variable degree of misery. There are no specific diagnostic tests; the symptoms usually provide the diagnosis. Treatment includes temperature control, fluids and whatever the child wants to eat. As for an adult, the child may prefer to remain in bed for a day or two although the illness is not as prolonged as in adults. Although influenza vaccinations are available, they are usually only given to patients who have other serious diseases.

Measles

There ought to be no reason for your child to have this illness, except perhaps in a very mild form, as there is an effective vaccine (see p. 253). However, when it is contracted, it starts with an obvious upper respiratory infection like a cold, and then is followed by a red rash which starts on the face or behind the ears and rapidly spreads to the trunk. Spots, which are separate to begin with, often join together and the child may look completely covered. After a few days it gradually fades, and may change to a brownish colour before it disappears. As the rash disappears the temperature, which may be quite high, will gradually improve and the child will feel better.

Sometimes measles is complicated by an infection of the throat, ears or chest, in which case antibiotics may be necessary. Other associated symptoms may include vomiting, diarrhoea, arthritis, and, very rarely, inflammation of the brain. There is no specific treatment other than encouraging the consumption of fluids, managing the temperature with paracetamol, and general support and care at home. A doctor's visit is not essential, but may be helpful if the parents are anxious or if secondary complications occur.

Meningitis

Meningitis is an infection around the brain. It is a very frightening illness because it sometimes leads to death or handicap. However, the type that is caused by viruses is often a mild illness, and that caused by bacteria can be completely cured if treated early with antibiotics.

The symptoms include fever, irritability, convulsions and drowsiness or unconsciousness. In a child over two years there is a characteristic stiffness of the neck, where the child is unable to move his chin down on to his chest. In babies, the signs of the disease are less obvious, but bulging of the fontanelle is very characteristic.

One particular type of meningitis is caused by a bacterium known as meningococcus. This can be very dangerous and causes a rash with tiny bruises anywhere on the body. If your child has a fever and such a rash contact your doctor urgently.

Mouth problems

Mouth infections are common and may be produced by herpes virus, causing ulceration around the mouth or on the tongue and inside the mouth, and bacterial infections which often cause crusting ulcers on the lips themselves. This may be a form of impetigo, which will need antibiotic ointment from your doctor.

Some mouth ulcers are small and not painful and older children may manage with simple analgesia. However younger children often find it difficult to eat, and more particularly, to drink, in the presence of these ulcers. A child may need admitting to hospital for a day or two if they are completely unable to take fluids.

Mumps

This illness produces a characteristic swelling of one or both of the salivary glands which are just in front of the ears. There is a swelling of the face in this area, which is tender and the child generally feels unwell. Parents often worry about inflammation of the testicles in boys, but this is very unusual in children and very rarely causes sterility, even if it does occur. There is no specific treatment for mumps and care is similar for the other infectious diseases. A vaccine is available for this illness, which is now being routinely introduced.

Common ailments in children

Recurrent abdominal pain

Abdominal pain is very common in later childhood – it usually occurs around the area of the navel. Urinary tract infection has to be ruled out before further investigations are made. Some people think that this sort of pain may be a form of migraine, especially when it recurs. It is common in families where migraine headaches occur and there may be food sensitivity involved such as cheese, chocolate, orange squash and some food additives. There may be episodes of diarrhoea which occur with the pain, and the attacks are provoked by periods of stress.

Treatment involves attempting to remove any offending food-stuffs, looking into possible psychological factors, and occasionally specific medication is indicated. Simple analgesia such as paracetamol is valuable.

Roseola infantum

This rather less common infection in children is characterized by a long period, usually five or six days, of high fever, without other symptoms. Parents and doctors are often worried during this period because of the absence of any other diagnostic sign. On the sixth day, a pale pink rash comes out over the whole trunk, and the temperature rapidly resolves.

The treatment involves control of the high temperature, but sometimes these children are seen by doctors or even admitted to hospital because of the difficulty in making early diagnosis. In young children a febrile convulsion (see p. 264) may occur during the fever period. There is no other physical treatment, and the illness has no serious after-effects.

Rubella (German measles)

This is a mild infection which may show itself only as a slight fever with a pale pink rash covering the face and trunk. There may be occasional large glands in the throat and a mild upper respiratory infection. Complications are rare. Again, treatment is supportive. It is important that the child does not come into contact with any women who may be in early pregnancy (see p. 13), and all girls and women should be vaccinated *before* they have children.

Scarlet fever

This is due to a bacterial infection, usually following a sore throat or tonsillitis. The child develops a fever and is rapidly covered with a continuous red rash which may last for a few days. It should be treated with antibiotics from your doctor.

Sinusitis

This is a relatively rare infection, usually seen in older children. The signs and symptoms are similar to adults: pain in the bone under the eyes or around the nose, with a high temperature and sometimes the production of thick mucus from the nose. Antibiotics are sometimes necessary, but more immediate relief may be given by steam inhalations, pain relief such as paracetamol, and nasal decongestant.

Skin problems

These are very common in children and include sunburn, boils, warts and chilblains. Many of these problems can be managed with a medication available over the counter at the chemist, which usually will do no harm and occasionally some good.

It is important not to make the condition worse, however, as many of these will improve if left alone. Warts in particular are often over-treated. They are common in children and usually resolve themselves over a period of years, but a doctor's advice is essential if these conditions prove troublesome – verrucas (plantar warts in the feet) can, for instance, be extremely difficult to eradicate.

Ringworm, which is not a worm infection but a fungal infection, occurs anywhere on the body, scalp or feet (athlete's foot). All these conditions are usually readily treated by prescribed medication.

Sore throats and tonsillitis

Like ear infections, a sore throat may be due to a virus infection or infection from a bacterium. It is very difficult for a doctor to decide by appearance which organism is responsible and if a child is unwell with fever, most doctors would prescribe an antibiotic.

Most children have enlarged glands in the neck. Sometimes they become very enlarged and painful during an illness like tonsillitis, but they usually resolve spontaneously. Abdominal pain may be present with a sore throat, and is

Common ailments in children

probably due to abdominal glands being infected with the same virus. This condition, called mesenteric adenitis, is sometimes confused with acute appendicitis, where abdominal pain is the major feature. The condition usually resolves on its own without treatment.

Tonsillectomy is performed far less often than it used to be. The usual indications are extremely infected or enlarged tonsils, tonsils which obstruct the mouth or airway, and when a child is missing long periods from school because of recurrent infection.

Glandular fever, a relatively common infection by a virus, sometimes produces very severe and prolonged tonsillitis. Other glands in the body are frequently enlarged at the same time. There is no specific treatment for this condition other than relief for pain and temperature. The long term symptoms may continue for several weeks or even months, although the disease usually resolves spontaneously.

Testicular pain

A boy's testicles may be damaged by external injury such as kicking or occasionally may become unexpectedly painful, swollen, and with a blue discoloration. Abdominal pain may also be present, however, and indeed may be the major symptom. It is important therefore that the testicles are examined if a boy has abdominal pain. If the testicle becomes severely painful, with or without injury, your child should be examined by a doctor at once, as sometimes the testis becomes twisted by itself (torsion), which may require an operation. If neglected, the testicle may be irreparably damaged.

Whooping cough

Unfortunately this condition is still prevalent. It is most serious in young babies and toddlers, although it may occur in children or even adults. The early stages are typical of a straightforward cold – runny nose and cough – but the cough gradually becomes worse, persistent and prolonged and eventually is followed by a characteristic 'whoop', or very noisy in-drawing of the breath. Babies and toddlers may become red in the face or even blue during the coughing episodes. The cough may be associated with severe and persistent vomiting immediately following an attack. An early serious complication is a coughing attack being followed by the baby stopping breathing.

Mild attacks may be managed at home, although it is as well to get your doctor's advice. Apart from that, control of the temperature and by feeding the baby immediately after a vomiting attack are all that is needed. Cough medicines are rarely helpful. In more severe cases, the baby may need to be admitted to hospital for other therapy, including feeding by tube, inhaled medication and sometimes oxygen.

Long term effects are serious in a small number of cases, and include fits, brain damage and perhaps damage to the lungs. There is no specific treatment, which is why universal immunization is so important. Young babies are particularly susceptible to this illness and should not be in contact with other children who may have the illness. Antibiotics given early in the disease, if another affected child in the family is diagnosed before the others, may prevent a severe attack.

Urinary infections

Infections in the urinary tract occur more commonly in girls although boys too may be affected. A child may complain of abdominal pain, vomiting, diarrhoea, or pain on passing urine, and may want to pass urine frequently. The urine may be rather smelly and occasionally have blood in it. Children who are normally dry both day and night may start wetting the bed again or become incontinent during the daytime. Infants may be unwell without any obvious cause for their illness.

It is important that your doctor is consulted early on in order that a urine test can be taken and appropriate antibiotic treatment started. As a general rule a child who has had more than one such infection should probably have some X-ray investigations at the local hospital to rule out any anatomical abnormality of the bladder or kidneys. An abnormality may require surgical correction.

If a child still has recurrent infections then there may be a place for regular antibiotic treatment over a long period of time. This should obviously be discussed with the doctor.

ALLERGIES

Allergy is an abnormal response to the body coming into contact with a substance foreign to it. The foreign substance may be swallowed, inhaled, or just in contact with the skin. An allergic person will react to this substance in a variety of ways which may be unpleasant or even harmful, and the symptoms produced may vary depending on which part of the body has come into contact with the foreign substance.

Allergy tends to occur in families, and most allergic patients are sensitive to more than one substance. Tests for allergy to specific substances are possible but in practice are not always useful. They often serve only to confirm the presence of general allergy, rather than providing a clue to precise identification. However in a small number of cases, where a patient is allergic to only one or two substances, it is useful to identify these so that contact with them may be avoided.

Desensitization, usually in a series of injections, may be undertaken in a few individuals where only one or two offending substances can be identified. Unfortunately, for the majority of people, this form of treatment is not useful.

ASTHMA

Asthma is a common condition probably more widespread than previously thought. It involves narrowing of the airways due to constriction of the small muscles in their walls and is made worse by the production of mucus. It is often provoked by an allergic reaction to a foreign substance, but it may also be provoked by changes in the weather, exercise, the effects of emotion, infection, or sometimes without any obvious cause. It is recognized as shortness of breath accompanied by a wheezing sound from the chest and also a cough. The particular difficulty is with breathing out, which produces the characteristic wheezing. Sometimes a cough alone, often during the night, is the only sign.

Although asthma can be serious, it is now very amenable to treatment by a number of medications available, and ordinary life should be interfered with as little as possible. Many children often tend to get less severe attacks as they grow older, and may in fact not have any further attacks beyond adolescence.

Treatment involves the use of medication prescribed by the general practitioner or a hospital paediatrician. Some of these drugs are used on a daily basis to prevent attacks from happening, and others are taken during an acute episode to control the symptoms. There are a number of drugs available and the combination of these will vary in each patient, so it is important to follow the doctors advice in this regard. The commonest drugs are those that relax the small muscles in the walls of the airways during an attack, such as Salbutamol, which is given by mouth or inhalation, often by a sort of spray. Other drugs are used to prevent asthma, usually by inhalation. These may be Theophylline, Intal, or a very small amount of steroid.

It is useful to identify any trigger factors so that these may be avoided. Taking medication before any exercise or during a cold may prevent symptoms developing. Many patients are allergic to house dust and a tiny creature, the house dust mite, which feeds on this dust. Exposure to this mite may be avoided by frequent vacuuming of the carpet and cleaning of the bed clothes.

Many parents learn to manage their child's asthma very well but it is also important to remember what to do if home management fails. A child may deteriorate rapidly in this situation. If your doctor knows the child well his advice may be useful, or alternatively take the child to the Accident and Emergency Department at your local hospital. Sometimes admission to hospital may be required for several days to treat the attack effectively.

Most districts have an Asthma Society which provides useful information for parents, holds meetings and discussion groups, and provides valuable support. It is well worth joining your local branch of the Society if your child is an asthma sufferer (see pages 296-299).

ECZEMA

Eczema is common in both infants and older children. While it may be due to allergy to a specific substance it is often difficult to identify this. The eczema may occur in small areas often behind the knees or on the elbows, but may also be widespread, covering the trunk, face and limbs. It is important that the treatment of your child's eczema is discussed in full with the doctor who advises on the appropriate regime. Treatment varies from the use of moisturizing creams and emollients in the bath to tar preparations and steroid preparations. Parents are often worried about the use of steroids but in practice these drugs are safe and extremely valuable if they are used correctly. Steroid creams come in a variety of strengths and most doctors will start with the most gentle preparation, gradually changing to more potent strengths if the eczema does not respond.

Allergy to food may play a very small role in the development of eczema (see below).

HAY FEVER

Hay fever is an allergic response of the lining of the nose to inhaled substances. In addition to the mucous membrane lining, the eyelids may also become inflamed. The symptoms produced include a runny nose, nasal stuffiness, itching of the nose and eyes, and eye redness.

Antihistamines may be useful to prevent these symptoms during the hay fever season which occurs in spring and early summer, because of the various pollens which are in the air at that time. Some people produce similar symptoms when in contact with cats or other furry pets. If antihistamines do not control symptoms, then other medication, usually applied directly to the eyes or the nose, may give some relief. Desensitization is only occasionally helpful.

URTICARIA

The response of the skin to an allergic substance, often swallowed, may be urticaria or hives. This fairly common reaction is shown as a sudden onset of itchy raised blotches or lumps on the skin. The commonest substances are fish, nuts, aspirin, some food colourings and fruit, and occasionally insect bites, particularly fleas. However, some specific allergies are difficult to identify. Very rarely, the mouth and throat may become swollen also, producing difficulty in swallowing and even breathing. In this situation a doctor's advice on referral to hospital is very important.

Where it is known that children are allergic to specific substances it is useful to keep an antihistamine at home to treat each episode when it occurs. However it is of course best to avoid contact with the substances altogether.

DRUG ALLERGIES

Many drugs may be responsible for producing allergy, and there is a wide variety of reaction which may occur. The commonest offender is penicillin but it is extremely important to be sure that true penicillin allergy has occurred. Penicillin-like drugs, such as ampicillin, may produce a mild rash which is not a true penicillin allergy. A true penicillin allergy usually shows itself as urticaria, sometimes associated with joint pains and a feeling of being unwell.

True penicillin allergy is unusual and unfortunately it is often overdiagnosed. Any other drugs which are known to provoke allergic reactions should of course be avoided. Parents and the child, when he is old enough, should know the names of these.

FOOD ALLERGY

Discussion of food allergy is widespread in the media. However our understanding of this allergy is still very limited. It may be a cause for a wide variety of disorders in children, including eczema, hyperactivity, diarrhoea, weight loss and many other symptoms. However, it is very difficult to prove such allergy and true food allergy is probably unusual.

There are no specific tests for food allergy. The only way of establishing allergy is by an exclusion diet which means removing various food-stuffs from the diet and gradually reintroducing them so that symptoms which may at first disappear, then recur with the re-introduction of the offending food.

The substances which are thought to be allergy-provoking include eggs, milk, preservatives and artificial colouring. It is sensible to avoid preservatives and colourings in any case, for all children. But it is also very important to avoid becoming too obsessive and end up by excluding everything from the child's diet. This may provoke unnecessary misery and tension between you and your child. Food allergy, if it does occur, is usually a minor problem. If parents are convinced that food allergy is important in a child's disease, the problem should first be discussed with your general practitioner or a hospital paediatrician.

The commonest symptom which is acknowledged to be due to food allergy is diarrhoea, probably due to cows' milk protein allergy. This is usually a condition which occurs in infancy, and which usually resolves by itself after the baby has been on a cows' milk free diet for six to twelve months. The management of this should be discussed with the doctor.

COT DEATH

Sadly, about one in every three or four hundred babies is found dead, usually in the cot, at home by one of his or her parents.

Considerable research is at present going on looking into the cause for these unexpected deaths, known medically as 'sudden infant death syndrome' (SIDS). Despite examination at autopsy, the majority of these babies have no obvious cause for their death. There are several theories which may explain these occurrences, however, and in fact there are probably several different causes which may be responsible for the death of a baby in this way. The possible causes include a congenital abnormality of heart function, a sudden drop in blood pressure for an unknown reason, a sudden and overwhelming infection, an abnormality of the breathing mechanism or other rare abnormalities of the control of body chemistry. Accidental suffocation by a pillow or blanket is extremely rarely, if ever, the cause of death.

The episodes tend to occur at weekends, and in the winter months, probably because of the increased likelihood of virus infections at that time of the year. The baby may occasionally have seemed slightly unwell in the day or two prior to the episode but frequently there is no evidence that the baby was at all unwell before the event.

Apart from the intense distress which most parents feel, they also have understandable feelings of guilt. They are often bewildered by what has happened, and their distress is compounded by questions from friends, neighbours, doctors and the police. However, all health workers who are likely to be involved with the parents are well aware of this reaction and are usually able to offer considerable support. Parents should feel that they are able to discuss the problem with their general practitioner, local paediatrician, health visitor, social worker or religious adviser.

If the baby has been taken to hospital, the parents will need to talk to doctors about the events which have occurred. Usually, an inquest is held, following a post-mortem examination. The findings of this should be discussed with the parents either by the coroner or by the hospital paediatrician. The doctor will be pleased to have several discussions over a period of time if the parents need this.

It is important to reassure parents that they are in no way responsible for the sudden death of their baby and, in fact, they are not alone in their experience. An organization called the Foundation for the Study of Infant Deaths may be contacted and will get parents in touch with families who have had a similar tragedy (see page 299). Support from others in this way is frequently a source of comfort and reassurance for recently bereaved parents.

THE RISK OF RECURRENCE

At a later stage many parents will want to discuss the risks of this happening again. At present the evidence from research studies is difficult to assess, but there is probably a small increase in risk of this episode happening to another baby. When a baby is born who is the sibling of a child who has died, the paediatric department at the hospital may offer to perform some investigations to assess the newborn baby's health.

Although there are alarm systems which detect when a baby stops breathing, the value of these is not yet proven. They are often troublesome and frequently sound without cause, but some parents are greatly reassured by their use in the first few months of their next baby's life.

The older siblings of a baby who has died will also need to talk about the death. Many children fantasize and may worry that a similar episode will occur to them. They should be reassured and allowed to talk about their feelings freely (see p. 291).

PREVENTION OF ACCIDENTS

Children have a natural curiosity which often overcomes their own fears, and indeed their own previous experience of life may be inadequate to prevent their exploration from becoming inappropriate or even dangerous. Children will eventually develop a sense of self-preservation but each child will do this at a different stage. Some children seem particularly accident-prone from early childhood, while others may rarely get involved in difficult situations.

It is important for parents to develop a balance between supervising adequately while avoiding over-protectiveness. If children have accidents, parents will of course feel guilty but it is probably worth realizing at the outset that children are bound to have accidents and indeed will probably injure themselves on numerous occasions, during the process of growing up.

It is however possible to limit the number of significant accidents occurring by making the house itself as accident-proof as possible. When a new baby arrives it is well worth while preparing the home for safety in anticipation of potential problems. (The tables of equipment in Chapters 12 and 13 will be helpful here.) In this way parents can, for the most part, keep one step ahead.

SAFETY OUT OF DOORS

It is essential to purchase prams and buggies which are stable and not likely to collapse unexpectedly. Make sure that strapping is available to keep the child in place. Although it is tempting, do not overload the handles with shopping bags as the stability may be affected. Be careful about allowing younger children to wheel a pram as their instinct for caring for the baby's safety may not be adequate.

IN THE CAR

A child or baby should *never* be carried on an adult's lap in the front seat as the forces in an accident can easily throw the child against the windscreen. Children should always be carried in either specially designed safety seats for the front and rear or, if the child is older, in conventional seat belts. Carry cots should be placed on the back seat and held in place with appropriate restrainer belts.

Children should never stand in a car or lean out of the window while it is in motion. Never allow a child to remain alone in a car. Make sure that the car doors are fitted with appropriate childproof catches. Older children should be dissuaded from playing games which may catch the attention of a driver following in a car behind. It is too easy to distract someone else's attention and thereby cause an accident.

ROAD SAFETY

Children should be taught road sense as soon as possible. These rules should be repeated on frequent occasions and every opportunity taken to reinforce them. However, it is not recommended that children under eight should have to cross roads on their own, and children under school-age should *never* be allowed on the road unaccompanied.

Make sure that gates to the house or driveway are securely locked to prevent children from wandering out on to the road. Take extra care when driving your own car from the house, such as reversing out of a garage, particularly if it is near a play area.

THE GREEN CROSS CODE

RoSPA (the Royal Society for the Prevention of Accidents) recommends that this simple code is taught to all children of school age. Even so, children under eight should not be allowed to cross roads on their own, and children under five should never be allowed on to the street unaccompanied.

☐ First find a safe place to cross, then stop.

☐ Stand on the pavement near the kerb.

☐ Look all round for traffic and listen.

☐ If traffic is coming, let it pass. Look all round again.

☐ When there is no traffic near, walk straight across the road.

☐ Keep looking and listening for traffic while you cross.

POISONING

Despite frequent and widespread warnings, children are still admitted to hospital daily having taken dangerous drugs and medicines. It is essential that drugs are kept high up in a locked cabinet; even quite mild proprietary medicines can cause severe poisoning if taken in quantity by a small child.

Children are extraordinarily versatile when it comes to gaining access to drugs. Don't keep drugs in the refrigerator – this is not safe. Make sure that all medicines are purchased in child-resistant bottles or preferably in blister packs.

Household and garden chemicals should similarly be kept well out of reach. *Never* put toxic substances in familiar bottles, such as lemonade bottles. If you live in an older house which may be covered with lead paint, remove paint in those areas which are accessible to the child. Make sure that toys are also lead free.

There are of course many poisonous plants some of which are particularly appealing to children, such as laburnum pods and trees with bright berries. Children should be warned frequently about the dangers of eating such berries.

ACCIDENTAL INJURIES

It is impossible to warn against the great many and varied injuries to children. Many precautions are commonsense such as purchasing safe toys, avoiding toys with small removable objects or which fall apart readily, and the need for keeping sharp objects such as knives, needles, pins, scissors and DIY tools well out of reach.

Children have a natural tendency to explore and a common danger is getting locked or trapped in a small enclosure such as a Wendy House, cupboard or wardrobe. Make sure the locks or latches do not only function on one side of a door, and make sure that your child cannot reach and open any door that leads into a street where traffic is passing.

Make sure children do not play near unsafe structures such as glass partition doors, removable screens or tall unstable objects. Place vases, pot plants, electrical equipment such as televisions and hi-fi on high and deep ledges, pushed well back out of reach. Warn children about running around with sharp objects in the mouth. Pencils and scissors are particularly dangerous and have often caused penetrating injuries to the face and inside of the mouth.

Supervise young children in playgrounds or by ladders or other high objects they might be tempted to climb. Many may not be able to get back down or may lose their balance and fall because they are not very aware of different heights.

FALLS

All equipment at home, including cots, prams, highchairs and harnesses must be stable. Most equipment these days is well designed and appropriate, but it may be necessary to have a close look at secondhand items to make sure the legs are even, the springs of prams are still firm and that the brakes work properly.

If a child is in a highchair or unstable pram it is important not to leave him alone, even if he is harnessed. Furniture must be securely fixed to avoid it being pulled down on top of the child. Stair-gates, either at the top or at the bottom of the stairs, should be fitted, and accessible windows should be locked or vertical bars placed across them. It is essential that a baby is never left alone on a table or high surface. Babies seem to have a knack of rolling off if left alone!

SUFFOCATION AND DROWNING

Pillows are unnecessary under the age of one year. Most babies will sleep happily without one and they are potentially dangerous. Other sources of suffocation include large or small plastic bags, old refrigerators where the door may close on an inquisitive child, and if you have a swimming pool or ornamental pond, it is essential that the child is not allowed access to these areas without supervision. Drowning is unfortunately still a common accident, and it does not take much depth of water for a child to drown. Cats and dogs should not be allowed direct access to a small baby as they may inadvertently lie on top of the child.

BURNS AND SCALDS

It is worth making a rule to always buy clothing, curtains and other fabrics which are fireproof. Most material should be appropriately labelled – the usual phrase is 'flame retardant'. Fireguards should be fixed across electric and gas fires, as well as open grates. Matches should always be kept out of reach. Other hot objects, including irons, cookers, fireworks, and DIY implements should similarly be kept safely. When the child is old enough to understand, the dangers of each potentially harmful object should be explained, several times over.

Never leave a child alone in the bathroom or indeed in the bath. When filling the bath add hot and cold water simultaneously, never hot water before the cold. Always test it yourself before putting the child in, and remember that a child's skin is much more delicate than an adult's.

Scalds very commonly occur in the kitchen from kettles or long-handled saucepans which are easily pulled off the cooker. Always turn the handles inwards, or provide a safety rack around the cooker itself. Beware of hot teapots which are unsafe on tablecloths or filled cups left on low tables in the living room.

ELECTRIC SHOCKS

Make sure your home has safe wiring – you can ask the local electricity board to check it if you are not sure. Choose sockets which have integral guards or provide socket covers. It is worth remembering not to leave the electric kettle disconnected from the flex if the flex is still plugged into its socket. It is too easy for the child to place the live end into his mouth.

CHOKING

A child's natural impulse to put something in the mouth frequently leads to choking. Small objects are easily inhaled and may lead to serious difficulty with breathing. Young children should never be given peanuts or other small hard food (peanuts can do particular damage if inhaled into the lungs), and be sure that toys do not have small removable parts.

Never leave a baby or small child alone while eating, and a baby should not be left lying or asleep with a bottle propped in the mouth. Apart from serious choking this often leads to small amounts of milk being inhaled eventually leading to lung damage. Furthermore, continuous sucking of sweet substances will certainly lead to damaged teeth.

THE ABC OF RESUSCITATION	
Check these points in an emergency, such as drowning, accident or electric shock.	
Airway	Is the child breathing? If not lay him on his back on a flat surface, gently open the mouth and look for foreign objects or vomit. Carefully remove obstruction with the finger.
Breathing	If the child still does not breathe, place your mouth over the child's mouth or mouth and nose, blow gently, observing the rise of the chest. Breathe at about 20 to 30 times per minute.
Circulation	Check for the pulse, feeling over the heart or the side of the neck. If you have been trained in resuscitation, start cardiac massage by pressing on the chest. If not, it is probably best at this point to call for help by ringing an ambulance or someone in the vicinity.
	It is important to keep trying to resuscitate the child until help arrives, or you can continue no longer.

Artificial respiration

This guide is for emergencies only. It is always better to be taught in a recognized First Aid class run by a reputable organization such as the Red Cross or the St John's Ambulance Brigade.
1 *If a child has stopped breathing, lay him flat, loosen all clothing and tip the head right back so that the chin is pointing up. Clear the mouth of any obstruction with a finger.*
2 *Pinch the child's nose between the thumb and forefinger of one hand and open the child's mouth wide with the other, holding it open with your thumb.*
3 *Lean right over the child and cover his mouth completely with your own, keeping the chin pulled down and the nose pinched shut. Breathe in through your nose and out through your mouth into the child's mouth in several smooth, long breaths, watching to see if the lungs inflate.*
4 *Then place two fingers from each hand crossed over the soft base of the breast bone. (The full weight of your hands on a young child's chest may be too strong and rupture internal organs.) Make fifteen compressions, then return immediately to mouth-to-mouth breathing. Continue with this sequence until the child takes over his own breathing, or until professional help arrives.*

A-Z of First Aid

Everyone facing an acute emergency at home will feel frightened and sometimes guilty. It is important, however, to keep calm and be reassuring, and to handle the first few minutes by following the guidelines listed alphabetically below. It is worth trying to memorize the principal points. It is also useful to make a list of the telephone numbers of your general practitioner and local hospital. Make sure all adults involved in the family, including child-minders or babysitters, know of the existence of this list, and also where to find the First Aid kit. Ideally, parents should join a First Aid course run by a reputable organization.

THE FIRST AID BOX

- ☐ 10 individually wrapped adhesive dressings
- ☐ Triangular bandage
- ☐ Large sterile covering (eg for burns)
- ☐ Sterile eye pad
- ☐ Wound dressings – 5 of various sizes
- ☐ Safety pins
- ☐ Cotton wool
- ☐ Crêpe bandage
- ☐ Antiseptic cleaner
- ☐ Antiseptic cream
- ☐ Calamine lotion
- ☐ Paracetamol (tablets or syrup)
- ☐ Scissors
- ☐ Tweezers
- ☐ Milk of magnesia

Artificial respiration
See the illustrations on the previous page.

Bites
Animal bites are common. If bleeding is slight then carefully wash out the bite with antiseptic solution and apply a dry dressing. If it is deep, it may need suturing and perhaps a tetanus booster (see p. 253).

Bleeding
If a bite or wound is freely bleeding, pressure on top will stop it. You may use either a dressing, piece of clothing or even a hand if necessary. Pressure should be continued for about five or ten minutes until the blood flow stops. The dressing should be placed on the wound as soon as possible afterwards. If the wound continues to bleed, place a second dressing on the top and continue pressure. Medical advice at this point will be necessary.

Broken bones, dislocations and sprains
Broken bones will require X-ray and treatment in hospital. If the fracture is an upper limb and the child is well enough, the limb should be placed in a sling and the child taken to hospital. If the fracture is elsewhere, particularly in the lower limb, the child should be moved as little as possible, and an ambulance called immediately. Do not attempt to straighten or splint the broken limb, as this will be done when the ambulance arrives. An open wound at the site of a fracture should be covered with sterile dressing, if possible; otherwise a freshly laundered handkerchief or table napkin which has been ironed can be used. If you suspect a fractured skull or spine the child should be moved only if absolutely essential to avoid further danger as more injuries may result.

Sprains and dislocations should be treated in much the same way, as it is difficult to tell the difference between sprains and fractures until an X-ray has been done. An upper limb or shoulder should be placed in a sling and an ankle should be left alone and the child taken to hospital immediately. If the parent or adult has trained First Aid experience then an ankle support bandage may be applied before going to hospital.

Burns and scalds
These should be treated immediately by holding the affected area under cold running water for at least five minutes, or covering the area with a bandage soaked in cold water, replacing the bandage regularly as it warms up, to keep the area cold. Do not break open blisters. Small burns can be kept covered with a dry dressing. Large burns should be lightly covered and the child taken to the Accident and Emergency department at your local hospital.

A-Z of First Aid

Choking

Choking is a common occurrence and usually implies that a piece of food or foreign body has become lodged in the airway. Most people will cough it out spontaneously, but if it is clear that the child is unable to breathe with development of blue or pale tinge to the lips and face and perhaps loss of consciousness, immediate treatment is essential. You may be able to reach in to the child's mouth and physically remove the object with your fingers, but if this is at all difficult don't pursue it as you may push it further down. A young child or baby may be held face downwards against your shoulder and several sharp slaps to the back are then given. The foreign body may then appear in the mouth where it can be removed by the fingers. If this does not help and further treatment does not dislodge the foreign body, call for help immediately, and attempt mouth to mouth resuscitation. An older child may be placed face down on the ground and slaps given to the back.

Convulsions (fits)

(See also p. 264). Place the child in the recovery position (see p. 279), and loosen the clothing. Do not put anything in the child's mouth as it may cause damage. Do not try and restrict the abnormal movements which occur during a fit: this may do the child harm. Most fits are brief; try to keep a clear head, even though it is a frightening experience for you. If the fit continues beyond ten minutes, then an ambulance should be called. If the child is known to be epileptic, and the fit not prolonged, then the child may not need to go to hospital. If, however, the fit is a new occurrence, then the child should be seen by a doctor.

Most children will sleep for a variable length of time, sometimes several hours, after a fit. They may be rather drowsy and perhaps have a headache for some time after the event. Make sure that no other injuries have occurred during the fitting episode.

Cuts and grazes

These are common in childhood and usually only require simple cleaning with antiseptic solution, and a small plaster or dry bandage placed on top. Check that tetanus immunization is up to date. If your child sustains a very deep cut or a cut on the head, then it is sensible to take him to the Accident and Emergency department of your local hospital. Young children frequently fall and bite their lips, which can bleed very profusely. However, there is not usually any need for the wound to be looked at by a doctor as it usually heals very quickly, although the lip may be swollen for a day or two.

Electric shock

If the child has obviously sustained an electric shock, and is unconscious, attempt to turn off the current at the main switch. If this is impossible, first move the child with a non-metal pole or thick piece of clothing so that he is no longer in contact with the electric circuit. Then call for help and commence artificial respiration (see p. 275).

A-Z of First Aid

Eye injuries

Eye injuries are best treated immediately in hospital. If there is an obvious foreign body which can readily be removed, do so and then place a clean eye pad over the eye and take the child immediately to hospital. If a substance has entered the eye causing irritation then wash immediately with running water, (for example, from a shower), for ten to fifteen minutes. The eye should then be seen in a hospital.

Fainting

Fainting is generally harmless, and it is important not to interfere with the natural process of recovery. Most people will wake up very soon after fainting but recovery can be hastened by making sure that the child is lying flat, perhaps with the feet higher than the body. Loosen the clothing and place the child in the recovery position (see illustration). If the child does not wake up quickly then an ambulance should be called.

Foreign bodies

If a foreign body, such as a splinter, is small and superficial, it may be readily removed. However deep foreign bodies are often best left in place for removal at hospital, as removal may cause injury, and its presence may also prevent more severe bleeding. A light dressing should be applied before the child is taken to the casualty department. Take care not to press down on the bandage or the object may be pushed further in.

A foreign body that has been pushed or inhaled into a nostril should not be tampered with as it may lodge further inside the nasal cavity. Take the child to the nearest Accident and Emergency department where the doctor will have the right instruments to remove it. This advice is also true for objects pushed into the ear canal, where further interference may damage the ear drum.

Head injuries

Most head injuries are minor and are not usually associated with loss of consciousness. Even a straightforward head injury will sometimes produce sleepiness in a younger child. If however there has been loss of consciousness or severe drowsiness following a head injury, the child should be seen in the Accident and Emergency department. If the child is unconscious from the moment of the injury, gently place him in the recovery position and call an ambulance.

Nose bleeds

Nose bleeds are common but can be frightening. There often seems to be far more blood than has in fact been lost. The child should be asked to sit slightly forward over a bowl and to spit out any blood which is present in the mouth. The front part of the nose should be squeezed tightly for about ten minutes and the child must be asked not to swallow the blood, or to blow his nose for sometime afterwards. If you've got one, put a cork between your child's teeth to keep his mouth open. A piece of ice held on the base of the nose can help reduce blood flow. If the bleeding continues or recurs then a doctor's advice is necessary.

A-Z of First Aid

Poisoning

If you suspect a child has swallowed some dangerous substance do not attempt to make the child vomit by putting the fingers down the throat or giving salt and water. Both of these procedures are potentially dangerous. Give the child milk to drink and take him immediately to an Accident and Emergency department. Make careful note of the substance which you suspect has been swallowed; if you are unsure what it is, perhaps because it was in an unmarked bottle, or a poisonous berry or plant, take a sample with you to the hospital. If the child is unconscious, then it is best to call an ambulance.

Stings

Bee and wasp stings are frightening and painful for the child but rarely cause serious illness, unless the sting has occurred in the mouth or throat. If the sting has been left in place remove it by scraping it out of the skin through pressure applied as close to the point as possible. Do not squeeze the outside of a sting as this may cause more poison to enter. The wound should be washed with antiseptic and a light dressing applied. An analgesia such as paracetamol may be necessary.

Shock

Shock is caused by a sudden drop in blood pressure after an accident or injury. The child will be pale, sometimes unconscious, with a fast heartbeat and shallow respiration. There may be associated injuries. Call an ambulance, loosen the clothing, and lightly cover the child. Reassurance is important both for the child and the parents. If the child is unconscious follow the instructions under 'Unconsciousness', opposite.

Unconsciousness

If the child is not breathing, follow the instructions for Artificial Respiration, p. 275. If the child is breathing normally but not responding, place him in the recovery position, below, and call for an ambulance. Continue to check that the pulse and breathing are regular, and make sure that no bleeding is occurring (see Bleeding, p. 276). Do not try to wake the child up by shaking or other stimulation. Do not give anything by mouth as this may cause choking.

The Recovery Position

CHAPTER SEVENTEEN

SPECIAL CHILDREN

Advice and reassurance for parents whose children have special physical, mental or emotional needs

Sometimes it happens that a child is born with problems. Sometimes these problems develop or become apparent as the child grows older. Some children have to cope with a lot of changes in their home life, either as the result of divorce, remarriage of their parents, adoption or being fostered. Sadly families sometimes have to cope with the death of a child. A parent may be trying to manage alone.

All the children in these circumstances have special needs, and you as their parents need and deserve a lot of support, advice and help. This chapter is about these situations and the professionals, voluntary organizations and statutory benefits that will help you.

Most important of all, your child, whatever his special situation, still wants to be a child and to have the same opportunities and love as other children. It is the teamwork of you the parents, your child and the professionals trained to help and understand, that together can minimize the difficulties you face and achieve maximum happiness and wellbeing for all involved.

THE HANDICAPPED CHILD

What do you do if you find your child is learning to walk and talk more slowly than other children? What do you do if your toddler has uncontrollable outbursts of temper and cannot seem to concentrate on playing? Where do you turn when your doctor tells you that your newborn baby suffers from Down's syndrome?

Whether suddenly, or over a period of months or even years, a significant minority of parents have to come to terms with the fact that all is not well with their child – that their child has a handicap. Whenever it happens, it is a devastating blow which leaves parents confused and frightened. But there is help at hand; there are teams of people working in your health district whose job is to help you and your child. Although nobody would deny that having a handicapped child is difficult and distressing, with proper support families can learn to come to terms with it and to bring their child to his or her full potential.

A handicapped child is a child suffering from a continuing disability of body, intellect or personality, severe enough to interfere with his normal growth, or development, or capacity to learn. These can take many forms; some of the most common are described below.

PHYSICAL HANDICAPS

The most important cause of physical handicap is damage to the central nervous system (the brain or spinal cord) during fetal life, at birth or in the first few years of childhood. The central nervous system is developing very rapidly at this stage so any damage is likely to have a profound effect, often causing delay in the normal development of body movement and control, speech, vision, hearing, social, emotional and learning skills.

CEREBRAL PALSY

A child with cerebral palsy has suffered some form of brain damage involving the nerve pathways which control movement. The problem may be mild, affecting tasks involving fine movement only, such as use of the hands, or it may be severe enough to prevent the child from ever learning to walk.

The layman's term for a child with cerebral palsy is 'spastic', but this is only one form of cerebral palsy. Damage to different parts of the brain causes the different patterns of cerebral palsy: spasticity, ataxia and dyskinesia. Spasticity is characterized by increased tone and weakness of the muscles; ataxia, by incoordination of the limbs and sometimes hand tremor; and dyskinesia by involuntary movements of the limbs or sometimes the whole body.

The initial damage to the brain is non-progressive, which means it does not get worse, but

Many Child Development Teams run toy libraries for handicapped children and their parents, where toys can be tried out and borrowed and problems discussed informally with the staff.

as the brain continues to mature during childhood, the symptoms of cerebral palsy may change, either because damage to some maturing part of the brain becomes more apparent, or because the brain develops and becomes better able to cope with the consequences of damage.

The child with cerebral palsy may also have damage to other parts of the brain, resulting in speech, hearing or visual problems, behaviour disturbances, epilepsy or specific learning problems. Children with cerebral palsy may have normal intelligence, but many are also mentally handicapped and are slower to learn to look after themselves.

SPINA BIFIDA

The brain and the spinal cord develop from the neural tube within the first 28 days of pregnancy (see p. 40). The two folds of the neural tube occasionally fail to fuse, which can also be associated with defective closure of the spinal column, resulting in spina bifida. The reason why the neural tube develops incorrectly is unknown, but it is thought to be connected with both genetic and environmental factors. Spina bifida is the most common defect present at birth in Britain, but its incidence is decreasing. Some spina bifida lesions may be surgically treatable. Spina bifida may be diagnosed during pregnancy by the measurement of alpha feto protein levels in the mother's blood, plus ultrasound scanning and amniocentesis (see p. 27).

Spina bifida does not always result in complete disability. In fact, the very mild form known as spina bifida occulta, where the outer part of one or more vertebrae is not completely joined, is only indicated by a dimple or small hair growth on the back and most people have no symptoms. Children with spina bifida cystica, however, have both the outer part of some of the vertebrae split and the meninges (lining of the spinal cord) pushed out through the opening to form a sac. If there is little involvement of the underlying spinal cord, the opening is termed a meningocele, and there will probably be only a few neurological signs in the body below the level of the opening. But if the spinal cord and nerve roots are also involved (a myelomeningocele), the consequences are much more serious. This usually means that movement and sensation in the lower part of the body are impaired or lost, often resulting in incontinence.

HYDROCEPHALUS

Maldevelopment of the neural tube can also be associated with defects at the base of the brain, interfering with the flow of cerebro-spinal fluid (CSF) through or around the base of the brain. This causes hydrocephalus, an accumulation of the cerebro-spinal fluid within the brain, shown by an abnormally fast growth rate of the head. Hydrocephalus may be apparent at birth, or after the surgical closure of the spina bifida back lesion.

Many babies with hydrocephalus are helped by the insertion of a 'shunt' to reduce the raised pressure inside the skull. The shunt drains away the cerebro-spinal fluid into a vein in the neck or into the abdomen. Hydrocephalus, with or without a shunt, may cause no disability.

EPILEPSY

A previously normal child may develop epilepsy, but it can also be a complication of maldevelopment of the brain, brain damage or brain surgery. The degree to which the child is disabled by seizures (convulsions or fits) will depend on the form that they take, their frequency and the child's response to anti-convulsant drug treatment, which can be very successful.

OTHER PHYSICAL PROBLEMS

The baby may be born with abnormalities which interfere with seeing or hearing. This will require referral to an opthalmologist or audiologist who will advise on treatment and special ways to help the clinical problem. There may be an abnormality of the heart which will limit normal activity and require surgery.

Cystic fibrosis is a serious inherited disorder affecting many tissues of the body, especially the lungs and the pancreas. There is no cure but a lot can be done through medication, nutrition and physiotherapy to improve the health of the child and delay the progression of the disease.

There are several different types of muscular dystrophy and a large number of other neuromuscular diseases. Many diseases are hereditary in nature, so that genetic counselling to reduce the likelihood of recurrence in further children is important (see p. 14). Some of these muscle diseases cause the child to become physically more disabled as the years pass and these children, and their families, need special help in coming to terms with this.

THE CHILD WITH A MENTAL HANDICAP

Mental handicap is a permanent disability that can happen in any family. Over the years names have varied from mental defect, subnormality, mental retardation to mental handicap, but all these terms have essentially the same meaning: the child has been born with a brain which does not mature as fast, or function as well as that of a normal child, so that the full mental capacities of a normal adult will not be reached. 'Developmental delay' is an acceptable term only while the diagnosis is in doubt. Sometimes it is important to understand that mental handicap is not the same as mental illness.

Causes of mental handicap include chromosome abnormalities, such as Down's syndrome; single gene defects, such as phenylketonuria; infection of the fetus during pregnancy by rubella, cytomegalovirus and other organisms (congenital infections) and damage to the baby's developing brain during pregnancy by alcohol or an underfunctioning thyroid gland. Babies starved of oxygen at birth, due to serious problems associated with the delivery, may develop cerebral palsy with or without mental handicap, but it is unusual for these children to develop mental handicap alone. Mentally handicapped children are often associated with a difficult pregnancy or birth, but it is likely that the obstetric problems are a consequence of the abnormally developing brain, rather than a cause of it. Sometimes the cause of a child's mental handicap cannot be discovered.

DOWN'S SYNDROME

Three-quarters of the children with a chromosomal abnormality have Down's syndrome. They have an extra chromosome in the nucleus of every cell in their body (47 instead of 46) as a result of abnormal cell division at the time of conception, and which interferes with normal development. Sometimes the extra chromosome is joined to another one (known as translocation), or appears after the formation of the zygote (see p. 39), resulting in mosaicism. The risk of the mosaic form of Down's syndrome increases with maternal age (see p. 27); if a parent is a translocation carrier, the risk of recurrence in subsequent pregnancies is high.

Down's syndrome babies have abnormal features recognizable at birth but the condition is confirmed by chromosome analysis. The potential for the baby's development cannot be predicted with any reliability in early infancy, though generally children with translocation or mosaicism are less severely handicapped. Down's children can be very loving and rewarding children, and many grow up to lead sheltered but independent lives. Some schools are beginning to introduce Down's syndrome children into classrooms with normal children of their own age. This has been beneficial for all concerned – children, parents and teachers – and is likely to become a more widespread practice as people's general acceptance and understanding grows.

CONGENITAL RUBELLA

There is a serious risk of damage to the fetus or of spontaneous abortion if a woman contracts rubella (German measles) during pregnancy (see p. 13). Although the incidence is falling due to immunization, rubella remains an important cause of handicap with damage occurring to the heart, eyes, ears or brain.

DIAGNOSING MENTAL HANDICAP

In many cases the diagnosis of mental handicap slowly emerges over the first few years of life, so that it may be only when a child starts school that the handicap becomes clearly apparent. Parents often accept the concept of developmental delay, but find it very hard to accept the not infrequent sequel of mental handicap.

Many parents in this situation may have read about autism or dyslexia and may believe, or have it suggested to them, that these terms could be more appropriate for their child than the label of mental handicap. Both autism and dyslexia seem to be socially more acceptable diagnoses, and where correctly applied, they require highly specialized teaching. Sadly, the use of these terms without professional verification may perpetuate the non-acceptance of the child's true problem, that of intellectual limitation.

THE HANDICAPPED CHILD'S PARENTS

Perhaps your child is handicapped. What do you feel? What support do you need? The effect on a family of a handicapped child can be profound and should never be under-estimated. Outwardly it may cause parents to seem aggressive and ungrateful for help and sympathy offered. Inwardly most parents experience guilt and worry as to who will care for their child when they are no longer able to do so; they are concerned for the effect of the handicapped child on normal brothers and sisters. Relationships between the two parents may become strained. All these feelings may occur even though you love your child and continue to try to give your best.

Where a handicap emerges slowly, parents have to cope with a long period of doubt about their child. They often withdraw from discussing their uncertainties with others and feel isolated. Sleepless nights and the child's antisocial behaviour may add to the enormous burden of these years.

If your child is handicapped, you need to be told what is wrong with your child, its cause, how it can be treated and what the future holds. If the handicap is due to chromosomal abnormality or some here-

Even quite young babies can benefit from the help of a physiotherapist, who will always involve the parents in physiotherapy sessions.

ditary defect, genetic counselling can help to alleviate the guilt by showing you that there was nothing you could have done to prevent what happened, and to assess the risk to future childen (see p. 14).

Many parents lack confidence in their ability to cope with the special problems likely to arise from their child's handicap. The support of your local Child Development Team (see below) will help you to gain confidence and learn the skills you need to become part-provider of your child's treatment, alongside the appropriate therapist. The paediatrician heading the team will guide you in possible courses of action, and will discuss your child's developmental progress. A key worker from the team will be assigned to you and you will be given his or her telephone number so that you will always have a quick and ready point of contact when problems arise. The key worker will probably be the therapist most closely involved in your child's treatment, or may be a social worker or special health visitor.

HELP FOR HANDICAPPED CHILDREN

In most health districts in Britain there are now multidisciplinary Child Development Teams who are responsible for the clinical care and co-ordination of management of handicapped children. The composition of the team is usually a paediatrician, specialist health visitor, social worker, clinical psychologist, physiotherapist, occupational therapist and speech therapist. Ideally there should also be a school teacher in the team as well.

In fact, in some well developed services, you may be bewildered by the number of professionals who are all eager to help your child. Don't be afraid to ask exactly what each person does, and remember that the key worker assigned to look after your child's progress will be happy to explain anything that is confusing or frightening.

The Child Development Team probably operates from a hospital-based Child Development Centre (CDC), allowing ready access to the specialist services necessary for each diagnosis, assessment and treatment. Some provide a day nursery or play group for young handicapped children, through which part of the assessment of the child's needs

The speech therapist is encouraging this two-year-old Down's syndrome child to recognize objects and match them to pictures. Speech therapy begins as early as possible with simple games to encourage listening and making sounds.

can be carried out. Most centres also run 'Toy Libraries' which enable parents to borrow and use toys which particularly help to stimulate their child's development. The therapists are there to advise you on the most suitable toys for your child.

REFERRAL TO THE CDC

If your child's development shows signs of delay or impairment, your health visitor, GP or clinic doctor will probably refer you to the Child Development Team. This is most likely to happen after one of the regular developmental checks but can happen at any time, especially if you have expressed anxiety through your own observations of your child's development. The child is seen first by the paediatrician who decides, through discussion with the team, which other members it is appropriate to involve in the assessment.

The children referred for assessment may have either mental, physical or behavioural handicaps, or a combination. They may be showing some delay in development or they may have certain learning problems which need investigation. The aim of the assessment by the different team members is to

recognize and define the handicap so that a diagnosis can be made and a plan formulated to help the child develop his full potential. The specialist health visitor liaises with the family health visitor and the special schools over a child's need, and is able to give information to the parents. The therapists involved devise treatment plans which they discuss with the parents. Therapy sessions may be arranged. All therapists work closely together and their roles with children often overlap.

TYPES OF THERAPY

The physiotherapist aims to help the child towards independent normal movement, paying particular attention to posture, movement and balance. She will advise parents on how to handle their children to encourage this by showing them the best way to carry, position and play with their child. Occasionally if there is a particular handicap, specific exercises may be given.

The occupational therapist assesses the quality of movement in general, but in particular, concentrates on the upper limbs, and the ease with which the child can use these in fine movement. She

One of the main aims of occupational therapy is to help children to gain independence in the ordinary tasks of daily life.

assesses difficulties the child may have with the activities of daily living (ADL) such as feeding, dressing, bathing and going to the toilet. She advises on the best positions for all of these activities, as well as for play.

The occupational therapist gives advice on the equipment necessary for the child, such as tables and chairs of the correct height and giving adequate support, and any special devices that may be required. In addition the occupational therapist will suggest suitable toys to develop hand function and perceptual skills, needed for activities such as writing or dressing. She helps you to obtain these aids.

ASSESSING THE CHILD'S NEEDS

The child's problems and ways to help them are then discussed at a special meeting ('case discussion') between the parents and the professionals involved. The child's teacher or health visitor may have been asked to come to the meeting. A date for reviewing the progress of the child is planned. This review may take a similar form to the initial assessment and re-occurs at varying intervals depending on the need. Wherever possible continuing therapy is planned to take place in the child's home or school.

The Child Development Centre is also an information base from which you can obtain advice about voluntary organizations that can help you and your child, financially, emotionally, through self-help groups, and with information about leisure activities. (Many useful addresses are listed on page 00.)

THE HANDICAPPED CHILD AT SCHOOL

As the handicapped child reaches school entry age, the focus for medical services shifts from the Child Development Centre to the school. This should not interrupt the continuity of care for your child's specific needs, for within the school health system is a similar team of health professionals as found in the Child Development Centre. They continue to review and make provision for the needs of the child and his family.

SPECIAL SCHOOLING

The need for special schooling for a child may have been apparent from a very early stage, or its suggestion may be the first time parents have had to face the fact that all is not well with their child. Nowadays the emphasis is on abolishing the sharp distinction between a handicapped and non-handicapped child, concentrating instead on the concept of children with 'special educational needs'. In Britain, there is now statutory backing for the consideration of each child's individual needs and suitable educational provision made to meet them, whether handicapped in the clinical sense of the word, or not.

illness, the effect it has had on the family in that time, the emotional repercussions with each phase of hopes raised and then crushed, leave their particular toll. The grief of family members may be out of step; some find it easier to talk of the event and their feelings than others. Family members may need help to understand each other.

THE DYING CHILD

Dying children need help too. Their degree of understanding will vary with age; younger children tend to accept events from day to day without too much looking into the future, while older children are comforted if they feel you are responding seriously to their anxieties. They will want to have their questions answered honestly and you will need to be frank in your replies. Children seldom talk about dying but may ask about death itself. You may wish to talk with your child about where this should happen. Normal events – friends visiting, new clothes, perpetuation of usual play by siblings within the home, should continue. At all times drugs will be adjusted by your doctor to ensure your child's comfort, yet allowing as much activity as possible.

THE REACTION OF BROTHERS AND SISTERS

Brothers and sisters of a dying child need the situation explained so that they have something to explain to others. Their reaction to the death will depend on how close they were to their brother or sister. Children under two years have little awareness beyond events directly concerning themselves. Between two and about six years they will interpret events at face value. This means that previous sibling rivalry may now leave them irrationally blaming themselves for the loss of their brother or sister. They may react in a similar way to the loss of a parent.

From seven or eight years old, the child more easily believes what he is told, even though deeper understanding of the event comes more slowly. But he is now more aware of the reactions of those around him and he will feel less excluded from your grief if you can show your feelings in front of him. He may need to talk through his own worries of whether a similar illness could happen to him. It is a valuable idea to give a photograph of the dead child to each of his brothers and sisters, and then to continue to talk about him whenever appropriate. The process of recovery is a long one. It is just as important for children to grieve as it is for parents. Ultimately the other children in your family will be grateful to have been fully involved.

DIVORCE

Year by year, the divorce rate is rising. There was a 400 per cent increase in the number of divorce decrees absolute in England and Wales between 1962 and 1982. It is inevitable that your marital difficulties will eventually have an effect on your children's feelings and perhaps behaviour. Your divorce will, however temporarily, result in a one-parent family situation. Between two-thirds and three-quarters of divorced parents marry again, perhaps to a partner with children, but this also means that yet another new family environment may arise for a child to adjust to. You may find yourself with step-children. It is a confusing, sometimes painful, time for children who lack the level of insight of an adult.

Prior to parental separation, your child may witness considerable verbal or physical abuse, and may react with minor but real physical symptoms; school performance may fall and bed-wetting return. Even if the separation is not accompanied by particularly dramatic or emotional scenes, or if the parents conceal them from their children, the children are bound to be affected. Children often have a greater awareness of what is happening than their parents realize.

Separation causes conflicting loyalties and is hazardous for any child. Too ready access to the parent who goes away may be damaging for the very young child, while those older may wish to reject their absent parent, at the same time as feeling rejected.

Divorce courts hold the welfare of the child as paramount, and have the power to place the child in the care of the local authority if they consider neither parent suitable for the continuing care. During the Hearing, the custody and care are discussed and formalized, and financial maintenance agreed. Access arrangements for the estranged parents are also discussed. A new family concept begins for the child which ironically may bring greater social, economic and emotional strains than the one which he had learned to tolerate. Loss of a parent can cause a child to become insecure, lack confidence, and be emotionally disturbed with reduced school performance.

Completion of divorce proceedings does however bring some positive consequences. There begins the opportunity for you all to return to a routine, and for peace and calm to prevail. It will take time for you and your children to forget the emotional bruising but with the greater stability you will all begin to feel more secure and your children will start to grow again mentally and physically within the new structure to your lives.

Many women are now in the position of bringing up children on their own, some even by choice. Although it can be hard work and sometimes lonely, there is the reward of a special closeness with the child.

ONE-PARENT FAMILIES

There has been a steady increase in the number of one-parent families over the last decade and now over 1,000,000 children are being brought up in this way. The largest rises have been in families headed by a divorced or single mother. Widowed parents or lone fathers form the remainder of the group. Most parents who find themselves in this situation don't do it from choice; however a significant minority of women choose to become mothers on their own.

If you are a one-parent family it is likely that you will already have discovered that one of the most acute problems is a shortage of money. Many two-parent families find it hard enough to manage, but statistics show that one-parent families have to manage on less than half the income of two-parent families. Sadly this can result in children of one-parent families suffering materially – they may be less well dressed, lack material possessions that they see other children with, and even be unable to participate in extra educational and leisure activities. In Britain, Child Benefit is currently available for all children, and a single parent can additionally claim an extra allowance for each child (DHSS Leaflet CH11). Family Income Supplement is a benefit available to the low paid and over half the families claiming it are one-parent families. (The administration of these benefits is changing in 1988 – see page 294.)

You may have found, as a single parent wanting to work rather than depend on state benefits, that this is difficult because of a lack of day nursery provision and good childminders. However, day nurseries often give priority to children from one-parent families, and the development of crèche facilities at some places of work is easing this problem a little. A very real difficulty for single parents can be a lack of friends or family to babysit and yet a lack of money to pay other people to do this. Adequate housing is another costly need, sometimes difficult to meet.

Single parents often do not know where to go or where to start to sort out the many, varied and inter-related problems. Your local social services will be able to help you. Also there is Gingerbread, an association for one-parent families (see page 299). They have local self-help groups through which single parents band together and provide each other with a mutual support system. An organization called Lone Fathers offers similar support. The National Council for One-Parent Families provides free and confidential advice on all issues relating to one parent families. They can also give you information about holidays for lone parents, and they maintain a list of Trusts who will give money directly to families such as yours in cases of special need. The DHSS produces a leaflet (FB3) on help for one-parent families.

Some situations cannot be changed and yet may not be ideal – you may feel that you and your children come into such a group. This is the time to look on the positive side of your circumstances. Your single parent state will mean that you will see more of your children which means the relationship between you all may be stronger than if you shared your time with a partner.

STEP-PARENTING

Step-parenting is an increasingly common situation. As divorce statistics rise, it is inevitable that more and more people contemplating marriage will be gaining a ready-made family as well as a partner, and the children will have been used to a different family pattern. Children can show a lot of love but they can also demonstrate their views without tact or tolerance. Even a baby gets used to distinguishing his carers, objecting if he wishes.

Step-parenting may succeed from the outset, but for some it may bring unanticipated stresses and problems. It takes time for a loving relationship to develop between step-parent and child, and in that time, when you are trying to reach out to your child, it can be very hurtful to be rebuffed, or to get little return of affection. If that is coupled with frank opposition, selfishness and difficult behaviour, enormous strains are put on the new marriage. On the other hand, the child may be offering affection, but the step-parent may be rejecting him.

PREPARING THE GROUND

Some problems of step-parenting may be avoided by careful thought and discussion beforehand. Couples need to agree on the standards they will expect in bringing up the children. All of you need to discuss what the children will call you, and they may have to be weaned gently off wayward ways which have developed in the period between their parent's two marriages.

Time spent getting to know the children before the re-formation of the family will help establish the new parent-child relationship. It is very important not to be so caught up as a new husband and wife that the childrens' feelings go unnoticed. Talk through where it is most appropriate to live with regard to the children's needs. Realize that a new baby may precipitate jealousy from the other children, particularly if favouritism is at all evident, and that it is not necessarily the answer to 'welding the two sides of the family together'.

There will have been pain for all parties through the broken marriage and that needs understanding. Children have feelings for the absent parent but may have difficulty talking about them. Few children are adult enough to cope with these divided feelings of loyalty. But if you can recognize them, it may explain behaviour in many situations and you will understand better. Access agreements need to be carefully worked through. Be prepared for being viewed with caution by grandparents, other relatives and neighbours that you are also taking on. Of course you have to clamp down on interference but equally grandparents should be able to contribute, so make them feel wanted.

HELP AND ADVICE

Patience, communication and enjoyment of each other will eventually lead towards family unity, for some more easily than others. The time will arrive when the pleasures and tribulations are very akin to those felt by the 'normal' family. The process of feeling just like any other parent may take years to reach, but is worth striving for.

However, if you are encountering difficulties and feel you need extra help, then you could get in touch with the Marriage Guidance Council (their telephone number is in your local telephone directory). They will offer you the opportunity to talk to a third person with experience of your sort of problems, and you can go and talk to them with your partner or on your own. Stepfamily, the national stepfamily association founded in 1983, offers a confidential telephone counselling service (details on p. 299). They also have local self-help groups and can put step-parents in touch with one another. Many towns have Family Centres – your local social services will tell you about them, and the Samaritans of course are an ever present help for those in real despair.

APPENDIX I

BENEFITS FOR PARENTS BEFORE AND AFTER THE BIRTH

The rules governing maternity leave and maternity pay are complicated, so it is well worth sorting them out early in pregnancy, especially since claims for benefit often have to be made well in advance of when they are due to be paid. The leaflet *Babies and Benefits* (FB 8), which is available free from post offices, the DHSS and branches of the Citizens Advice Bureau, gives most of the information you need. There are a number of forms and leaflets explaining your rights which the midwife at the booking clinic will give you. One of the most important forms is the maternity certificate, form Mat B1, which shows when your baby is due. You need it to claim most benefits. It can be obtained when you are 26 weeks pregnant, but not before.

Statutory Maternity Pay

The most substantial payments are those made to women who are working. These payments are made by the employer and are called Statutory Maternity Pay or SMP. You are entitled to SMP and to have your job back after your baby is born if you can satisfy the following conditions:

☐ you must have been in the same employment for at least 6 months without a break up to the 26th week of pregnancy; this is known as the *qualifying week* and is actually 15 weeks before the week in which your baby is due

☐ your average weekly earnings were at or above the level where you have to start paying National Insurance contributions

You do not have to intend to return to work to get SMP.

Statutory Maternity Pay can be paid for a maximum 18-week period. The 'core' period of 13 weeks starts 6 weeks before your baby is due, and goes on to include the week in which the baby arrives and the 6 weeks afterwards. The remaining 5 weeks can be taken at the beginning or the end of the core period. In other words the earliest time it can begin is 11 weeks before your baby is due, but you can carry on working until 6 weeks before if you want. At this point, that is week 34 of your pregnancy, you must stop work, or you may lose part of your SMP.

There are two rates of pay. The higher rate is 90 per cent of your normal wages, the lower rate is currently £32.85 a week. The rate to which you are entitled depends on how long you have been in your job. If you have been in the same employment for at least 2 years by the qualifying week, or part-time for 5 years and working at least 8 hours a week, you can get the higher rate for the first 6 weeks of your leave; you get the lower rate for the remaining 12 weeks. If you have been in the same employment for between 26 weeks and 2 years you will get the lower rate for the whole of the 18-week period. You may have to pay tax and National Insurance contributions on SMP.

In order to get SMP you must tell your employer in writing that you plan to stop work because of your pregnancy. Do this at least 3 weeks before you actually stop work. It's a good idea to inform him or her much earlier than this to avoid losing pay for keeping antenatal appointments. When you are 26 weeks pregnant, give your employer your form Mat B1.

Statutory Maternity Pay is a benefit to which certain women are entitled by law; but some employers have agreements which are better than SMP. You can find out about these from your personnel officer or trade union official. These are also the people who can help you if for some reason you think that your right to SMP is not being fulfilled.

Employment Rights

As with SMP, your right to return to work is subject to certain conditions. Your employer can write to you any time up to 7 weeks after the week in which your baby was due asking you to confirm that you are going back to work. You must reply in writing within 2 weeks or you lose your right to return. As well as this you must write to your employer at least 3 weeks before you plan to return to work to inform him of the date on which you wish to return. Having done this, you can return to work at any time up to 29 weeks from the week of your baby's birth. Your employer can only delay your return for up to a further four weeks and he has to let you know in writing. If you are ill you can postpone your return to work for four weeks after the 29-week period has run out, as long as you give your employer a medical certificate issued by a doctor (not a midwife). Twenty-nine weeks from the birth is the latest time by which you have a right to go back to your job.

The dates in this may seem complicated but the law insists that you follow them. If you do not, you may find yourself deprived of maternity pay and of the right to return to work.

You have the right to go back to the job in which you were employed previously, so it may be important to check before taking maternity leave exactly what you are coming back to. Your job is defined in your contract of employment, which can consist of verbal agreements and formal documents. If your employer has a number of places of business and your contract of employment obliges you to work at any of them, he or she might be able to move your place of employment even if you don't want to work there. It is always advisable to negotiate these matters before you leave work. Equally, if it is not reasonably practicable for your employer to offer you exactly your old job back he can offer you an equivalent job without being in breach of his obligations.

If you find that you have been made redundant while on maternity leave, you must be offered alternative employment where a suitable vacancy exists, or redundancy pay if not. If this happens take advice from a solicitor, your trade union or the Citizens Advice Bureau. You are entitled to any improvements in the rate of pay or holiday entitlement which may have been introduced for your class of work during your absence.

Maternity Allowance

If you cannot get SMP you may nevertheless be eligible for Maternity Allowance from the DHSS if you have recently given up your job, changed jobs or have recently been self-employed. To qualify you must have paid standard-rate National Insurance contributions for at least 26 of the

52 weeks that end with the qualifying week (15 weeks before your baby is due).

Maternity Allowance is currently £30.05 a week and is payable for up to 18 weeks. The payment period starts 11 weeks before your baby is due, but if you are still employed at that time it may start later. You cannot get the allowance for any week in which you are working. Payment is normally made for the core period of 13 weeks, beginning 6 weeks before your baby is due and ending 6 weeks afterwards; the remaining 5 weeks can be taken before or afterwards – it's up to you. You can divide the time up if you like and have 2 weeks before and 3 at the end, giving you a total of 8 weeks before, then the week in which your baby arrives, then 9 weeks more. But if you work any later than week 34 of your pregnancy you may lose part of your allowance.

To claim the allowance fill in form MA 1, available from your Social Security office or antenatal clinic. Send it with your maternity certificate (form Mat B1) to your Social Security office as soon as you reach the qualifying week. If your employer has refused to pay you SMP he or she should give you form SMP 1, and you should also enclose this with your application.

Low income benefits
Check with your Social Security office as soon as possible during your pregnancy to see if you or your family are entitled to any other benefits, such as Family Income Supplement (FIS). If you qualify for FIS you will get a weekly payment for 52 weeks whether or not your income changes. You may be able to claim Supplementary Benefit

if you or your partner do not have enough money to live on. In April 1988 FIS was replaced by Family Credit and Supplementary Benefit by Income Support. Information will be available at the post office and Citizens Advice Bureau and you should check to make sure you claim what is on offer.

If you or your partner is getting FIS or Supplementary Benefit you may be able to get a Maternity Payment of £80 from the Social Fund to help pay for things for your new baby. To apply, get a claim form from your Social Security Office and send it in after you are 29 weeks pregnant, but no later than 3 months after the birth. You may be entitled to other benefits as well, such as free milk and vitamins, or help with fares to hospital.

Child Benefit
Whatever your income, child benefit is a tax-free cash benefit paid for each of your children and is currently £7.25 a week (normally paid monthly). Ask your Social Security Office for an application form (there is a coupon for this purpose in the leaflet *Babies and Benefits*), fill it in and send it off with your baby's birth certificate. Single parents should apply at the same time for One Parent Benefit. This is currently £4.70 a week.

Other benefits
While you are pregnant, and for a year after your baby's birth, you are entitled to free dental treatment and free prescriptions, no matter what your income and regardless of National Insurance contributions. Ask your midwife for form FW 8.

APPENDIX II
SUPPORT FOR PARENTS OF SPECIAL CHILDREN

Information Services
The Disability Rights Handbook produced by the Disability Alliance Educational & Research Association (ERA), and the booklet entitled 'Help Starts Here' produced by the Voluntary Council for Handicapped Children, provide a very comprehensive guide to the rights, benefits, services and voluntary organizations available to the disabled and their families. Additionally, the Disability Alliance (ERA) plans in 1987 to publish a Guide dealing specifically with children's needs, and also to update its main Guide annually, with four-monthly interim bulletins. MENCAP publishes a very comprehensive London directory of services called Interlink, which gives information relating to each London borough as well as national provision for the mentally handicapped. MENCAP also produces a quarterly publication on welfare, legal and counselling services.

The Department of Health and Social Security publishes many leaflets relating to benefits; one in particular, 'Help for Handicapped People' (DHSS HB1) covers details about cash benefits and health social services. Social Security Offices are listed in the telephone directory under 'H' for Health, or your local post office can tell you their address. DHSS leaflets can also be obtained from the DHSS Leaflet Unit. Local Authority Social Services Departments, Housing or Education Departments can be contacted by telephone. The telephone number is listed under the first letter of the name of your local council. The

Citizens Advice Bureau provides free, confidential and impartial advice for the public.

Community Health Councils exist to improve the quality of the Health Services in your district, so do contact them if you have comments or questions. The FREEPHONE DHSS Service (available by dialling 100 and asking the operator for it) can give you general advice or information on benefits, but it does not deal with specific problems.

Voluntary Organizations
There are many national voluntary organizations with an interest in specific handicaps, which provide support to families. Information about these agencies is available through your local Child Development Centre and also through the services mentioned above. Many have local groups which you can join, where parents find that others with similar experiences can offer much good advice and support. The national organizations also work to generate greater public awareness about certain conditions, and can provide you with much helpful information about your child's condition. In addition, they can often provide special holiday opportunities. Many of these organizations are listed under Useful Addresses on pages 297-299.

Some organizations are particularly concerned with the promotion of leisure, sporting and holiday activities for the handicapped. Gateway and PHAB (Physically Handicapped and Able Bodied) Clubs provide local weekly social events and activities for mentally and physically handicapped children respectively, while the organization Contact a Family provides a link for parents of handicapped children.

RADAR (Royal Association for Disability and Rehabilitation) has published much useful material on housing, holidays and employment opportunities, and also administers REMAP, which adapts day-to-day items to meet the specific needs of the handicapped.

ACCESS is concerned with advising on building design to aid the handicapped person. The Disabled Living Foundation has a permanent display of appropriate aids and equipment.

NETWORK for the Handicapped is a free Law and Advisory Centre for disabled and handicapped people and their families.

NAWCH (National Association for the Welfare of Children in Hospital) represents children's interests in hospital, covering design, care and welfare.

MEDICALERT offers necklaces or bracelets engraved with medical details and the appropriate course of action in an emergency.

SPOD (Sexual and Personal Relationships of the Disabled) has local self-help groups which give advice on building relationships and matters such as masturbation and sexual precocity.

Are you still searching for some specific sort of help?
If you cannot find what you need, write to The Voluntary Council for Handicapped Children and they will try to put you in touch with the appropriate resource.

BENEFITS FOR PARENTS OF SPECIAL CHILDREN

The Attendance Allowance (DHSS Leaflet N.I.205)
This is a tax-free allowance payable to individuals over the age of 2 years who are severely disabled either mentally or physically, and who have needed considerable supervision for at least 6 months. It is not means tested and there are no contribution tests. The allowance is paid at one of two rates: a lower rate for those requiring continual supervision throughout the day, or who need frequent help with going to the toilet, washing or feeding; or a higher rate, where one of these conditions is also applicable during the night. The attendance allowance does not prejudice other benefits, and is ignored as income for Supplementary Benefit (with two exceptions), Housing Benefit and Family Income Supplement. It can, therefore, make a significant difference to the family income. If you qualify for both the Attendance Allowance and Supplementary Benefit, you are automatically entitled to a weekly payment for heating. If a claim for the Attendance Allowance is refused for a non-medical reason, you have the right to appeal within 28 days to a Social Security Appeal Tribunal. Similarly, you can request a review if the application is turned down on medical grounds.

The Mobility Allowance (DHSS Leaflet N.I.211)
The Mobility Allowance is also a non-means tested, tax-free weekly cash benefit designed to help severely disabled people become more mobile. A child is not eligible until aged 5, but it is possible to submit the claim in advance so that the allowance can be received from the 5th birthday. The allowance is for spending on outdoor mobility of any form: taxis, a wheelchair, buying or hiring a car. It is the parent or adult looking after the child who claims. In order to qualify, the child must be unable, or virtually unable, to walk, or the exertion required to walk constitute a danger to life or lead to a serious deterioration in health. The walking difficulty must be caused by a physical handicap, but it may be possible to qualify if it is accepted that a mental handicap has a physical cause.

Motability is a voluntary organization set up on the initiative of the Government to advise people how to make the best use of their Mobility Allowance.

The Family Fund
Any family caring at home for a severely mentally or physically handicapped child under the age of 16 years, may apply for help from The Family Fund. This fund is run by the Joseph Rowntree Memorial Trust and is financed by the Government. It can provide a grant for specific items which arise from the care of the child. The fund is discretionary, but works within general guidelines agreed with the Government. There is no means test but social and economic circumstances are taken into account in assessing applications. The fund's aim is to relieve stress arising from the day-to-day care of a handicapped child. It does not replace the help available from a local authority.

Invalid Care Allowance (DHSS Leaflet N.1.212)
Since July 1986 it has been possible for women as well as men to claim this allowance if they are looking after a severely disabled person at home. This follows the EEC directive on Equal Treatment for Women. For you to qualify, your child must be eligible for the Attendance Allowance, and there are certain conditions to be met about your age, status and income. ICA counts as taxable income, but you can also be claiming Mobility Allowance and Supplementary Benefit although the latter will be reduced when you also claim ICA.

Additional Weekly DHSS Benefits
Additional weekly allowances are available if you are on Supplementary Benefit and your handicapped child is less than 16 years old. These weekly payments are to meet needs over and above those designed for your basic weekly benefit. They are for heating, diet, bathing, laundry costs, wear and tear on clothing or special clothing, hospital fares and domestic help. You may also be eligible for a single payment for a particular expense.

Housing Improvement Grant
A home improvement grant may be given by the DHSS Housing Department to make your home more suitable for the needs of a handicapped child.

Vaccine Damage (DHSS Leaflet HB3)
This scheme provides a tax free lump sum of £10,000 for a person who has suffered permanent and very severe damage under a routine vaccination programme against diphtheria, tetanus, pertussis, measles, rubella, smallpox or tuberculosis. The claimant must be 2 years or over when the claim is made, and the claim be made within 6 years of the vaccination.

USEFUL ADDRESSES

GENERAL

BRITISH PAEDIATRIC ASSOCIATION
5 St Andrew's Place
London NW1 4LB
01-486 6151

CITIZENS ADVICE BUREAU
The address of your local CAB can be found through your telephone directory under 'Citizens'

COMMUNITY SERVICE VOLUNTEERS (ADVICE CENTRE)
237 Pentonville Road
London N1 9NJ
01-278 6601

DHSS (DEPARTMENT OF HEALTH & SOCIAL SECURITY)
Alexander Fleming House
Elephant and Castle
London SE1 6BY
01-407 5522

DHSS LEAFLETS UNIT
P.O. Box 21
Stanmore, Middx HA7 1AY

LOCAL AUTHORITY: SOCIAL SERVICES, HOUSING & EDUCATION DEPARTMENTS
Look in your telephone directory under the first letter of the name of your local council

NATIONAL ASSOCIATION FOR MATERNAL & CHILD WELFARE
1 South Audley Street
London W1Y 6JS
01-491 2772

NATIONAL ASSOCIATION FOR THE WELFARE OF CHILDREN IN HOSPITAL (NAWCH)
Argyle House
29-31 Euston Road
London NW1 2SD
01-833 2041

NATIONAL CHILDMINDING ASSOCIATION
8 Masons Hill
Bromley, Kent BR2 9EY
01-464 6164

NATIONAL SOCIETY FOR THE PREVENTION OF CRUELTY TO CHILDREN (NSPCC)
67 Saffron Hill
London EC1N 8RS
01-242 1626

OPUS (Organisation for parents under stress)
106 Godstone Road
Whyteleafe
Croydon, Surrey CR3 0EB
01-645 0469

PATIENTS ASSOCIATION
Room 33
18 Charing Cross Road
London WC2H 0HR
01-240 0671

CONCEPTION, PRENATAL CARE, CHILDBIRTH & FEEDING

ACTIVE BIRTH MOVEMENT
18 Laurier Road
London NW5 1SG
01-267 3006

ASSOCIATION FOR BREASTFEEDING MOTHERS
131 Mayow Rd
London SE26 4HZ
01-778 4769

ASSOCIATION FOR IMPROVEMENTS IN THE MATERNITY SERVICES (AIMS)
163 Liverpool Road
London N1 0RF

FAMILY PLANNING ASSOCIATION
27-35 Mortimer Street
London W1N 7RJ
01-636 7866

FORESIGHT
(The Association for Pre-conceptual Care)
Mrs E Mervyn-Smith
The Old Vicarage
Church Lane
Witley
Godalming, Surrey GU8 5PN
0428 794 500

GENETIC COUNSELLING
Every GP should have a list issued by the DHSS relating to this service

INDEPENDENT MIDWIVES ASSOCIATION
8A The Drive
Wimbledon
London SW20
01-505 2010

LA LECHE LEAGUE
(Breastfeeding Advice)
BM 3424
London WC1N 3XX
01-242 1278

MATERNITY ALLIANCE
15 Britannia Street
London WC1X 9JP
01-837 1265

NATIONAL CHILDBIRTH TRUST
9 Queensborough Terrace
London W2 3TB
01-221 3833

NIPPERS (National Information for Parents of Prematures: Education, Resources & Support)
c/o Perinatal Unit
St. Mary's Hospital
Praed Street
London W2 1NY
01-725 6666

SOCIETY TO SUPPORT HOME CONFINEMENTS
Lydgate
Lydgate Lane
Wolsingham
County Durham DL13 3HA
0388 528044

GENERAL FOR HANDICAPPED CHILDREN

ATTENDANCE ALLOWANCE UNIT
DHSS
North Fylde Centre Office
Norcross, Blackpool FY5 3TA
0253 856123

CONTACT A FAMILY*
16 Strutton Ground
London SW1P 2HP
01-222 2695/3969

THE DISABILITY ALLIANCE EDUCATIONAL & RESEARCH ASSOCIATION
25 Denmark Street
London WC2H 8NJ
01-240 0806

DISABILITY INFORMATION SERVICE
10 Warwick Row
London SW1E 5EP
01-630 5994

THE FAMILY FUND
P.O. Box 50
York YO1 1UY
0904 21115

HANDICAPPED PERSONS RESEARCH UNIT
Newcastle upon Tyne Polytechnic
1 Coach Lane
Newcastle Upon Tyne NE7 7TW
0912 664061

IN TOUCH*
10 Norman Road
Sale, Cheshire M33 3DF
061-962 4441

NATIONAL BUREAU FOR HANDICAPPED STUDENTS (B.H.S.)
336 Brixton Road
London SW9 7AA
01-274 0565

VOLUNTARY COUNCIL FOR THE HANDICAPPED CHILD
National Children's Bureau
8 Wakley Street
London EC1V 7QE
01-278 9441

*Both of these organizations help to bring together families with physically or mentally handicapped children, locally and nationally, sometimes with rare disorders.

VOLUNTARY ORGANIZATIONS/ INSTITUTIONS WITH A SPECIAL INTEREST
(Listed alphabetically by interest, not necessarily first word of name)

ALLERGY SUPPORT SERVICE
Chris Dowsett SRN
Seven Trees
62 Marshals Drive
St Albans, Herts AL1 4RF
0727 58705

AL-ANON FAMILY GROUPS
61 Great Dover Street
London SE1 4YF
01-403 0888

ASTHMA RESEARCH COUNCIL & ASTHMA SOCIETY
300 Upper Street
London N1 2XX
01-226 2260

NATIONAL SOCIETY FOR AUTISTIC CHILDREN
276 Willesden Lane
London NW2 5RB
01-451 3844

ROYAL NATIONAL INSTITUTE FOR THE BLIND
224 Great Portland Street
London W1N 6AA
01-388 1266

BRITTLE BONES SOCIETY
Unit 4
Block 20
Carlunie Rd
Dundee DD2 3QT
0382 817771

NATIONAL CAESAREAN SUPPORT ASSOCIATION
72 Perry Rise
London SE23 3QL
01-699 8399

CLEFT LIP AND PALATE
ASSOCIATION (CLAPA)
Speech Therapy Department
Hospital for Sick Children
Great Ormond Street
London WC1N 3JH
01-405 9200

COELIAC SOCIETY OF THE
UK
(Post-Diagnosis Support)
P.O. Box 220
High Wycombe
Bucks HB11 2HY
0494 37278

COLOSTOMY WELFARE
GROUP
38 Eccleston Square
London SW1V 1PB
01-828 5175

CRY-SIS (Support Group for
Parents of Crying Babies)
B.M. Families
London WC1N 3XX
01-404 5011

CYSTIC FIBROSIS RESEARCH
TRUST
Alexandra House
5 Blyth Road
Bromley, Kent BR1 3RS
01-464 7211

ROYAL NATIONAL
INSTITUTE FOR THE DEAF
105 Gower Street
London WC1E 6AH
01-387 8033

NATIONAL DEAF
CHILDREN'S SOCIETY
45 Hereford Road
London W2 5AH
01-229 9272/4

BRITISH DIABETIC
ASSOCIATION
10 Queen Anne Street
London W1M 0BD
01-323 1531

DOWN'S SYNDROME
ASSOCIATION
12-13 Clapham Common
South Side
London SW4 7AA
01-720 0008

THE DH (DIAPHRAGMATIC
HERNIA) CLUB
4 Ladywood Road
Sturry, Kent CT2 0LB

THE DYSTONIA SOCIETY
66 Turnpike Lane
London N8 0PR
01-881 3827

THE DYSAUTONOMIA
SOCIETY OF GREAT BRITAIN
c/o Mrs Pinnick
22 Oakwood Avenue
Borehamwood
Herts WD6 15R
01-953 5900

BRITISH DYSLEXIA
ASSOCIATION
98 London Road
Reading, Berks RG1 5AU
0734 668271

NATIONAL ECZEMA SOCIETY
Tavistock House North
Tavistock Square
London WC1H 9SR
01-388 4097

BRITISH EPILEPSY
ASSOCIATION
Anstey Office
40 Hanover Square
Leeds LS3 1BE
0532 439393

FRIEDREICH'S ATAXIA
GROUP
The Common
Cranleigh, Surrey GU6 8SB
0483 272741

NATIONAL ASSOCIATION
FOR GIFTED CHILDREN
1 South Audley Street
London W1Y 5DQ
01-499 1188/9

GIFTED CHILDREN'S
INFORMATION CENTRE
Hampton Grange
21 Hampton Lane
Solihull, West Midlands
021-705 4547

HEADWAY
(Support Group for Head
Injured Patients & their
Relatives)
17 Clumber Avenue
Sherwood Rise
Nottingham NG5 1AG
0602 622382

HYPERACTIVE CHILDREN'S
SUPPORT GROUP
59 Meadowside
Angmering
Littlehampton, West Sussex

THE FAMILIAL
HYPERCHOLESTEROLAEMIA
ASSOCIATION (FHA)
P.O. Box 612
London W2 2EE

HAEMOPHILIA SOCIETY
123 Westminster Bridge Road
London SE1 7HR
01-928 2020

INCONTINENTIA PIGMENTI
ASSOCIATION
98 Dynes Road
Kemsing
Sevenoaks, Kent TN15 6RF

INVALID CHILDREN'S AID
NATIONWIDE (ICAN)
198 City Road
London EC1V 2PH
01-608 2462

LEUKAEMIA CARE SOCIETY
P.O. Box 82
Exeter EX2 5DP
0392 218514

LINK (Neurofibromatosis
Association)
1 The Alders
Hanworth, Middx TW13 6NU

MENCAP
Royal Society of Mentally
Handicapped Children and
Adults
123 Golden Lane
London EC1Y 0RT
01-253 9433

THE SOCIETY FOR
MUCOPOLYSACCHARIDE
DISEASES
30 Westwood Drive
Little Chalfont, Bucks

MILK ALLERGY SELF-HELP
(MASH)
4 Queen Anne's Grove
Enfield, Middx EN1 2JP

MOTHERS APART FROM
THEIR CHILDREN (MATCH)
c/o BM Problems
London WC1N 3XX

MUSCULAR DYSTROPHY
GROUP OF GREAT BRITAIN
Nattrass House
35 Macaulay Road
London SW4 0QP
01-720 8055

MULTIPLE SCLEROSIS SOCIETY
25 Essie Road
London SW6 1EE
01-381 4022

MIND
National Association for
Mental Health
22 Harley Street
London W1N 2ED
01-637 0741

NAEVUS SUPPORT GROUP
(Melanocytic, Strawberry and
Port Wine Stain Birthmarks)
58 Necton Road
Wheathampstead
Herts AL4 8AU
058 283 2853

NATIONAL ASSOCIATION
FOR CHILDREN WITH
STOMAS (NASPCS)
55 Peverall Road
Bowthorpe
Norwich, Norfolk NR5 9AT
0603 744912

OESOPHAGEAL ATRESIA
AND TRACHEO-
OESOPHAGEAL FISTULA
(Parent Support Group)
4 Woolam Hill
Main Street
Burstwick
Hull, North Humberside

PARTIALLY SIGHTED
SOCIETY
206 Great Portland Street
London W1N 6AA
01-387 8840

NATIONAL SOCIETY OF
PHENYLKETONURIA AND
ALLIED DISORDERS
Mr J Goss
Worth Cottage
Lower Scholes
Pickels Hill, Keighley
West Yorkshire BD20 6BD
0535 44865

LADY HOARE TRUST FOR
PHYSICALLY HANDICAPPED
CHILDREN
7 North Street
Midhurst
West Sussex GU29 2DJ
0730 813696

PLAY IN HOSPITALS LIAISON
COMMITTEE
41 York Mansions
Prince of Wales Drive
London SW11 4BP
01-622 1524

ASSOCIATION FOR POST-
NATAL ILLNESS
c/o Institute for Obstetrics &
Gynaecology
Queen Charlotte's Hospital
Goldhawk Road
London W6
01-731 4867

RADAR
Royal Association for
Disability and Rehabilitation
25 Mortimer Street
London W1N 8AB
01-637 5400

UK Rett's Syndrome
Association
(Parent Support Group)
Freepost
Orpington, Kent BR5 1SZ

SENSE
National Association for the
Deaf/Blind & Rubella
Handicapped
311 Grays Inn Road
London WC1X 8PT
01-278 1000

SHAFTESBURY SOCIETY
Shaftesbury House
2A Amity Grove
London SW20 0LH
01-946 6635

THE SPASTICS SOCIETY
12 Park Crescent
London W1N 4EQ
01-636 5020

SICKLE CELL SOCIETY
Green Lodge
Barretts Green Road
London NW10 7AP
01-961 7795/8346

**ASSOCIATION FOR ALL
SPEECH IMPAIRED
CHILDREN (AFASIC)**
347 Central Markets
London EC1A 9NH
01-236 3632/6487

**ASSOCIATION FOR SPINA
BIFIDA AND
HYDROCEPHALUS**
22 Upper Woburn Place
London WC1H 0EP
01-388 1382

**SPINAL INJURIES
ASSOCIATION**
Yeoman House
76 St James Lane
London N10 3DF
01-444 2121

Steps
(Support Group for parents of
children with congenital
abnormality of the lower
limbs)
8 Princes Road
Urmston
Manchester M31 3SS
061-747 7014

**TUBEROUS SCLEROSIS
ASSOCIATION OF GREAT
BRITAIN**
Little Barnsley Farm
Catshill
Bromsgrove, Worcs B61 0NQ
0527 71898

**TURNERS SYNDROME
SOCIETY**
Sandywood
Woodside Road
Cobham, Surrey KT11 2QR

TWINS CLUB ASSOCIATION
Pooh Corner
54 Broad Lane
Hampton
Middlesex TW12 3BG
01-941 0641

**ASSOCIATION OF PARENTS
OF VACCINE DAMAGED
CHILDREN**
2 Church Street
Shipston-on-Stour
Warks CV36 4AP
0608 61595

LEISURE

**BRITISH SPORTS
ASSOCIATION FOR THE
DISABLED**
Hayward House
Barnard Crescent
Aylesbury, Bucks HP21 9PP
0296 27889

**UK SPORTS ASSOCIATION
FOR PEOPLE WITH MENTAL
HANDICAP**
c/o The Sports Council
16 Upper Woburn Place
London WC1H 0QP
01-388 1277

**RIDING FOR THE DISABLED
ASSOCIATION**
Avenue R
National Agricultural Centre
Kenilworth, Warks CV8 2LY
0203 56107

HOLIDAY CARE SERVICE
2 Old Bank Chambers
Station Road
Horley, Surrey RH6 9HW
0293 774535
(Information Service only)

HORTICULTURAL THERAPY
Goulds Ground
Vallis Way
Frome, Somerset BA11 3DW
0373 64782

**NATIONAL FEDERATION OF
GATEWAY CLUBS**
117 Golden Lane
London EC1Y 0RT
01-253 9433

**NATIONAL TOY LIBRARIES
ASSOCIATION (NTLA)**
c/o Play Matters
68 Churchway
London NW1 1LT
01-387 9592

ONE O'CLOCK PLAYROOMS
Parent and Toddler Groups
The Play Office
Strakers Road
Peckham Rye Common
London SE15 6HU
01-299 2860

**PALACE PLAYGROUND FOR
HANDICAPPED CHILDREN**
Bishops Avenue
London SW6 6EA
01-731 2753

**PHYSICALLY HANDICAPPED
& ABLE-BODIED CLUB
(PHAB)**
Tavistock House North
Tavistock Square
London WC1H 9HX
01-388 1963

**PRE-SCHOOL PLAYGROUPS
ASSOCIATION**
Alfred House
Aveline Street
London SE11 5DJ
01-582 8871

**TALKING BOOKS FOR THE
HANDICAPPED**
National Listening Library
12 Lant Street
London SE1 1QH
01-407 9417

**AIDS, APPLIANCES,
MOBILITY etc**

**DISABLED LIVING
FOUNDATION**
380-384 Harrow Road
London W9 2HU
01-289 6111

MEDIC ALERT FOUNDATION
11/13 Clifton Terrace
London N4 3JP
01-263 8597

MOTABILITY
Gate House
West Gate
Harlow, Essex CM20 1HR
0279 635 666

**MOBILITY ALLOWANCE
UNIT**
DHSS
Norcross
Blackpool, Lancs FY5 3TA

LEGAL

CHILDREN'S LEGAL CENTRE
20 Compton Terrace
London N1 2UN
01-359 6251

**NETWORK FOR THE
HANDICAPPED (LEGAL
ADVICE)**
16 Princeton Street
London WC1R 4BB
01-831 8031/7740

EDUCATION

**ADVISORY CENTRE FOR
EDUCATION (ACE)**
18 Victoria Park Square
London E2 9PB
01-980 4596

**NATIONAL COUNCIL FOR
SPECIAL EDUCATION**
1 Wood Street
Stratford-Upon-Avon
Warks CV37 6JE
0789 205332

SEXUAL PROBLEMS

**SEXUAL & PERSONAL
RELATIONSHIPS OF THE
DISABLED (SPOD)**
286 Camden Road
London N7 0BJ
01-607 8851/2

ADOPTION AND FOSTERING

**BRITISH AGENCIES FOR
ADOPTION AND FOSTERING**
11 Southwark Street
London SE1 1RQ
01-407 8800

**NATIONAL ASSOCIATION
FOR THE CHILDLESS (NAC)**
318 Summer Lane
Birmingham B19 3RL
021-359 4887

**NATIONAL FOSTER CARE
ASSOCIATION (NFCA)**
Francis House
Francis Street
London SW1P 1DE
01-828 6266

POST-ADOPTION CENTRE
Gregory House
48 Mecklenburgh Square
London WC1N 2NU
01-833 3214

**PARENT-TO-PARENT
INFORMATION ON
ADOPTION SERVICES (PPIAS)**
Lower Boddington
Daventry
Northants NN11 6YB
0327 60295

**BEREAVEMENT AND THE
DYING CHILD**

**THE COMPASSIONATE
FRIENDS**
6 Denmark Street
Bristol BS1 5DQ
0272 292778

**FOUNDATION FOR THE
STUDY OF INFANT DEATHS**
15 Belgrave Square
London SW1X 8PS
01-235 0965

MISCARRIAGE ASSOCIATION
18 Stonybrook Close
West Bretton
Wakefield, Yorks WF4 4TP
092-485 515

**THE STILLBIRTH AND
NEONATAL DEATH SOCIETY**
28 Portland Place
London W1N 3DE
01-436 5881

DIVORCE

**NATIONAL MARRIAGE
GUIDANCE COUNCIL**
Herbert Grey College
Little Church Street
Rugby, Warks CV21 3AP
0788 73241

**NATIONAL COUNCIL FOR
DIVORCED AND SEPARATED**
13 High Street
Little Shelford
Cambs CB2 5ES
0533 708880

ONE-PARENT FAMILIES

GINGERBREAD
35 Wellington Street
London WC2E 7BN
01-240 0953

**NATIONAL COUNCIL FOR
ONE-PARENT FAMILIES**
255 Kentish Town Road
London NW5 2LX
01-267 1361

STEP-PARENTING

**THE NATIONAL STEP-
FAMILY ASSOCIATION**
162 Tennyson Road
Cambridge CB1 2DP
0223 460312

INDEX